Drug Treatment
of Respiratory Disease

MONOGRAPHS IN CLINICAL PHARMACOLOGY
Volume 5

General Editor
Daniel L. Azarnoff M.D.
Senior Vice President
Worldwide Research and Development
G.D. Searle & Co.
Chicago, Illinois
Formerly Professor of Medicine and Pharmacology
University of Kansas

ALREADY PUBLISHED

Clinical Pharmacology of Psychotherapeutic Drugs   Leo E. Hollister M.D.
Drugs and Renal Disease   William M. Bennett M.D.
Drug Treatment of Gastrointestinal Disorders   Norton J. Greenberger M.D.,
    Constanti Arvanitakis M.D. and Aryeh Hurwitz M.D.
Clinical Neuropharmacology   Henn Kutt M.D., Fletcher McDowell M.D.,
    Henry Masur M.D. and Henry W. Murray M.D.

FORTHCOMING VOLUMES IN THE SERIES

Pediatric Clinical Pharmacology   Lars O. Boreus M.D.
Clinical Cardiovascular Pharmacology   David Shand M.B., Ph.D.
Drugs for Rheumatic Disease   Carl M. Pearson M.D., Harold Paulus M.D. and
    Daniel Furst M.D.
Clinical Pharmacology in Dermatology   David Bickers M.D.

Drug Treatment
of Respiratory Disease

R.B. COLE, M.D., F.R.C.P.

Consultant Physician
North Staffordshire Hospital Centre
Stoke-on-Trent
Senior Lecturer
Department of Postgraduate Medicine
University of Keele
Staffordshire, England

CHURCHILL LIVINGSTONE
New York   Edinburgh   London   Melbourne   1981

Distributed in the United Kingdom by Churchill Livingstone, Robert Stevenson House, 1-3 Baxter's Place, Leith Walk, Edinburgh EH1 3AF and by associated companies, branches and representatives throughout the world.

First published 1981
Printed in USA
ISBN 0 443 08012 7

9 8 7 6 5 4 3 2 1

Library of Congress Cataloging in Publication Data
Cole, Robert B.
    Drug treatment of respiratory disease.
    Bibliography: p.
    Includes index.
    1. Anti-infective agents. 2. Respiratory
organs—Diseases—Chemotherapy. 3. Repira-
tory agents. I. Title. [DNLM: 1. Respira-
tory tract diseases—Drug therapy. WI
M0567KP v. 5 / WF 145 D793]
RM388.C64   616.2'00461   81-10055
ISBN 0-443-08012-7   AACR2

General Editor's Foreword

This is the first volume in the monograph series to provide an extensive discussion on the sources of variation in the response of humans to drugs. The chapter that deals with these variations relates to all drugs, not just to those used to treat pulmonary disorders. Dr. Cole's discussion is understandable and well done.

The therapy of pulmonary diseases is frequently based on intuition and dogma, since few well-controlled trials are available to document the effectiveness of various procedures and therapies. Dr. Cole has made clear the lack of such studies for some drugs—for example, expectorants.

The physician will also find useful the chapters on the use of drugs in the treatment of infections of the pulmonary system, as well as the discussions of bronchodilators, anticoagulants and antithrombotic agents, and respiratory stimulants.

This volume is replete with practical suggestions for the care and treatment of patients with pulmonary disorders. I recommend it to you.

Daniel L. Azarnoff, M.D.

Preface

Clinical pharmacology has become increasingly important to the practising clinician in recent years because it has begun to reveal a great deal of practical information about the behaviour of drugs and the factors which determine their therapeutic success. Yet clinical pharmacology is a facet of medicine which has had a relatively minor place in most medical school curricula, and I believe that drugs are sometimes used uncritically and often ineffectively. This book is about the drugs which are commonly used in the treatment of patients with respiratory diseases, and it is written with the threefold aim of describing the way each drug works, the special characteristics which determine how it should be used, and the practical problems of treatment. I hope that this approach will help to explain some of the pitfalls and difficulties of drug therapy and to enable clinicians to treat respiratory illnesses in an effective and logical way.

Drug Treatment of Respiratory Disease has been written against the background of a very busy hospital practice in chest medicine in one of the great industrial cities of England. My natural tendency has therefore been to describe drugs as they are commonly used in the United Kingdom, but I have done my best to modify this bias by presenting both the American and British points of view where these differ significantly, as in the treatment of pulmonary tuberculosis. I have included some drugs which are not available for general use in the United States, such as salbutamol (that is, albuterol) and sodium fusidate, because in Britain and elsewhere they are widely judged to make a valuable contribution to therapy.

Many people have helped me. I am deeply grateful to my family for their understanding and for tolerating my unsociability while I have been writing the book; without my wife's constant support and encouragement it would never have been completed. I owe sincere thanks to Susan Forster for her expert secretarial help, to Brian King for his skill in preparing the diagrams, and to Dr. Leslie Bowcock and the staff of the Department of Medical Photography and Audio-Visual Aids at the North Staffordshire Hospital Centre for the photographic work. I appreciate Jean Wheeler's assistance in preparing the references, and I acknowledge with gratitude the invaluable help I have been given by the medical librarians at the North Staffordshire Medical Institute, Mrs. Ruth Woosnam and Mrs. Elizabeth Bell, and by Mr. Stanley Jenkins of the Barnes Library, University of Birmingham. I particularly appreciate the helpful criticism of my clinical colleagues who read the manuscript and gave me valuable advice: Dr. John Gray, Dr. R. M. Ibbotson, Dr. John Mucklow and Dr. Warren Perks from the North Staffordshire Hospital Centre; and Dr. Ian Green from the Selly Oak Hospital, Birmingham.

R.B. Cole, M.D.

Contents

Drug Treatment
of Respiratory Disease

1

Sources of Variation in the Response to Drugs

The great majority of people respond to a given drug in a similar way so that it is generally possible to devise a standard therapeutic regimen which will have a reasonably predictable effect, provided that appropriate adjustments to dosage are made for age, weight, and mode of administration. This is perhaps surprising in view of the complexity of the processes which result in the drug exerting its effect on biological function. In brief, most drugs act by combining reversibly with specific receptors located on or within the cells of the target tissue, and as a result, this drug-receptor combination alters the biochemical and physiological function of the cell and brings about the drug's biological effect. Only a tiny proportion of the total dose administered reaches the receptor, while the remainder of the drug is "lost" in the processes of absorption, distribution, and elimination—which together determine the drug concentration in a given tissue at any particular time after administration. The term *pharmacodynamics* commonly applies to the study of those aspects of drug behaviour which relate to its action or effect, and the term *pharmacokinetics* applies to the study of the factors that determine its effective concentration at the site of action.

Although accepting that most patients will respond satisfactorily to standard treatment, one must also recognise that misjudgements in therapy are responsible for considerable morbidity from drug toxicity[36,69] and no doubt for an equal amount of totally ineffective prescribing. A description of the major factors causing variability of response to drugs is therefore considered to be of practical value in introducing this account of the use of drugs in respiratory disease. This description follows the sequence of drug behaviour in man from the process of administration to the point at which the drug takes biological effect.

THE DOSE ADMINISTERED

Errors of Compliance

The assumption that patients follow their doctors' advice in taking prescribed medication is not always justified,[52,53] and an unexpected failure of response to treatment should prompt a tactful enquiry into any problem the patient may have experienced in adhering to the treatment regimen. Nevertheless, the diagnosis of non-compliance as the cause of therapeutic failure or adverse effects is not always easy, since patients are often unwilling to acknowledge it openly.

Common reasons for failure of drug compliance are (1) deliberate discontinuation of drugs when symptoms are improved, (2) misunderstanding of the regimen or forgetfulness due to the multiplicity of drugs, and (3) insufficient warning of unpleasant side-effects. Clearly the avoidance of compliance errors depends very much upon simplifying treatment and reducing the frequency of doses as much as possible, and on a careful explanation of the nature, objectives, and likely duration of therapy, including appropriate information about the possible side-effects which may be encountered. Much depends upon the authority of the doctor and the understanding which he establishes with the patient.[9] Patients may be helped by written instructions which should be provided when the treatment regimen is complex,[78] and particularly when attention to correct dosage is critical for avoiding serious side-effects, for example, with oral anticoagulant therapy. The help of the spouse or a relative in supervising the administration of treatment is invaluable, particularly in the case of elderly patients.

Drug Interactions *In Vitro*

Interactions between drugs prior to their administration may result from pharmaceutical incompatibility. Inactivation of parenteral preparations has often been produced unwittingly when incompatible drugs are mixed in the syringe or the infusion bottle before they are given to the patient. Drugs should not be mixed prior to parenteral administration if it can be avoided but instead should be given by bolus injection into the infusion line.[61]

PHARMACOKINETIC VARIABLES

Much of the variability of response to drugs is due to differences in their blood and tissue concentrations from one person to the next and depends upon the wide variation in the manner in which individual drugs are handled and the rate at which this occurs. Some of the factors which contribute to these pharmacokinetic differences are described in this section, including brief descriptions of the ways in which drug interactions may affect response.

Absorption Variability

Parenteral administration of drugs has the great advantage that absorption problems are minimised, and in the case of intravenous administration, are eliminated altogether. Absorption of subcutaneous and intramuscular preparations, however, is affected by changes in blood flow at the injection site, whether due to muscle activity, circulatory disturbance, or the simultaneous administration of vasconstrictor drugs. Although it is generally assumed that drugs injected intramuscularly or subcutaneously are completely absorbed into the systemic circulation, this has been shown not to be true for certain drugs such as digoxin[30] and may be equally untrue for other important drugs, probably because of such factors as local inactivation or drug insolubility at the pH of the tissue.

Ineffectual drug delivery is a particular problem which arises in the treatment of bronchial asthma by topical application with inhaled pressurised aerosols. The rationale for such treatment is that the bronchodilator agent is applied directly to the effector tissue, allowing dosage to be reduced and the unwanted effects to be minimised. When severe bronchospasm develops, however, access to the bronchial mucous membrane by the aerosol is prevented because of impaired and uneven gas flow, and this form of therapy becomes ineffective, necessitating the administration of the drug by an alternative route.

Most drugs are taken orally for convenience, safety of administration, and economy, although this route clearly cannot be used for drugs which are susceptible to alteration or degradation by the processes of digestion. The oral route is also very difficult to use in the case of drugs which are gastrointestinal irritants, such as aminosalicylic acid (para-aminosalicylic acid, PAS). Drugs taken by mouth must necessarily progress through a number of stages in the process of absorption before reaching the systemic circulation; this discussion will give an account of the factors which may affect the rate or completeness of absorption and which in turn may introduce variability in drug response.

In the course of absorption the factors which are most liable to be a source of variability in the individual response to a drug are:

1. Pharmaceutical formulation.
2. Rate of gastric emptying.
3. "First-pass" metabolism.
4. Concurrent gastrointestinal disease.
5. Drug interactions.

Pharmaceutical Formulation   This may have an important influence on the rate and extent of drug absorption, particularly those which are poorly soluble and slowly absorbed. Differences in the particle size, crystal form, inclusion of other ingredients (excipients) besides the active agent, and many other variables are likely to affect the disintegration and dissolution of solid dosage forms. These factors are often critical in determining the rate at which drugs are liberated into the gastrointestinal contents prior to absorption across the mucosa, and they may result in therapeutic non-equivalence between different preparations containing chemically equivalent doses of the same drug. Such preparations are said to differ in their *bioavailability*, that is, the percentage of the dose that enters the systemic circulation unchanged. Differences in bioavailability between different preparations is a matter of practical significance in the use of many important drugs, of which the cardiac glycosides, tetracyclines, anticonvulsants, antihypertensives and anticoagulants are notable examples.

Rate of Gastric Emptying   This affects the absorption of different drugs in different ways. As a general rule, factors which reduce the rate of gastric emptying also reduce the rate of drug absorption, because the main absorptive area for drugs is the mucosa of the small intestine; thus a low gastric pH, nausea, pain, the simultaneous ingestion of food, or the administration of drugs with anticholinesterase effects all retard absorption by delaying gastric emptying. The opposite effect occurs following a rise in gastric pH, after a gastrectomy, or after the administration of metoclopramide, which increases the gastric emptying rate. However the absorption of some drugs, like digoxin, is *favoured* by slow gastric emptying—probably because the drug remains longer at its optimum site of absorption.

Generally speaking, reduction in the *rate* of absorption has little effect on the therapeutic response to drugs administered regularly by multiple dosing provided that the total dose absorbed is constant. A reduced absorption rate does, however, reduce the peak plasma drug levels, a factor which may be important in determining the therapeutic response to some antibiotics. In the case of a drug given in a single dose such as a hypnotic or an analgesic preparation, the reduction and delay in peak plasma blood level may diminish the intensity of its effect because the minimum effective concentration of the drug at its site of action may never be reached.

First-Pass Metabolism   Certain drugs are metabolised as they traverse the gut wall and liver before gaining access to the general circulation, and even if gastrointestinal absorption is complete, individual variation in metabolic activity of the intestinal mucosa or liver may lead to considerable variation in the plasma level of the unchanged drug in the systemic circulation. For example, extensive metabolism of isoproterenol occurs in the small intestinal mucous membrane, and metabolism of propranolol and nitroglycerine (glyceryl trinitrate) occurs in the liver. The process is subject to marked differences between individuals and is therefore a significant source of variability in the response to drugs.

Concurrent Gastrointestinal Disease   Reduction in gastric acidity due to achlorhydria or to antacid ingestion may affect the absorption of weakly acidic drugs such as aspirin or cephalexin. Any drug which is a weak acid or a weak base exists in both ionised and non-ionised forms, the extent of ionisation depending upon the ionisation constant, or pKa, which is defined as the pH at which the drug is 50 percent ionised. Since non-ionised substances are lipid-soluble and since they diffuse readily across cell membranes while ionised substances do not, the extent of ionisation of a drug at its site of absorption affects its diffusibility through the cells of the gastrointestinal mucosa. For example, in the case of aspirin which has a pKa of 3.5, most of the drug is non-ionised in the stomach where the pH is 1–2, and absorption from this site is therefore theoretically favoured by gastric acidity. In practice the absorption of salicylates occurs mainly from the upper part of the small intestine and is enhanced by rapid gastric emptying which increases when the intragastric pH is raised. In addition ingested salicylates are more readily soluble, and thus more readily absorbed, at higher pH. The net effect of these different influences on aspirin absorption is therefore likely to vary between individuals, and this explains the conflicting results which have been obtained in studies of drug absorption in patients with achlorhydria.

This example illustrates how individual responses to drugs may vary because of interacting pharmacokinetic factors which lead to variability in the rate or completeness of drug absorption. Physiological or pathological changes in gastrointestinal function are most likely to alter the absorption of drugs which are incompletely absorbed even under the most favourable circumstances, such as digoxin, bishydroxycoumarin, and guanethidine.

Diseases which affect the gastric emptying rate may influence drug absorption. In gastrectomised patients this effect is well-documented for several drugs such as digoxin, levodopa, and sulphonamides. Whether alterations in intestinal transit time associated with small bowel disease have similar effects on absorption is less easy to determine, since loss of absorptive capacity due to diminished mucosal surface area, changes in intraluminal pH, alterations in bowel flora, increased permeability of the gut wall, and several other factors may influence drug absorption in malabsorption syndromes such as coeliac disease, jejunal diverticulosis, and Crohn's disease. In these conditions it is of practical importance to be aware that the absorption of many commonly used drugs such as antibacterial agents is unpredictable and may be responsible for therapeutic failure or drug resistance.[60]

Drug Interactions which Affect Drug Absorption   As mentioned earlier, a distinction must be made between factors which influence the *rate* of drug absorption and those which affect the *total amount* of drug absorbed; the latter effect is more likely to cause clinically important variations in drug response. Drug interactions which affect the total amount of the drug absorbed include the following:

1. Effect on gastrointestinal pH: for example, sodium bicarbonate reduces the absorption of tetracycline, which is more soluble in acid solution.[5]
2. Binding or chelation: for example, adsorption of lincomycin by kaolin; chelation of tetracycline by iron preparations or by calcium-, aluminium-, or magnesium-containing antacids; binding of many drugs, including warfarin, by cholestyramine. All these reactions produce poorly-absorbed drug complexes.
3. Competition for pathways of active absorption: for example, by enzyme inhibition, as has been postulated to occur between chlorpromazine and levodopa.

The above interactions are likely to occur only if the interacting drugs are given within 30–60 minutes of each other, and may be avoided by timing their administration with care.

4. A direct toxic effect on the small intestine causing morphological changes to the mucosa, as may occur with colchicine or neomycin. Decreased absorption of penicillin[16] and of digoxin[45] have been reported during neomycin administration.

Distribution Variability

Once absorbed into the systemic circulation, drugs are distributed in the tissues and body fluids in a way which depends upon the inter-reaction of a number of variables, of which the following are the major ones:

1. Regional blood flow.
2. The lipid solubility of the drug, which is related to the extent of its ionisation at physiological pH values, and which determines to a high degree its rate of diffusion through cell membranes.

3. Active transport processes across cell membranes that apply to some drugs which utilise specialised "pump" mechanisms to exert their effect (for example, the guanidinium antihypertensive agents), or to those which are eliminated by the renal tubules or the biliary canaliculi.
4. Preferential concentration of drugs in particular plasma or tissue constituents which act as reservoirs by virtue of their capacity for selectively binding the drug.

Variability in the individual response to a drug may be related to one or more of the above factors.

Variability in Distribution Volume In the case of a macromolecular compound which is injected intravascularly and is unable to penetrate the vascular endothelium, the volume of distribution is equal to that of the plasma. Most drugs diffuse through vascular walls very easily, however, and the extent to which a drug is distributed outside the circulation is usually assessed by determining its apparent volume of distribution (V_D), that is, the volume in which it would appear to be distributed in a steady state, if it existed throughout that volume at the same concentration as in the plasma. Thus V_D relates the total amount of drug in the body to its plasma concentration:

$$V_D = \frac{\text{total amount of drug in the body}}{\text{plasma concentration of the drug}}$$

Variability in distribution volume between individuals has been described for certain drugs, notably nortriptyline, oxazepam, and diazepam, and some studies suggest that such differences may have a partial genetic basis.[2]

Plasma Protein Binding Many drugs are reversibly attached to plasma proteins in the circulation, most frequently to albumin. Only unbound drug is diffusible and available for tissue distribution or elimination, so that the bound drug in effect forms an inert reservoir which is in equilibrium with the unbound drug in the plasma. The degree of plasma protein binding is relevant when comparing the relative merits of different antimicrobial agents, for example, the cephalosporins. At first sight the achievement of high plasma levels may appear to indicate a drug's therapeutic effectiveness, but it is not informative if the drug is highly protein bound since the high level simply reflects the reservoir of protein-bound drug which exerts no direct antibacterial effect in the tissues.[40]

The degree of binding is influenced by the amount of drug in the circulation, its affinity for albumin, and the amount of circulating albumin.

Hypoalbuminaemia, which may be a consequence of several diseases such as advanced cirrhosis of the liver, nephrotic syndrome, and malnutrition, leads to reduced drug binding and to an increased risk of toxicity. In *renal failure* there is reduced albumin binding of certain drugs, including warfarin, salicylates, sulphonamides, and some penicillins, apparently because of qualitative changes in the binding protein and also partly because available binding sites are occupied by acidic metabolites.

Displacement from protein binding sites may be due to endogenous substances such as hormones and bilirubin. It arises commonly as a practical problem to be foreseen and avoided in the use of such drugs as coumarin anticoagulants or sulphonylurea antidiabetic agents, which may be displaced from their protein binding sites by other drugs, leading to loss of anticoagulant or diabetic control.

Drug Interactions which Affect Drug Distribution   One drug may interact with another by displacing it from its usual binding site, thereby increasing its unbound concentration and hence its effect at the site of action. This type of interaction is particularly important with regard to drugs which are bound to plasma proteins (principally albumin), because many drugs have common binding sites on albumin, and a small displacement of a highly protein-bound drug will represent a disproportionately large increase in the amount of active, unbound drug. However, unless the unbound fraction has a small volume of distribution, the displaced drug will be distributed to the various body tissues, and the wider the distribution the less will be the absolute increase in the concentration of unbound drug. Hence displacement drug interactions of this type will only be of clinical importance if the displaced drug is more than 80–90 percent protein bound and has a small volume of distribution. Warfarin is a drug which meets both of these criteria, and a number of drugs are potentially capable of displacing warfarin, causing an unexpected increase in its anticoagulant effect which may have serious consequences by causing hypoprothrombinaemia and bleeding. In practice, probably only phenylbutazone and chloral hydrate are of definite importance in this respect, although salicylates in high dosage may have a similar effect. It must also be appreciated that displacement of warfarin from its albumin binding sites increases its liability for biotransformation and elimination, so that the increased anticoagulant effect is a temporary one, lasting only until a new equilibrium is established with the same concentration of unbound active drug which existed prior to the administration of the displacing drug.

Variability in Drug Metabolism

The termination of drug effects on biological function is brought about either through the excretion of the drug by the kidney or through deactivation of the drug. Deactivation occurs mainly in the liver and is followed by direct excretion in the bile or excretion of its metabolites in the urine. Hepatic metabolism of drugs usually, but not invariably, leads to loss of pharmacological activity[18]; in the case of some drugs such as prednisone it is the metabolite, prednisolone, which is responsible for the pharmacological activity of the parent drug.[37]

Although there are several biochemical mechanisms responsible for deactivation, the predominant effect of these metabolic processes is to decrease the lipid solubility of the drug by making the metabolite more polar, that is, more highly ionised than the parent drug, so as to reduce its capacity for diffusion into cells or for reabsorption from the renal tubules. The net result is conversion of the active drug into a pharmacologically inert compound which can be readily excreted.

Metabolic Processes　Deactivation of drugs by the cells of the intestinal mucosa has already been mentioned as one aspect of first-pass metabolism, and the biotransformation of drugs may occur in a number of sites which include plasma, brain, and kidney tissue. However, by far the greatest number of such chemical reactions occur in the liver. Biotransformation can be divided into two main categories, the non-synthetic types of reaction which include oxidation, reduction, and hydrolysis; and the synthetic or conjugation reactions in which there is synthesis of a derivative of the drug.

Non-synthetic drug metabolism is usually the first stage of drug biotransformation, and the resultant metabolite may be, but is not necessarily, pharmacologically inactive. Indeed, this process may convert an inactive drug into an active agent, as has been mentioned above in the case of prednisone, or may change an active drug into another pharmacologically active compound which may be more or less active, or more or less toxic, than the parent drug.

The great majority of oxidations and reductions are catalysed by non-substrate-specific enzymes located in liver cells where they are associated with the smooth-surfaced endoplasmic reticulum and are known as *microsomal enzymes*. The activity of these drug-metabolising microsomal enzymes depends upon the presence of molecular oxygen, a haemoprotein known as cytochrome P450, and reduced nicotinamide adenine dinucleotide phosphate (NADPH). Because of the very low substrate specificity of the microsomal P450-dependent system, numerous drugs may compete with each other for oxidation and, by inhibiting each other's metabolism, may cause increased pharmacological activity and potential toxicity.

Synthetic drug metabolism, or conjugation, is usually an energy-requiring process which involves the coupling of the drug with, for example, a hydroxyl, amino, or sulphydryl radical. The most important of these reactions are glucuronide synthesis, amino-acid conjugation, acetylation, sulphate conjugation, and methylation, and they result almost invariably in the pharmacological inactivation of the original compound.[25] Usually the conjugated metabolites are less lipid soluble, more highly ionised, and hence more readily excreted in the urine or bile.

Factors Affecting the Metabolic Processes   A number of factors influence drug metabolism. They include genetic factors, the effect of dosage on the way some drugs are handled (dose-dependent kinetics), age, nutritional status, smoking and drinking habits, the effects of other diseases (particularly hepatic disease), and the influence of other drugs administered previously or concurrently. Some of these factors are discussed below.

Genetic differences   Among normal subjects, wide differences in the rate at which drugs are metabolised have been attributed to genetic variation.[75] This source of variability in drug response is unpredictable, and in any individual there is little correlation between the elimination rate of different oxidised drugs; for this reason it is not possible to use the rate of oxidative metabolism of one drug as a basis for predicting the rate of oxidative metabolism of another.[68]

In contrast, individuals who acetylate one drug slowly will also be slow acetylators of other drugs which are metabolised in the same way.[21] Genetic differences in the rate of drug acetylation are an important source of variability in response to certain drugs, notably isoniazid and hydrallazine. It is possible to divide populations into two groups—slow and rapid acetylators—depending on the incidence of an autosomal recessive gene for slow acetylation.[21] Population studies have shown a wide range in the frequency of the slow acetylator gene, obtaining the lowest incidences among Eskimos and oriental people and a high incidence among Scandinavians. The incidence among Caucasians in the United States and Britain is between 50 and 60 percent for the slow acetylator gene.[20] This genetic variability has important consequences in the use of isoniazid for treating tuberculosis, since slow acetylators are more likely to accumulate the drug and develop neuropathy, but they respond better than rapid acetylators to widely-spaced isoniazid dosage regimens.

Dose-dependent kinetics   As a general rule drugs are metabolised at a rate which is directly proportional to their concentration in the body: the higher the concentration of the drug, the more rapid is its rate of metabolism. This behaviour is an example of first-order kinetics, and since the metabolism of drugs is mediated by enzymes, it implies that the enzyme system has sufficient capacity to cope with whatever concentration of substrate is imposed on it, at least within the limits of normal therapeutic usage of the drug. In the case of a few substances, however, including ethyl alcohol, salicylates, bishydroxy-coumarin (dicoumarol), and diphenylhydantoin (phenytoin), the enzyme systems become saturated at relatively low concentrations of the drug; if the concentration is increased by the administration of higher dosages, the rate of metabolism follows zero-order kinetics, and metabolism proceeds at a constant rate, independent of the concentration of the drug in the body, until it has been reduced sufficiently to follow the pattern of first-order kinetics. The clinical use of such drugs is complicated because small dosage increments may result in a disproportionate increase in plasma concentration, thereby causing toxic effects. Moreover, the threshold for enzyme saturation varies from one individual to the next so that it is difficult to predict the critical dose.

AGE   The metabolism of drugs is reduced in the elderly, compared with patients of other age groups. In neonates, particularly the premature, drugs such as diazepam, barbiturates, sulphonamides, chloramphenicol, and salicylates are metabolised slowly. Reduced hepatic metabolism in old age has been demonstrated for a number of drugs including phenylbutazone, amylobarbital, propranolol, and meperidine (pethidine).

EFFECT OF CONCURRENT DISEASE   Hepatic disease might reasonably be expected to influence the individual response to drugs, since the liver is responsible to a very large extent for their biotransformation and deactivation, and such indeed proves to be the case. The elimination half-lives of propranolol and phenylbutazone, for example, are prolonged in chronic liver disease, and decreased first-pass metabolism of labetalol has also been demonstrated.[35] However, prediction of variability in drug responsiveness in the individual patient with liver disease is not easy, because defects in drug metabolism correlate poorly with routine liver function tests, except possibly with reduced serum albumin levels and prolongation of the prothrombin time—both of which may reflect impaired synthesis of proteins, including the drug metabolising enzymes.[12] A further factor influencing first-pass metabolism significantly but unpredictably is the presence of portosystemic shunts in chronic cirrhosis, which may greatly increase the bioavailability of orally-administered drugs that are normally highly extracted by the liver.[34]

Thus, although a great deal of progress has been made in identifying the effects which liver disease may have on drug disposition, the problem of quantifying these effects is complicated by several variables.

1. Not all drugs involved in the same biochemical pathway are equally affected.
2. Induction of drug metabolising enzymes by other drugs or alcohol may lead to relatively normal drug clearance, even in liver disease.
3. The extent of impaired drug metabolism does not correlate with the results of routine liver function tests.

4. Intrahepatic and extrahepatic portosystemic shunts may have a profound influence on the bioavailability of highly-extracted drugs.

In the drug treatment of patients with liver disease it is therefore necessary to be cautious in the use of drugs known to be deactivated by the liver, to use plasma-level monitoring where indicated, and to adjust the dosage carefully according to the patient's response. It should also be borne in mind that hepatic function and blood flow may be temporarily but seriously affected by diseases of other systems, such as congestive heart failure or respiratory failure, with the result that the metabolism of certain drugs such as lidocaine (lignocaine) and theophylline may be altered during the acute illness, causing unexpected toxicity.[62,72]

Drug Interactions which Affect Drug Metabolism   There is much evidence from experimental work in animals and man that the drug-oxidising system of the liver may be stimulated or "induced" by a variety of compounds, which includes insecticides, food additives, alcohol, environmental chemicals, dyes and, most importantly, numerous drugs when administered in normal therapeutic dosage. The process known as *enzyme induction* results from stimulation of the synthesis of microsomal enzymes involved in drug oxidation and an increase in the activity of the cytochrome P450 system, leading to enhanced elimination rates of drugs metabolised by this pathway and to consequent decrease in therapeutic effect. It usually takes several days or weeks for the development of induction, which persists for a similar duration after the inducing agent is withdrawn. Barbiturates have been widely studied for their enzyme-inducing properties, and the use of phenobarbital as an inducer of glucuronyl transferase in neonatal hyperbilirubinaemia is well known as a method for increasing the conjugation and excretion of bilirubin, and so for reducing the risk of kernicterus.

The long-term administration of an enzyme-inducing drug such as a barbiturate will clearly affect the elimination of other drugs metabolised by the same pathway. This is particularly relevant to maintenance therapy with drugs which require control of plasma levels within fairly narrow limits, such as coumarin anticoagulants or oral hypoglycaemic agents. For example, a patient in the hospital with pulmonary thromboembolism may receive nightly treatment with a barbiturate hypnotic, which increases his requirement for warfarin to obtain an appropriate level of anticoagulation; on discharge from the hospital the barbiturate may be discontinued, with the result that the rate of warfarin metabolism gradually declines so that after several days there is a risk of haemorrhage from hypoprothrombinaemia.

Some drugs induce their own metabolism so that their pharmacological activity is reduced after a period of treatment. This type of decreased responsiveness has been described, for example, in the use of corticosteroids[19] and rifampin.[22]

ENZYME INHIBITION   The lack of specificity of the cytochrome P450-dependent enzyme system permits a drug to inhibit the metabolism of other drugs, which may be structurally unrelated, either by depression of the metabolising enzymes or by competition for the enzyme by the new drug substrate. The effect of inhibition is to prolong and intensify the biological activity of the affected drug, leading to toxic effects even when conventional doses are used. The time course of enzyme inhibition is determined by the time taken for sufficient concentration of the inhibitor to accumulate at the site of metabolism, and it is much shorter than that for enzyme induction. A number of drugs exert their effects by enzyme inhibition, including the xanthine oxidase inhibitor, allopurinol, the monoamine oxidase inhibitor, phenelzine, and the carbonic anhydrase inhibitor, sulthiame. The use of such agents may interfere with drug metabolism and lead to an unexpected exaggeration of the pharmacological effects of other drugs administered coincidentally, although this phenomenon may not be of clinical importance except where it affects drugs having a narrow margin of safety, such as anticoagulants, oral hypoglycaemics, or anticonvulsants. The glucuronidation pathway is also liable to inhibition if two drugs which are both eliminated by this route, such as acetaminophen and salicylate, are given simultaneously, resulting in prolongation of the effect of both drugs.

HEPATIC BLOOD FLOW   Because hepatic function has such a profound effect on the metabolism of many drugs, it is not surprising to find that changes in hepatic blood flow induced by disease or by drugs such as propranolol, phenobarbitone, and isoproterenol may influence the effect of drugs which are highly extracted by the liver, such as lidocaine.[55] The clinical importance of these experimental observations has still to be assessed.

Variability in Drug Excretion

Many drugs are excreted by the kidneys, either unchanged or after hepatic biotransformation. The mechanisms of renal drug excretion are the following:

1. Glomerular filtration, which permits the passage of free drug molecules while retaining drug bound to albumin.
2. Proximal tubular secretion, in which there are two active, carrier-mediated processes responsible, respectively, for the transport of acidic and basic compounds.
3. Passive tubular reabsorption, which occurs in both proximal and distal

tubules and is due to passive diffusion down a concentration gradient created by the progressive reabsorption of water and electrolytes from the tubular fluid. Drug reabsorption here depends upon lipid solubility and the degree of ionisation, and hence on the pH of the tubular fluid.
4. Active tubular reabsorption takes place for certain inorganic ions, amino acids, glucose, and some pharmacological agents such as lithium.

These processes are reasonably consistent between normal individuals, and variations in the mechanisms of renal drug excretion do not appear to contribute significantly to the variability of drug response in the presence of normal renal function. Where renal function is impaired, however, profound changes are seen in the elimination of drugs which follow renal excretory pathways. The main factors responsible for the variability of drug response attributable to excretion problems are age, renal disease, disease of other systems affecting renal function, and interactions between drugs excreted by the kidneys.

Effect of Impaired Renal Function   OLD AGE is associated with a fall in glomerular filtration rate and reduced renal tubular function, leading to a parallel reduction in drug excretion. Impaired excretion in old age is well recognised for such widely-used drugs as digoxin, chlorpropamide, and aminoglycoside antibiotics, causing increased risk of toxicity which severely curtails or prevents the use of such drugs in the elderly. *In the newborn* renal function is relatively poorly developed, and some accumulation may occur, for example, of acetaminophen (paracetamol), salicylates, and penicillins, which requires that dosage regimens be carefully regulated.

DISEASE AFFECTING RENAL FUNCTION   Most drugs are metabolised to pharmacologically inactive compounds before excretion, and for them the "elimination route" is biotransformation, since subsequent excretion of inert metabolites is of little pharmacological importance. But for those drugs which are excreted unchanged or are transformed to pharmacologically active metabolites which are subsequently excreted by the kidneys any impairment of renal function will have a material effect on their elimination, and therefore upon their pharmacological effect and toxicity. This is of minor significance for drugs with a high therapeutic index (or margin of safety) such as the penicillins, or for which alternative routes of elimination are available (for example, the biliary excretion of ampicillin), but is of overriding importance for drugs with a low therapeutic index such as the aminoglycosides.

Modification of dosage, either by reducing each dose or by increasing the dosage interval, is therefore necessary in treating patients with functional renal impairment. As a first approximation, the reduction in renal clearance of a drug is proportional to the reduction in creatinine clearance. This is therefore commonly used as a guide to dosage adjustments, since even in renal failure drug elimination rates are fairly predictable provided that renal function is stable. Tables and nomograms indicating the required dosage corrections for renal impairment of different grades of severity have been prepared for many drugs, and these data have great practical value.[8,15,50] Patients with impaired renal function are unusually susceptible to the toxic effects of some drugs, including nitrofurantoin in causing peripheral neuritis, ethacrynic acid in causing deafness, and most tetracyclines (but not doxycycline) in aggravating the deterioration in renal function. Such drugs are best avoided altogether if renal disease is known or suspected to be present.

Renal blood flow and glomerular filtration rate are diminished in cardiac failure and shock with resulting impairment in the clearance of drugs excreted by the kidneys.

Drug Interactions Affecting Renal Drug Excretion   Alteration in urine pH alters the passive tubular reabsorption of drugs which are weak electrolytes and are therefore only lipid soluble in their non-ionised form. Reduction in lipid solubility decreases their diffusion across tubular epithelial cells, decreases their reabsorption, and enhances their elimination. Urinary alkalinisation of weak acids such as salicylates causes them to become more ionised and increases their elimination, while urinary acidification enhances the excretion of weak bases such as amphetamine or quinidine. Therapeutic use of such interactions is employed in forced alkaline diuresis of salicylate and phenobarbital.

Competition for the common proximal tubular pathway for secreting acidic drugs or drug metabolites may allow one drug to interfere with the secretion of another, leading to accumulation and toxicity. Drugs which are secreted in this manner include salicylates, probenecid, penicillins, cephalosporins, phenylbutazone and thiazide diuretics, and the interference with penicillin excretion by probenecid is an example of the therapeutic use of this type of drug interaction.

PHARMACODYNAMIC VARIABLES

Up to this point the sources of variability in the response to drugs have been ascribed to factors which influence the concentration of the drug at its point of action. At this site the drug molecule becomes reversibly attached to a receptor which is usually rather specific for that drug, although other molecules of similar conformation may sometimes occupy the same receptor. The essential feature of the drug-receptor reaction site is that it forms a link in the chain of some biological system so that interaction at the site brings about a change in the rate at which that system functions: that is, drugs do not create biological actions, but they alter the rate at which such actions occur. To take a common example, the effect of a beta-adrenergic agent such as isoproterenol on bronchial smooth muscle is to stimulate the activity of the enzyme adenylcyclase, resulting in an increased concentration of the active molecule cyclic AMP, which produces bronchodilatation.[74] In considering the possible sources of pharmacodynamic variation in response to drugs it is necessary to ask whether two individuals, each with precisely the same concentration of drug at their respective drug-receptor interaction sites, may show different physiological responses; and if so, what the mechanism of this variation in response may be.

Genetically-determined Differences in Pharmacodynamic Response

A brief account has been given earlier in this chapter of variation in the biotransformation of certain drugs, for example, isoniazid. Genetic factors are also responsible for variations in tissue response to drugs, which can be categorised into quantitative and qualitative differences.

Quantitative Differences   Quantitative differences in tissue responsiveness are seen in the ways in which different individuals respond to warfarin. A striking variation is seen in patients with warfarin resistance, a condition described in two families, many of whose members required twenty or more times the usual dose and much higher plasma levels of anticoagulant to obtain the usual clinical response. Measurements of half-life and protein-binding indicate that the pharmacokinetic behaviour of warfarin is normal in these individuals.[56,57] The pattern of inheritance and the rarity of this abnormal response to warfarin suggests that it is transmitted by an autosomal dominant gene. Another instance of quantitative variability between individuals is the response to vitamin D, which is diminished in patients with vitamin D-resistant rickets characterised by retarded growth, hypophosphataemia, hypophosphaturia, and normocalcaemia. These abnormalities fail to respond to the usual doses of vitamin D but very large doses, more than one thousand times the normal amount, are effective. The condition is familial, inherited as a sex-linked dominant trait,[27] but its precise mechanism remains uncertain.

These examples of quantitative differences in individual responses to drugs are striking but rare, depending on single genes of major effect; it is likely that more commonly observed biological variations in the responsiveness to drugs have a genetic basis which may be due to several genes of small effect influencing tissue response. The seven-fold range of variation in heart rate response to a bolus injection of intravenous isoproterenol is an instance of the differences in drug sensitivity which may be encountered in an unselected population.[24]

Qualitative Differences   Qualitative differences among individuals in their response to drugs may also have a genetic basis. One of the best known is the deficiency of glucose-6-phosphate dehydrogenase (G6PD) in the red cell, which is quite common among some Mediterranean and Middle Eastern races, Indian and Indonesian subjects, and in dark-skinned peoples originating in Africa. It is determined by an X-linked gene which leads to a deficit of reduced sulphydryl (–SH) groups and impaired reduction of glutathione in the erythrocyte due to lack of an essential cofactor $NADPH_2$. Deficiency of –SH compounds in the red cells is conducive to haemolysis which is therefore enhanced by drugs or other agents that bind or oxidise – SH groups, such as a number of antimalarials, sulphonamides, other antimicrobial agents, and analgesics.[49] Estimates of the incidence of G6PD deficiency suggest that about one hundred million people are at risk of drug-induced haemolysis in the world population.

Another genetically-determined abnormality characterised by an unexpected response to a number of drugs is acute porphyria, which is due to excessive activity of the enzyme delta-aminolaevulinic acid synthetase (ALA-synthetase) in the liver. A third example is hereditary methaemoglobinaemia. Methaemoglobin is present in normal erythrocytes but in a concentration of less than 1 percent. This low concentration is maintained by the activity of intracellular enzymes which reduce methaemoglobin as soon as it is formed by spontaneous oxidation from ferrous to ferric ions in the haemoglobin molecule. The most important of these enzymes is methaemoglobin reductase which is absent in hereditary methaemoglobinaemia, a trait transmitted as an autosomal recessive allele. The administration of drugs which are oxidising agents causes the concentration of methaemoglobin to increase, leading to cyanosis and impaired oxygen-carrying capacity by the red cells. This disorder can be induced in normal people by excessive ingestion of substances such as phenacetin, nitrites and nitrates, aniline and its derivatives, and sulphonamides, but is much more prone to occur in individuals with the inherited enzyme deficiency.

Acquired Tolerance to Drugs

One mechanism which causes tolerance to the action of drugs is the phenomenon of induction, described earlier in this chapter, which leads to increased metabolism and therefore to more rapid clearance from the body of enzyme-inducing drugs such as corticosteroids or barbiturates when administered on a long-term basis (*pharmacokinetic tolerance*).

Another form of decreased drug responsiveness is the slow development of tolerance to drugs which affect mood and behaviour, such as opiates, barbiturates, alcohol, and amphetamine, apparently causing some sort of decreased sensitivity of the target cells in the brain, which is associated with drug dependence or addiction. It is sometimes referred to as *pharmacodynamic* or *cellular tolerance*. A third form of tolerance of some interest to the specialist in respiratory diseases is that of acute tolerance or *tachyphylaxis,* which has long been recognised in experimental animals and in man particularly with regard to the sympathomimetic amines such as ephedrine, amphetamine, and tyramine, which bring about their pharmacological effect indirectly by stimulating the release of norepinephrine from storage sites at adrenergic nerve endings. Repeated administration leads to norepinephrine depletion with loss of responsiveness to the administered drug. A similar tachyphylactic phenomenon can be seen in the vasodilator effects of morphine, which are due to morphine-induced histamine release from tissue storage sites. Whether refractoriness to sympathomimetic agents in asthmatic patients is due to tachyphylaxis is a matter of controversy, although the mechanism was considered to be a possible contributory factor in the epidemic of asthma deaths in Britain in the 1960s which coincided with an increase in the sale of isoproterenol-containing pressurised aerosol preparations.[70] Resistance to the chronotropic effect of isoproterenol has been observed in normal subjects infused with low doses intravenously[17]; and a few reports suggest that some of the adrenergic effects of the beta-sympathomimetic agent terbutaline may be reduced by chronic administration of the drug.[38] *Cross tolerance* to the effect of different sympathomimetic agents has also been demonstrated, for example, a reduction in the metabolic and circulatory responses to one agent (epinephrine) following the chronic administration of another (ephedrine).[54]

Drug Resistance

Drug resistance is the term used to describe partial or complete loss of sensitivity to chemotherapeutic agents which normally inhibit cell growth or cause cell death. In the field of respiratory disease, the phenomenon of drug resistance has a profound influence on the way antimicrobial agents are used for treating infections; a brief description of the more important mechanisms whereby micro-organisms develop resistance is given in Chapter 3.

Tissue Responsiveness to Drugs in the Elderly

For a variety of reasons drug therapy in the elderly is more liable to failure than in younger patients.[76] Failures of compliance are common because memory and comprehension are less dependable, especially when multiple pathologies lead to complex medication. In addition, the greater prevalence of multiple drug therapy increases the likelihood of adverse drug reactions and interactions. Alterations in drug disposition are probably the most important source of undesired drug effects, since declining renal function in old age limits the rate of excretion of many drugs, and coincidental chronic diseases, particularly those affecting renal and hepatic function, are likely to influence the time course of absorption, distribution, and elimination. The elderly are also often less able to metabolise drugs than younger patients, perhaps partly because the incidence of two important enzyme-inducing factors, smoking and alcohol consumption, is reduced in this age group. In contrast to numerous clearly recognised causes of variability in drug response which are largely pharmacokinetic in nature, it is surprisingly difficult to find well-documented instances of altered pharmacodynamic response to drugs which are related to age, even though there is a widely held clinical impression that the elderly are unduly sensitive to the therapeutic and toxic effects of many drugs.

The most convincing evidence of age-related alterations in tissue sensitivity comes from studies on drugs which act on the central nervous system. For instance, increased sensitivity of the ageing brain to benzodiazepines has been demonstrated in a comparison of the effects of nitrazepam in elderly and young subjects by relating its pharmacological effects on psychomotor performance to the plasma concentration.[14] This conclusion is supported by data from patients who received diazepam as sedation for elective cardioversion, showing increased sensitivity of the central nervous system in the elderly to the depressant effects of the drug.[63] Age was shown to be the most important variable in a study of post-operative pain relief with morphine and pentazocine which demonstrated an enhanced analgesic effect on the older patients, apparently due to age-related differences in pain perception.[7]

Other examples of age-related variability in tissue sensitivity are not so well-substantiated. Evidence for increased sensitivity to heparin in elderly women has been put forward,[39] but it is not possible to differentiate between pharmacokinetic or pharmacodynamic explanations for this observation. Inhibition by warfarin of vitamin K-dependent clotting-factor synthesis is more marked in the elderly,[67] but whether this is due to decreased affinity to vitamin K or to altered pharmacokinetics of the vitamin remains uncertain. The increased sensitivity of the elderly to antihypertensive drugs may be conditioned by the postural hypertension of old age, which is due to an impaired baroceptor response[32] and reduced peripheral venous tone.[13] It seems likely that this contributes to the high incidence of postural hypotension in elderly patients treated with thiazides, beta blocking agents, tricyclic antidepressants, and phenothiazines. And finally, there is recent laboratory evidence which suggests a correlation between increasing age and reduced sensitivity to isoproterenol[46] and propranolol,[76] using change in heart rate as a measure of the response to these drugs. It seems likely that as measurements of drug levels in plasma come to be applied more widely in the investigation and control of therapy, the significance of age-related variability in tissue responsiveness to drugs will be more clearly defined.

Disease-induced Differences in Tissue Sensitivity to Drugs

Most instances of disease-induced variation in the pharmacological effects of drugs can be attributed to the influence of the disease on drug disposition. However, there are several well-recognised clinical situations in which the liability to side-effects from a drug is greatly increased because a disease-induced pathophysiological change in a tissue alters its sensitivity to the drug. Examples include the increase in myocardial sensitivity to cardiac glycosides, which results from potassium depletion and leads to an increased risk of cardiac arrhythmias; and the sensitivity of patients with myasthenia gravis to the neuro-muscular blocking effect of aminoglycoside and polymyxin antibiotics which have a weak curare-like action, inapparent in normal individuals.

In the field of respiratory disease there are at least two examples of altered tissue sensitivity in disease which materially influence therapeutic practice. It is widely recognised that patients with chronic obstructive pulmonary disease are more liable to develop respiratory failure if they are given hypnotic or sedative drugs, and measurements of the effect of nitrazepam on central respiratory drive suggest that patients with chronic hypercapnia are unduly sensitive to the central depressant action of the drug.[66] This observation emphasises the need to avoid sedation not only in patients with acute hypercapnia due to an exacerbation of chronic bronchitis but also in those with chronic stable respiratory failure. The other example is related to the incautious use of beta-adrenoceptor blocking agents for the treatment of cardiac arrhythmias, hypertension, or angina in patients with co-existent bronchoconstrictive disorders such as asthma or chronic obstructive pulmonary disease. It appears that in most of these patients bronchial patency is maintained by an underlying increase in sympathetic tone which is abolished by non-selective beta blockers such as propranolol.[64]

Some of the clinically more important instances of variability in tissue sensitivity to drugs in disease states are summarised in Table 1-1; others are reviewed in greater detail by Lowenthal.[47]

Pharmacodynamic Drug Interactions

Pharmacodynamic drug interactions are those in which one drug interferes with the action or effect of another. The interfering drug may do this in one of three ways:

Table 1-1 / Examples of Disease-induced Variation in Tissue Sensitivity to Drugs

Disease	Tissue affected	Physiological or pathological abnormality	Drug	Undesired effect of drug	References
Conditions leading to hypokalaemia (such as chronic renal disease)	Cardiac muscle	Hypokalaemia	Digitalis	Enhanced sensitivity to arrhythmogenic effects	71
Chronic respiratory disease	Cardiac muscle	Hypoxia plus other factors (?)	Digitalis	Enhanced sensitivity to arrhythmogenic effects	29
Conditions leading to chronic hypercapnia, e.g. chronic obstructive pulmonary disease, severe kyphoscoliosis	Respiratory "centre"	Hypercapnia	Benzodiazepines (such as nitrazepam)	Depression of central respiratory drive	66
Asthma, chronic obstructive pulmonary disease	Bronchial smooth muscle	Increased sympathetic tone maintaining bronchodilatation	Non-selective β-adrenoceptor blockers, (such as propranolol)	Abolition of sympathetic tone	64
Myasthenia gravis	Neuromuscular end-plate	Reduced acetylcholine release, decreased responsiveness of end-plate (?)	Aminoglycoside and polymyxin groups of antibiotics	Neuromuscular blockade	73
Hepatic encephalopathy	Cerebral	"Cerebral depression" leading to hepatic coma	Morphine	Drowsiness with EEG evidence of hepatic pre-coma	41

1. It may prevent the primary drug from reacting with its tissue receptor.
2. It may alter the responsiveness of the tissue to the primary drug.
3. It may act independently on the same physiological system as the primary drug, either potentiating or antagonising its effect.

These three types of pharmacodynamic interaction are illustrated by the following examples.

Interference at the Site of Drug–Receptor Interaction   A classic example is the interaction between guanidinium antihypertensive agents such as guanethidine, bethanidine, and debrisoquine, and trycyclic antidepressant drugs. These antihypertensive agents act by blocking the release of norepinephrine from the sympathetic nerve ending, but are prevented from doing so by the tricyclics (for example, amitriptyline, nortriptyline) which interfere with the uptake of the antihypertensive drug.[51] This interaction leads inevitably to loss of blood pressure control. Another example of this type of drug interaction is that of direct competition for drug receptor sites, which occurs between the narcotic antagonists nalorphine, levallorphan, and naloxone, and the opiates such as morphine. This interaction is used therapeutically to antagonise opiate overdosage.

Alteration of Tissue Responsiveness   Potassium depletion increases the sensitivity of cardiac muscle to the dysrhythmogenic effect of cardiac glycosides, and it also antagonises the antiarrhythmic actions of diphenylhydantoin, lidocaine, procainamide, and quinidine. Potassium-losing diuretics such as the thiazides, furosemide, and ethacrynic acid are therefore liable to interact with these drugs through their indirect influence on the potassium content of cardiac tissue. Hypokalaemia also causes hyperpolarisation of the motor end-plate, thereby antagonising the action of acetycholine and hence prolonging paralysis by non-depolarising muscle relaxants such as tubocurarine; here again, potassium-losing drugs such as diuretics and carbenoxolone are a possible source of drug interaction if potassium depletion is allowed to occur.

Effect on the Same Physiological System   There are many examples of interactions due to two drugs influencing the same physiologic function and so antagonising or potentiating each other's effects. Indeed, this type of mutual interaction is often used to obtain an enhanced therapeutic effect such as in the concurrent use of thiazide diuretics and beta-adrenergic blocking agents for the control of hypertension, and it is wise to anticipate such interactions when one of the actions of a drug is upon the same system or is of the same kind as another drug with which it is being administered.

As a rather non-specific example one can cite the mutual potentiation which occurs between alcohol and other central nervous system depressants such as barbiturates, phenothiazines, sedative antihistamines, and benzodiazepine derivatives. The interaction between coumarin anticoagulants such as warfarin and salicylates has the effect of increasing the liability to haemorrhage from the gastrointestinal tract, partly because salicylates may act synergistically with coumarins by direct or indirect mechanisms to augment anticoagulant-induced hypoprothrombinaemia and also because salicylates are apt to cause local bleeding from the gastric mucosa.

One illustrative example of this type of drug interaction is that between beta-adrenergic blocking drugs and hypoglycaemic agents; the blood-sugar-lowering effect of the latter leads to catecholamine secretion, which normally stimulates glycogenolysis—a response which is blocked by propranolol, causing prolonged hypoglycaemia.[1]

DRUG ALLERGY[59]

Although allergic reactions to drugs are difficult to predict, they are a source of significant morbidity and rarely are a cause of death. It is therefore important that prescribers should be conscious of the possibility of an allergic response, should make appropriate enquiries for any allergic history before the drug is administered, and should ask themselves whether the drug is really necessary. The importance of this question is emphasised in an account of thirty fatal reactions to penicillin wherein it is suggested that the indications for penicillin therapy were doubtful in thirteen cases and not apparent at all in five of the cases.[65]

The incidence of allergic drug reactions is low although difficult to assess with precision, because it is not always possible to distinguish between allergic and idiosyncratic (that is, genetically-determined hypersensitivity) reactions. Assessments of incidence are based on hospital studies, and mild reactions—which are undoubtedly more common than severe ones—are usually unreported. From drug surveillance studies carried out in hospitals it appears that well under 10 percent of all adverse reactions to drugs had an allergic basis,[10] that the rate of allergic skin reactions is approximately 3 per 1,000 courses of drug therapy,[4] and that drug-induced anaphylaxis (which included reactions to the administration of blood and blood products) is even less common, occurring with an incidence of 0.6 per 1,000 medical inpatients.[11] Penicillin and its semi-synthetic derivatives account for a large share of allergic drug reactions, and it appears that relatively few drugs are allergenic.

Pathogenesis

Antigenicity of Drugs   The allergic response occurs as the result of a reaction between the allergen, which like a protein is a macromolecular structure, and the antibody which is a specific immunoglobulin produced in response to an earlier exposure to the same allergen. Most drugs do not have a macromolecular structure but are simple chemicals which produce allergic reactions because they are able to combine with endogenous macromolecules—mainly with proteins, but possibly with polysaccharides and polynucleotides as well. Simple chemicals which are incomplete antigens are called haptens, and the hapten-protein conjugation that creates the active antigen is formed irreversibly by covalent bonds. As a general rule, drugs themselves do not react with protein; the hapten-protein conjugation takes place only after the drug has been metabolised *in vivo* to an active derivative. A drug such as penicillin produces a number of haptenic determinants, the major one being the penicilloyl group which probably stimulates the production of penicillin antibodies in all persons who receive penicillin; but it is important to stress that the presence of an immunological response does not necessarily mean production of the clinical manifestations of allergy.

Cross-allergenicity occurs between drugs of similar chemical structure, for example, among all penicillin derivatives which differ from each other in their side chain but have the same 6-aminopenicillanic acid nucleus; and between penicillins and cephalosporins, which have a rather similar nucleus. This potential for cross-reactions has obvious clinical importance in relation to the choice of antibiotic therapy in persons for whom a previous history of drug allergy is suspected.

Types of Immunological Response   This classification of the types of immunological response is based on the mechanism of its production. *Type I* describes the immediate, anaphylactic kind of reaction which is due to interaction between the antigen and tissue cells previously sensitised by cell-bound antibody, leading to the abrupt release of pharmacologically active substances. The antibody, originally known as reagin, is circulating IgE which becomes fixed to tissue mast cells. In the *Type II* reaction the antigen is located on the surface of a target cell, usually one of the formed elements of the blood, and reacts with a circulating antibody with resulting agglutination of cells, or lysis in the presence of complement. The *Type III* response is the immune complex reaction, and this includes serum sickness, urticarial and maculopapular rashes, nephropathy and polyarthritis, due to circulating antigens which remain in the circulation for long periods of time and form soluble circulating antigen-antibody complexes. These localise in vascular walls and surrounding tissues where they cause damage to cells and blood vessels in the presence of complement. The *Type IV* reaction describes a delayed hypersensitivity which results from the interaction between the antigen and previously sensitised lymphocytes, causing tissue injury. Examples of Type IV reactions include tuberculin sensitivity and contact dermatitis.

The risk of Type I reactions is increased in atopic individuals,[43] but other allergic reactions seem to occur equally in atopic and non-atopic people.

Clinical Manifestations

The typical reaction of *anaphylaxis* develops within a few minutes following the administration of an offending drug, most commonly when it is given by the intravenous or intramuscular route, although in highly sensitive people the reaction may occur as a result of oral, subcutaneous, or even respiratory administration. Anaphylaxis is characterised by bronchospasm; hypotension; angioneurotic oedema; skin reactions involving pruritus, urticaria, and erythema; and sometimes cardiac arrhythmias and hyperperistalsis. These symptoms may occur singly or in combination. Penicillin is by far the commonest cause of anaphylactic reactions, but other causative agents include streptomycin, local anaesthetic agents, cephalosporins, cromolyn sodium, demethylchlortetracycline, radio-opaque organic iodides, and protein-containing preparations such as blood or its derivatives. Drug-induced anaphylaxis is rare, being shown to occur in only 8 of 11,526 consecutively monitored medical hospital cases, with one fatality.[11]

Skin reactions are the commonest manifestation of allergic drug reactions, and they may take any of the following forms: urticaria; morbilliform, maculopapular, vesicular, bullous, exfoliative, and eczematous eruptions; purpura; contact dermatitis; fixed eruptions; erythema nodosum; erythema multiforme; photosensitivity; and pruritus. Sometimes the diagnosis may be helped by observing that skin and visceral manifestations occur together, but none of the above patterns in themselves are diagnostic of drug allergy. Urticaria is a common manifestation of immediate, Type I sensitivity, and contact dermatitis is particularly characteristic of the delayed hypersensitivity reaction, Type IV.

Fever is a common manifestation of drug allergy which may occur with other symptoms or in isolation. It is associated with many antibiotics and chemotherapeutic agents and the unexplained occurrence or persistence of fever during a course of therapy for an infectious illness, for example, a therapeutic trial of antituberculosis drugs, may mask a favourable response to treatment. It also occurs in relation to treatment with iodine, quinidine, procainamide, thiouracils, and anticonvulsants.

The onset of *serum sickness* usually occurs 7–12 days after the initiation of therapy with the offending drug, and it is mediated by antigen, complement, and IgG antibody. The main features of the syndrome are fever, joint pains, lymphadenopathy, and urticaria, sometimes with the development of polyar-teritis nodosa and other collagen disorders. Nephropathy, vasculitis, myocar-ditis, polymyositis, and neuropathy may all occur in association with the serum sickness syndrome. Drugs which may produce serum sickness include some commonly used chemotherapeutic agents such as penicillin, streptomycin, aminosalicylic acid, and sulphonamides.

Immunologically-mediated *blood disorders* are an important manifesta-tion of drug allergy and are due to Type II reactions, in which a great variety of drugs may cause agglutination or lysis of erythrocytes, leucocytes, or platelets. Drug-induced allergic haemolytic anaemia is caused by a number of agents, which includes penicillin, aminosalicylic acid, quinidine, sulphonamides, cephalosporins, and acetophenetidin (phenacetin). Immunologically-mediated thrombocytopenia causes purpura, fever, and other allergic manifestations, and may be precipitated by acetaminophen (paracetamol), quinidine, chlor-othiazide, chloramphenicol, the sulphonamides and, classically, Sedormid (apronalide). Allergic granulocytopenia may be produced by phenylbutazone, phenothiazines, sulphonamides, thiouracil, anticonvulsants, gold, organic arsenicals, and tolbutamide.

Drug-induced inflammatory reactions in organs such as the kidneys, the liver, and the lungs are poorly defined and may be due to direct toxicity rather than to an allergic reaction. However the association of hepatitis with fever, eosinophilia, rashes, and lymphadenopathy certainly suggests an allergic aetiology, especially if symptoms recur on readministration. Such hepatic reac-tions may follow the administration of a number of drugs, including phe-nothiazines, sulphonamides, aminosalicylate, and isoniazid. Pulmonary eosin-ophilia, with fever, recurrent pulmonary infiltration, and hilar lymphadeno-pathy is an allergic manifestation of treatment with nitrofurantoin, and may occur infrequently as a reaction to other drugs such as penicillins, aspirin, sulphonamides, and aminosalicylic acid. Interstitial nephritis associated with severe renal dysfunction and eosinophilia in blood and urine may be induced by therapy with methicillin and other semi-synthetic penicillins.[23]

Vasculitis and connective tissue diseases as a manifestation of drug allergy are other poorly defined sources of variability in the individual response to drugs. Vascular lesions which affect mainly small arteries and arterioles can lead to syndromes which may be classified as hypersensitivity vasculitis or polyarteritis nodosa, or may even resemble giant-cell arteritis. The drugs which are most frequently thought to cause these complications are penicillins, phenytoin, sulphonamides, tetracyclines, thiouracil, thiazides, busulphan, phenylbutazone, and iodides. A clinical syndrome similar to systemic lupus erythematosus has been described in connection with prolonged hydrallazine therapy and less frequently with anticonvulsant agents, procainamide, isoniazid, tetracyclines, sulphonamides, thiouracil, iodides, heavy metals, and oral contraceptive agents. In addition to a positive LE cell reaction and antinuclear factors, a positive Coombs test and occasionally haemolytic anaemia may be associated with the syndrome. It usually resolves promptly when the drug is stopped.

Management

Most allergic drug manifestations respond simply to withdrawal of the offending drug and substitution of another, but the prescribing physician must take care to ensure that there is no likelihood of cross-reactivity with the alternative chosen. Symptomatic treatment with antihistamines may be necessary to relieve urticaria and itching, and corticosteroids may be indicated for severe skin reactions, vasculitis, hepatitis, interstitial nephritis, and sometimes for drug-induced haemolytic anaemia and thrombocytopenia.

Acute anaphylactic reactions are best treated with subcutaneous epinephrine 0.5–1 ml of 1:1,000 aqueous solution, given without delay. Antihistamines are not helpful in treating an acute reaction, but supportive therapy to control cardiac arrhythmias, sustain blood pressure, and maintain an adequate airway may be essential. The resources for providing these emergency measures are unlikely to be available outside the physicians office or clinic, and since parenteral penicillin is the most likely cause of an acute anaphylactic reaction outside the hospital, the administration of penicillin by mouth is normally the procedure of choice.[58] The possible risks of acute anaphylactic reactions can be minimised by seeking for a history of atopy or previous drug allergy before the parenteral administration of a potentially lethal drug such as penicillin, by considering the possibility of cross-reactivity, for example, between penicillins and cephalosporins or between different aminoglycosides, and by administering the drug under the safest possible conditions.

If no satisfactory alternative to the offending drug is available and its use is essential, *hyposensitisation* may be attempted. Beginning with the oral route, very small quantities of the drug are given by mouth with gradually increasing dosage over a period of four to twenty-four hours until therapeutic levels are reached. At this stage parenteral administration is introduced, beginning intradermally or subcutaneously with a minute dose and increasing this progressively while the oral preparation is continued at the previous maximal dose. A suggested procedure for penicillin hyposensitisation is described in Chapter 4, but it is hazardous and can lead to death of the patient.[33] This procedure, therefore, should only be attempted for a life-threatening condition when no alternative therapy is available and with all of the necessary emergency medications and resuscitative equipment ready for immediate use.

THE PLACEBO RESPONSE

Placebos in Clinical Practice

In a revealing study on a group of asthmatic subjects,[48] it was shown that a proportion of the subjects could be induced to develop asthma after inhaling normal saline which they believed to be an allergen, and afterward could be "cured" by inhaling the same saline which they then believed to be isoproterenol. This observation is one example of the suggestibility of sick people who believe they are receiving potent pharmacological preparations, and it illustrates the degree of variability in the patient's response to medication which can be attributed simply to the placebo effect.

The placebo response is a well-substantiated phenomenon which must have been largely responsible for the success of physicians until the end of the nineteenth century, before the application of scientific method and pharmacological knowledge began to provide a rational basis for drug therapy. Nevertheless, the contribution of the placebo effect to the total therapeutic response remains significant to the present day and can sometimes be quantified in comparison with pharmacologically-active drugs by applying appropriate investigative techniques (see reference 26, for example). Symptomatic relief has been provided by placebo medication for a wide variety of illnesses, including angina pectoris,[3] asthma,[26] cough,[28] pulmonary tuberculosis,[42] and essential hypertension.[31] Studies suggest that at least a third of patients will respond to placebo medication, and an even higher proportion with psychological symptoms such as anxiety and sleeplessness will be helped.[6] There is, however, no specific group of subjects who can be categorised as "placebo responders," since at one time or another any subject may respond to a placebo.

The placebo response seems to depend to a great extent upon the relationship between the patient and doctor and upon their individual attitudes toward the treatment. The term "placebo" (Latin for "I shall please") seems to imply that the preparation is given simply to satisfy the patient's wishes, without any expectation of success on the part of the doctor; but there is ample evidence to show that pharmacologically inert compounds can relieve symptoms, particularly when the patient has high expectations of success from the treatment[44,80] or if the doctor is optimistic.[79] Nevertheless it would be wrong to suppose that placebo effects are imaginary since real changes in physiological function such as alteration in bronchial calibre or change in blood pressure and pulse rate can readily be demonstrated.

A beneficial response to therapy may therefore occur independently of the pharmacological action of the drug, and a clear understanding of the placebo effect is necessary if treatment is to be assessed critically.

Placebos in Clinical Drug Trials

Because the placebo effect has such an unpredictable influence on the individual's response to drug therapy it is of the utmost importance that due allowance be made for it in assessing the pharmacological efficacy of drugs. In order to determine whether a drug has a significant effect on a measured physiological or pathological variable (for example, on the bronchodilator effect of a new beta-sympathomimetic agent or the pain-relieving effect of an analgesic preparation) it is necessary to administer the drug to a group of patients with the abnormality and to measure the change which follows the administration. But to avoid the possibility that the measured change is due to a placebo effect, a companion study must be performed on a similar group of patients who receive not the drug but an inert placebo preparation which is indistinguishable to the patient from the active drug, and a comparison must be made between the two groups. Since the doctor may by his attitude influence the patient's response to the drug or the placebo, he too should remain ignorant of which preparation each patient receives until the trial is completed. This is the essential nature of the *double-blind trial,* which may sometimes be further refined by repeating the experiment on a different occasion but under the same conditions, only ensuring that each individual who received the active preparation on the first occasion receives the placebo preparation on the second, and vice versa. By this means, each patient serves as his own control, a manoeuvre which minimises the effect of individual variability and increases the likelihood of detecting a difference between the effect of the drug and the effect of the placebo.

Such an experiment is called a *double-blind crossover* trial which lends itself to stringent statistical analysis provided that appropriate care is taken in randomising the allocation of drug and placebo preparations to each individual to ensure that the order in which each preparation is administered is randomly but equally distributed throughout the whole group.

The use of a placebo in drug trials provides a standard with which the drug on trial may be compared. It may sometimes be more appropriate to use another drug of known characteristics as the standard instead of a placebo, so that the efficacy of the new drug is required to stand comparison with a well-tried preparation. Experimental designs of this nature allow observations to be made not only on the desired pharmacological effect of the drug but also on important incidental aspects of its use, such as its acceptability to the patient, administration problems, and the incidence of unwanted effects. Probably one of the greatest practical problems lies in the selection of cases, to ensure that the patients studied form a homogeneous but representative group, allowing deductions drawn from the test sample to be applied to a wider population.

REFERENCES

1. Abramson EA, Arky RA, Woeber KA: Effects of propranolol on the hormonal and metabolic responses to insulin-induced hypoglycaemia. Lancet 2: 1386–1389, 1966.
2. Alexanderson B, Borga O: Interindividual differences in plasma protein binding of nortriptyline in man—a twin study. Eur J Clin Pharmacol 4: 196–200, 1972.
3. Amsterdam EA, Wolfson S, Gorlin R: New aspects of the placebo response in angina pectoris. Am J Cardiol 24: 305–306, 1969.
4. Arndt KA, Jick H: Rates of cutaneous reactions to drugs. JAMA 235: 918–923, 1976.
5. Barr WH, Adir J, Garretson L: Decrease of tetracycline absorption in man by sodium bicarbonate. Clin Pharmacol Ther 12: 799–784, 1971.
6. Beecher HK: The powerful placebo. JAMA 159: 1602–1606, 1955.
7. Bellville JW, Forrest WH, Miller E, Brown BW: Influence of age on pain relief from analgesics. JAMA 217: 1835–1841, 1971.
8. Bennett WM, Singer I, Golper T, Feig P, Coggins CJ: Guide-lines for drug therapy in renal failure. Ann Intern Med 86: 754–783, 1977.
9. Blackwell B: The drug defaulter. Clin Pharmacol Ther 6: 841–848, 1972.
10. Borda IT, Slone D, Jick H: Assessment of adverse reactions within a drug surveillance program. JAMA 205: 645–647, 1968.
11. Boston Collaborative Drug Surveillance Program: Drug-induced anaphylaxis. JAMA 224: 613–615, 1973.
12. Branch RA, Herbert CM, Read AE: Determinants of serum antipyrine half-lives in patients with liver disease. Gut 14: 569–573, 1973.
13. Caird FI, Andrews GR, Kennedy RD: Effect of posture on blood pressure in the elderly. Br Heart J 35: 527–530, 1973.
14. Castleden CM, George CF, Marcer D, Hallett C: Increased sensitivity to nitrazepam in old age. Br Med J 1: 10–12, 1977.
15. Cheigh JS: Drug administration in renal failure. Am J Med 62: 555–563, 1977.
16. Cheng SH, White A: Effect of orally administered neomycin on the absorption of penicillin V. N Engl J Med 267: 1296–1297, 1962.
17. Connolly, ME, Davies DS, Dollery CT, George CF: Resistance to β-adrenoceptor stimulants (a possible explanation for the rise in asthma deaths). Br J Pharmacol 43: 389–402, 1971.
18. Drayer DE: Pharmacologically active drug metabolites: Therapeutic and toxic activities, plasma and urine data in man, accumulation in renal failure. Clin Pharmacokinet 1: 426–443, 1976.
19. Dwyer J, Lazarus L, Hickie JB: A study of cortisol metabolism in patients with chronic asthma. Australasian Ann Med 16: 297–303, 1967.
20. Ellard GA: Variations between individuals and populations in the acetylation of isoniazid and its significance for the treatment of pulmonary tuberculosis. Clin Pharmacol Ther 19: 610–625, 1976.
21. Evans DAP, White TA: Human acetylation polymorphism. J Lab Clin Med 63: 394–403, 1963.

22. FURESZ S: Chemical and biological properties of rifampicin. Antibiotica and Chemotherapia 16: 316–351, 1970.
23. GALPIN JE, SHINABERGER JG, STANLEY TM, BLUMENKRANTZ MJ, BAYER AS, FRIEDMAN GS, MONTGOMERIE JZ, GUZE LB, COBURN JW, GLASSOCK RJ: Acute interstitial nephritis due to methicillin. Am J Med 65: 756–765, 1978.
24. GEORGE CF, CONOLLY ME, FENYVESI T, BRIANT RH, DOLLERY CT: Intravenously administered isoproterenol sulfate dose-response curves in man. Arch Intern Med 130: 361–364, 1972.
25. GLAUSER SC: Drug metabolism: conjugation and multiple pathways. Med Clin North Am 58: 945–949, 1974.
26. GODFREY S, SILVERMAN M: Demonstration of placebo responses in asthma by means of exercise testing. J Psychosom Res 17: 293–297, 1973.
27. GRAHAM JB, McFALLS VW, WINTERS RW: Familial hypophosphatemia with vitamin D-resistant rickets. 2: Three additional kindreds of the sex-linked dominant type with a genetic analysis of four such families. Am J Hum Genet 11: 311–332, 1959.
28. GRAVENSTEIN JS, DEVLOO RA, BEECHER HK: Effect of antitussive agents on experimental and pathological cough in man. J App Physiol 7: 119–139, 1954.
29. GREEN LH, SMITH TW: The use of digitalis in patients with pulmonary disease. Ann Intern Med 87: 459–465, 1977.
30. GREENBLATT DJ, DUHME DW, KOCH-WESER T, SMITH TW: Evaluation of digoxin bioavailability in single dose studies. N Engl J Med 289: 651–654, 1973.
31. GRENFELL RF, BRIGGS AH, HOLLAND WC: Antihypertensive drugs evaluated in a controlled double-blind study. South Med J 56: 1410–1416, 1963.
32. GRIBBON B, PICKERING TG, SLEIGHT P, PETO R: Effect of age and blood pressure on baroreflex sensitivity in man. Circ Res 29: 424–431, 1971.
33. GRIECO MH, DUBIN MR, ROBINSON JL, SCHWARTZ MJ: Penicillin hypersensitivity in patients with bacterial endocarditis. Ann Intern Med 60: 204–216, 1964.
34. GUGLER R, LAIN P, AZARNOFF DL: Effect of portacaval shunt on the disposition of drugs with and without first-pass effect. J Pharmacol Exp Ther 195: 416–423, 1975.
35. HOMEIDA M, JACKSON L, ROBERTS CJC: Decreased first-pass metabolism of labetalol in chronic liver disease. Br Med J 2: 1048–1050, 1978.
36. HURWITZ N, WADE OL: Intensive hospital monitoring of adverse reactions to drugs. Br Med J 1: 531–536, 1969.
37. JENKINS JS, SAMPSON PA: Conversion of cortisone to cortisol and prednisone to prednisolone. Br Med J 2: 205–207, 1967.
38. JENNE JW, CHICK TW, STRICKLAND RD: Induction of betareceptor tolerance by terbutaline. J Allergy Clin Immunol 55: 96, 1975.
39. JICK H, SLONE D, BORDA IT, SHAPIRO S: Efficacy and toxicity of heparin in relation to age and sex. N Engl J Med 279: 284–286, 1968.
40. KUNIN CM: Drugs, receptors and serum protein binding. N Engl J Med 281: 1188–1189, 1969.
41. LAIDLAW J, READ AE, SHERLOCK S: Morphine tolerance in hepatic cirrhosis. Gastroenterology 40: 389–396, 1961.
42. LASAGNA L, LATIES VG, DOHAN JL: Further studies on the "pharmacology" of placebo administration. J Clin Invest 37: 533–537, 1958.
43. LEVINE BB: Immunological mechanisms of penicillin allergy. A haptenic model

system for the study of allergic diseases in man. N Engl J Med 275: 1115–1125, 1966.

44. LIBERMAN R: An analysis of the placebo phenomenon. J Chronic Dis 15: 761–783, 1962.

45. LINDENBAUM J, MAULITZ RM, SAHA JR, SHEA N, BUTLER VP: Impairment of digoxin absorption by neomycin. Clin Res 20: 410, 1972.

46. LONDON GM, SAFAR ME, WEISS YA, MILLIEZ PL: Isoproterenol sensitivity and total body clearance of propranolol in hypertensive patients. J Clin Pharmacol 16: 174–182, 1976.

47. LOWENTHAL DT: Tissue sensitivity to drugs in disease states. Med Clin North Am 58: 1111–1119, 1974.

48. LUPARELLO T, LYONS HA, BLEECKER ER, McFADDEN ER: Influence of suggestion on airway reactivity in asthmatic subjects. Psychom Med 30: 819–825, 1968.

49. MARKS PA, BANKS J: Drug-induced haemolytic anaemias associated with glucose-6-phosphate dehydrogenase deficiency: a genetically heterogeneous trait. Ann NY Acad Sci 123: 198–206, 1965.

50. MAWER GE, AHMAD R, DOBBS SM, McGOUGH JG, LUCAS SB, TOOTH JA: Prescribing aids for gentamicin. Br J Clin Pharmacol 1: 45–50, 1974.

51. MITCHELL JR, CAVANAUGH JH, ARIAS L, OATES JA: Guanethidine and related agents, 3. Antagonism by drugs which inhibit the norepinephrine pump in man. J Clin Invest 49: 1596–1604, 1970.

52. MOHLER DN, WALLIN DG, DREYFUS EG: Studies in the home treatment of streptococcal disease. I. Failure of patients to take penicillin by mouth as prescribed. N Engl J Med 252: 1116–1118, 1955.

53. MOULDING T, OVSTAD GD, SBARBARO JA: Supervision of outpatient drug therapy with the medication monitor. Ann Intern Med 73: 559–564, 1970.

54. NELSON HS, BLACK JW, BRANCH LB, PFUETZE B, SPAULDING H, SUMMERS R, WOOD D: Subsensitivity to epinephrine following administration of epinephrine and ephedrine to normal individuals. J. Allergy Clin Immunol 55: 299–309, 1975.

55. NIES AS, SHAND DG, WILKINSON GR: Altered hepatic blood flow and drug disposition. Clin Pharmacokinet 1: 135–155, 1976.

56. O'REILLY RA: The second reported kindred with hereditary resistance to oral anticoagulant drugs. N Engl J Med 282: 1448–1451, 1970.

57. O'REILLY RA, AGGELER PM, HOAG MS, LEONG LS, KROPATKIN ML: Hereditary transmission of exceptional resistance to coumarin anticoagulant drugs. N Engl J Med 271: 809–815, 1964.

58. PARKER CW: Practical aspects of diagnosis and treatment of patients who are hypersensitive to drugs. in Samter M and Parker CW (eds) International Encyclopaedia of Pharmacology and Therapeutics. Section 75: Hypersensitivity to Drugs, Vol 1. p. 367–394. Oxford, Pergamon, 1972.

59. PARKER CW: Drug allergy. N Engl J Med 292: 511–514, 732–736, and 951–960, 1975.

60. PARSONS RL: Drug absorption in gastrointestinal disease with particular reference to malabsorption syndromes. Clin Pharmacokinet 2: 45–60, 1977.

61. POOLE HH: Drugs in infusion fluids. Adverse Drug Reaction Bulletin 62: 216–219, 1977.

62. POWELL JR, VOZEH S, HOPEWELL P, COSTELLO J, SHEINER LB, RIEGELMAN S: Theophylline disposition in acutely ill hospitalised patients. The effect of smoking, heart failure, severe airways obstruction and pneumonia. Am Rev Resp Dis 118: 229–238, 1978.

63. REIDENBERG MM, LEVY M, WARNER H, COUTINHO CB, SCHWARTZ MA, YU G, CHERIPLCO J: The relationship between diazepam dose, plasma level, age, and central nervous system depression in adults. Clin Pharmacol Ther 23: 371–374, 1978.

64. RICHARDSON PS, STERLING GM: Effects of beta-adrenergic receptol blockade on airway conductance and lung volume in normal and asthmatic subjects. Br Med J 3: 143–145, 1969.

65. ROSENTHAL A: Follow-up study of fatal penicillin reactions. JAMA 167: 1118–1121, 1958.

66. RUDOLF M, GEDDES DM, TURNER JAM, SAUNDERS KB: Depression of central respiratory drive by nitrazepam. Thorax 33: 97–100, 1978.

67. SHEPHERD AMM, HEWICK DS, MORELAND TA, STEVENSON IH: Age as a determinant of sensitivity of warfarin. Br J Clin Pharmacol 4: 315–320, 1977.

68. SMITH SE, RAWLINS MD: Prediction of drug oxidation rates in man: Lack of correlation with serum gamma-glutamyl transpeptidase and urinary excretion of D-glutamic acid and 6 β-hydroxycortisol. Eur J Clin Pharmacol 7: 71, 1974.

69. SMITH JW, SEIDL LG, CLUFF, LE: Studies on the epidemiology of adverse drug reactions. Ann Intern Med 65: 629–640, 1966.

70. SPEIZER FE, DOLL R, HEAF P, STRANG LB: Investigation into use of drugs preceding death from asthma. Br Med J 1: 339–343, 1968.

71. SURAWICZ B: Role of electrolytes in etiology and management of cardiac arrhythmias. Prog Cardiovasc Dis 8: 364–386, 1966.

72. THOMSON PD, MELMON KL, RICHARDSON JA, COHN K, STEINBRUNN W, CUDIHEE R, ROWLAND M: Lidocaine pharmacokinetics in advanced heart failure, liver disease and renal failure in humans. Ann Intern Med 78: 499–508, 1973.

73. TOIVAKKA E, HOKKANEN E: The aggravating effect of streptomycin on the neuromuscular blockade in myasthenia gravis. Acta Neurol Scand 41 (Suppl 13): 275–277, 1965.

74. TRINER L, NAHAS GG, VULLIEMOZ Y, OVERWEG NIA: Cyclic AMP and smooth muscle function. Ann NY Acad Sci 185: 458–476, 1971.

75. VESELL ES: Polygenic factors controlling drug response. Med Clin North Am 58: 951–963, 1974.

76. VESTAL RE: Drug use in the elderly: a review of problems and special considerations. Drugs, 16: 358–382, 1978.

77. VESTAL RE, WOOD AJJ, SHAND DG: Reduced beta-adrenoceptor sensitivity in the elderly. Clin Res 26: 488A, 1978.

78. WANDLESS I, DAVIE JW: Can drug compliance in the elderly be improved? Br Med J 1: 359–361, 1977.

79. WHEATLEY D: Influence of doctors' and patients' attitudes in the treatment of neurotic illness. Lancet 2: 1133–1135, 1967.

80. WOLF S: Effects of suggestion and conditioning on the action of chemical agents in human subjects: the pharmacology of placebos. J Clin Invest 29: 100–109, 1950.

2
Cough and Sputum

Like breathlessness or pain, cough is a symptom which has to be investigated and explained so that appropriate curative treatment can be given for the underlying disease. There are occasions, however, when symptomatic treatment is necessary for those who seek relief from the irritation of a distressing cough or complain of difficulty in expectorating viscid sputum, and this short chapter provides a critical appraisal of the pharmacological agents which are either effective or, though of uncertain value, are widely used in the suppression of cough or the encouragement of expectoration.

STRUCTURE AND FUNCTION

Bronchial secretion and foreign particles deposited within the tracheobronchial tree are removed by three physiological processes: mucociliary clearance, cough, and alveolar clearance. Consideration of alveolar clearance[35] is outside the scope of this book, since it relates to the phagocytic activities of alveolar macrophages which are not currently amenable to pharmacologic manipulation. Mucociliary clearance and cough, however, are protective mechanisms responsible for keeping the conducting airways clear of inhaled foreign particles and the debris of secretion, and are influenced by a wide range of physicochemical and pharmacological agents which are used, sometimes uncritically, in the treatment of respiratory disease.

Mucociliary Clearance

In the normal individual the tracheobronchial tree is lined with an epithelium consisting of several cell types, and among them are the ciliated columnar cells and the goblet cells which contribute directly to mucociliary function. The relative numbers of these two types of cell decrease from the trachea toward the peripheral airways, but in chronic bronchitis the goblet cells and sub-mucosal mucous glands hypertrophy and extend peripherally into the smaller airways. Approximately two hundred cilia project from the surface of each ciliated columnar cell. Sensory nerve endings penetrate into the epithelium in the neighbourhood of goblet cells, which seem to secrete on direct irritation, while the submucosal glands are predominantly innervated by efferent post-ganglionic parasympathetic fibres. Cilia too may be under cholinergic influence,[23] but they possess intrinsic activity and rhythmicity, and they beat independently of the central nervous system.[33]

The epithelium is covered by a surface fluid layer consisting of a pericili-ary sol layer in which the cilia beat, their tips projecting into the overlying gel layer which consists of mucus. The continuity of the mucous layer throughout the airways is a matter of debate, but some convincing arguments suggest that the mucus is sparsely distributed and discontinuous,[86] although estimates of the total volume of tracheobronchial mucus vary widely, from approximately 35 ml[83] to 355 ml[86] secreted in 24 hours. In spite of these differences in estimate there seems little doubt that normal bronchial secretion is dealt with entirely by the mucociliary mechanism which transports it to the pharynx where it is swallowed; productive cough is an indication of abnormal mucus secretion and is related to mucous gland hypertrophy.[64]

Approximately 95 percent of normal human respiratory secretion is water, while the remainder is largely macromolecular material consisting of glycopro-tein, proteins, and fats. *In vitro* studies of mucociliary transport[46] indicate that one of the essential requirements of mucus is that it have a gel-like structure, but that a variety of gels with different chemical compositions, including gela-tin, agarose, and polyacrylamide, can be effective substitutes. It would appear that the interaction between ciliary activity and mucus is a function of its rheological properties rather than of its biochemical characteristics.

Normal functioning of the mucociliary transport process depends upon the integrity and activity of the cilia, the presence of a periciliary fluid layer, and the physical properties of respiratory mucus. The ciliary beat comprises a fast, effective "power" stroke followed by a slow recovery wave, projections on the tips of the cilia coming into contact with the mucous layer only during the effective stroke. Transport of particles fails in the absence of mucus[69] even though the cilia continue to beat, a consequence which emphasises this specif-ic interaction as the determinant of effective mucociliary function. Mucus transport rates decrease from central to peripheral airways, possibly in relation to the reduction in ciliary beating frequency, ciliary length, and the number of ciliated cells, all of which decline toward the periphery.

Several methods are available for measuring tracheobronchial mucociliary function in man such as the clearance of radioactive particles from the lungs and airways, the clearance of radio-opaque tantalum powder and the rate of movement of discrete markers in the trachea. These methods show that many factors commonly depress the rate of mucociliary clearance including disease of the airways, such as chronic bronchitis, cystic fibrosis and bronchial asthma, inhaled pollutants which include cigarette smoke, sulphur dioxide and nitrogen dioxide, anaesthesia or the administration of high concentrations of inspired oxygen, and physiological variables such as sleep, the state of hydration, and the humidity of the inspired air.

Adequate hydration and high relative humidity of inspired gas are often presented as fundamental tenets of effective physiotherapy for airway disease, but both have to be considered critically. Variations in the humidity of inspired air has no effect on the mucociliary transport in humans,[3] and in view of the remarkable efficiency of the nasal humidification system, it may be inferred that changes in humidity have little or no effect on mucus transport in the lower airways as long as nasal breathing continues. The use of water or saline aerosols may, however, increase pulmonary mucus clearance by increasing the effectiveness of coughing.[59,60] The situation is different in mouth-breathing individuals or those who breathe through artificial airways, for experimental studies reveal that gross reduction in tracheal mucus transport occurs in dogs exposed to dry air[37] which also causes histological changes in the respiratory mucosa. Water deprivation has been shown to produce a pronounced decrease in nasal and tracheal mucus flow in birds,[5] but no change in tracheal mucociliary clearance was observed in dogs dehydrated by 14 percent of body weight[31]—suggesting that in a clinical context dehydration would have to be of considerable severity before it affected mucociliary clearance of sputum.

Clinicians and physiotherapists tend to feel intuitively that the clearance of sputum in patients with obstructive pulmonary disease is likely to be aided if the sputum can be "liquified" with aerosol therapy. There is some experimental evidence to suggest that because mucus transport depends largely upon the elastic properties of the mucous gel, effective mucociliary clearance is maintained in the presence of large increases in mucus viscosity but may actually be diminished if mucus is diluted with water or if its gel structure destroyed with mucolytic agents, decreasing its elastic modulus beyond the optimal value.[73]

Cough

The cough reflex consists of three components: the sensory nerves, the cough centre, and the motor nerves. Specialised cough receptors are concentrated at the main carina, at points of bronchial branching, and in the trachea where they are mainly located in the posterior wall. There are two types of receptor, each of which responds preferentially to mechanical or to chemical stimulation. Receptors of the first type are concentrated mainly in the carina and in the trachea, and are particularly sensitive to mechanical deformation of the tracheal epithelium, while receptors of the second type are distributed throughout the tracheobronchial tree and are more responsive to irritating chemical stimuli.[89]

Excitation of the cough receptors transmits afferent impulses via the vagus nerve to a cough centre which animal experiments suggest is located in the dorso-lateral region of the medulla.[19] Clearly it is under the influence of higher centres since cough can be voluntarily initiated, postponed, or suppressed. Efferent impulses originating from the cough centre are transmitted through cholinergic pathways to the abdominal and intercostal muscles and to the diaphragm.

The effect of the cough reflex is to expel foreign particles which have entered the bronchial tree and to expectorate sputum from the bronchial lumen by promoting vigorous expiratory efforts. Cough is preceded by a deep inspiration which increases lung volume, and by closure of the glottis with contraction of the expiratory muscles, which leads to a transient increase in intrathoracic pressure up to 300 mmHg. Sudden opening of the glottis with continued contraction of the thoracic and abdominal muscles results in the cough itself, an explosive release of air with peak gas flows of 6 litres per second and peak tracheal velocities which have been estimated to approach the speed of sound.

Repeated coughing exhausts the patient, disturbs sleep, and causes crippling breathlessness in those whose respiratory reserve is already seriously diminished by chronic lung disease. But promotion of cough may be an essential element in the therapy of patients who have respiratory failure due to airflow obstruction. Choice of treatment for cough therefore depends very much on making a correct interpretation of the physiological and pathological state of the patient to determine whether his cough should be suppressed or whether expectoration should be encouraged.

COUGH SUPPRESSANTS

Although the greatest value of the narcotic drugs such as morphine, codeine, and the semi-synthetic derivatives of opium lies in their use as analgesics, they also have other important therapeutic applications which include the suppression of cough. A number of other structurally distinct chemical classes of drugs share the properties of the opiates in producing analgesia, cough suppression, gastrointestinal spasm, respiratory depression, and physical dependence, and it seems likely that they share a structure which includes or can simulate a piperidine ring and which has affinity for the opiate receptors in the nervous system.[32] The antitussive effect of the more potent narcotic drugs such as morphine and diamorphine is frequently used in the treatment of distressing cough due to malignant disease of the respiratory tract, but often this use is considered a benefit supplementary to the main objective of relieving pain and fear, and it is never adopted without giving due weight to the risks of respiratory depression and drug dependence. Except in terminal disease, it is better to avoid the potent narcotics and instead to use those opiates with less potential for addiction, such as codeine, dihydrocodeinone, pholcodine, and possibly methadone. Because of the addictive properties of the narcotic antitussive agents and the consequent limitation on their widespread use, much effort has been spent in devising or synthesising drugs with effective cough suppressant properties but devoid of addiction potential, respiratory depression, or analgesic effects. These constitute the non-narcotic antitussive group.

Narcotic Antitussive Agents

In the past the phenanthrene alkaloids of opium, particularly codeine, have been the standard agents employed for suppressing troublesome cough, and they are still widely used in many parts of the world. The opiates act by depressing the cough centre; and although the precise mechanism whereby they exert their effects is uncertain, they appear to react with a variety of receptors which have been identified at numerous sites in the central and peripheral nervous systems. The actions of all the morphine-like drugs are similar and include analgesia; respiratory depression due to a direct effect on the brain stem respiratory centre; nausea and vomiting due to stimulation of the vomiting centre in the medulla; increase in tone but reduction in propulsive peristaltic contractions in the small and large bowel; and depression of the cough centre. Other effects include slight bronchoconstriction and possibly drying of the respiratory tract mucosa, both of which may be relevant in the treatment of gas flow disorders such as bronchial asthma or chronic bronchitis.

The development of tolerance and physical dependence is the major drawback to the morphine-like drugs, and for this reason their use as antitussive agents tends to be discouraged.[88] Narcotic antitussive drugs do however play a valuable part in the treatment of some types of cough and their usefulness in the individual case should be considered dispassionately, neither disregarding nor overemphasising their potential for abuse. An important drug interaction which is common to all the narcotic antitussives is liable to occur on concurrent administration of phenelzine or other monoamine oxidase inhibitors. Excitatory and depressant effects on the central nervous system may occur, leading to deep coma and death. This type of reaction is especially liable to occur with meperidine (pethidine)[52] but all narcotics should be used with caution in the presence of monoamine oxidase inhibitors.

Narcotic Antitussives with High Addiction Potential (Morphine, Heroin, and Methadone) Because of their potential for abuse these drugs should only be used as antitussives in patients with severe distressing cough which cannot be relieved with less potent agents. Their use as antitussive agents should be confined to patients with terminal disease such as bronchial carcinoma, often to relieve pain and anxiety as much as for cough suppressant effect. All cause sedation, respiratory depression, and constipation—side-effects which must be taken account of in assessing the suitability of one or other of these drugs in the individual case. Heroin cannot be used legally for any purpose in the United States, but in Britain its use is sometimes preferred to morphine because it seems less likely to cause nausea or vomiting.

Narcotic Antitussives with Low Addiction Potential Codeine has been widely studied for its cough suppressant effect,[27] and for many years it has been used as the standard for comparison against which the pharmacological and clinical effects of other and newer drugs have been measured (Figure 2-1). Codeine has good analgesic and antitussive activity when given orally and is usually administered in this way. A single oral dose of 15–60 mg has been shown to be an effective remedy for patients with persistent cough, and it lasts from 4 to 6 hours.[71] The usual adult dose is 10–30 mg in a single dose which may be repeated after 3 or 4 hours. Many clinicians find that fairly frequent doses of 10–15 mg are more effective than larger doses at longer intervals. For children the normal antitussive dose is 1.5–2.5 mg per kg body weight over 24 hours, divided into 4 to 6 doses.

A small proportion of absorbed codeine is metabolised in the liver to morphine or norcodeine, but the majority is excreted in the urine either free or conjugated with glucuronic acid,[26] most of the excretion products appearing in the urine within 6 hours. On the basis of electroencephalographic changes which appear to reflect susceptibility to hepatic encephalopathy it has been argued that morphine is contraindicated in patients with severe liver disease,[48] but there is no pharmacokinetic evidence to show whether the metabolism of either morphine or codeine is altered when liver function is reduced. In view of the well-documented impairment of disposition of the related narcotic analgesic, meperidine, in liver disease,[54] it is advisable to use codeine cautiously in patients with severely diminished hepatic function. Codeine can be used with-

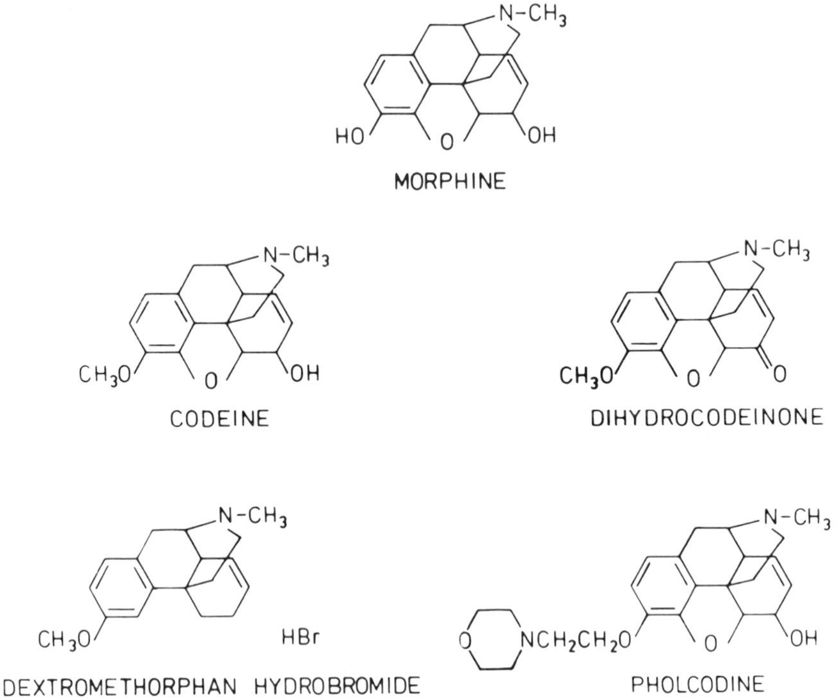

Figure 2-1   *Chemical structure of antitussive agents, illustrating their structural similarities.*

out dose modification in patients with renal failure, and dosage supplementation is not necessary during dialysis.[6]

Codeine has a considerably lessened respiratory depressant effect than morphine, but this possibility must not be overlooked when seeking to relieve cough or control diarrhoea (which may occur as an unwanted effect of antibacterial chemotherapy) in a patient with inadequate respiratory function; its use may be just enough to tip the balance and precipitate respiratory failure. The side-effects most commonly seen when codeine is used therapeutically are constipation, drowsiness, nausea, and vomiting, but they are relatively untroublesome with usual dosage regimens. Allergic cutaneous reactions such as erythema multiforme and urticaria occur rarely. Prolonged use of codeine in high dosage leads to dependence in a very few cases, but the consensus of informed opinion appears to be that the abuse potential of codeine is low.[88]

Dihydrocodeinone is similar in its action to codeine (Figure 2-1) and is used in some proprietary antitussive preparations in combination with a variety of other ingredients. It is a potent analgesic and narcotic rather more addictive than codeine, and its effectiveness as an antitussive agent has been demonstrated in a number of experimental and clinical studies.[8] It appears to have no particular advantages over codeine.

Pholcodine is not available in the United States, but it is widely used as an antitussive agent in Britain and elsewhere as an alternative to codeine (Figure 2-1). It has little or no analgesic effect, although it has some sedative action, and its respiratory depressant effect is equal to that of codeine. Pholcodine is effective in suppressing experimentally-induced cough in man[10] and in relieving cough due to acute and chronic respiratory illness.[74] It is said to be at least as effective as codeine in clinical practice and to have less liability to codeine's side-effects,[56] but the possibility of physical dependence must be kept in mind.

Pholcodine is given by mouth in an adult dose of 5–15 mg which may be repeated every 4 to 6 hours. For children the dose is 5 mg for those over 2 years and 2.5 mg for those younger than 2 years of age. Side-effects from pholcodine administration appear to be uncommon, although nausea, constipation, and drowsiness are complained of occasionally.

Controlled experimental evidence that pholcodine is as effective an antitussive agent as codeine is meagre, although what there is suggests that there is little to choose between these two drugs in the management of everyday respiratory illness, and both appear to be equally acceptable to patients. In countries where both drugs are available the choice seems to depend upon the personal experience and preference of the prescriber.

Non-narcotic Antitussive Agents

The search for antitussive agents which lack the side-effects and abuse potential of the narcotics has led to the production of a number of synthetic drugs which are claimed to be as effective as codeine in controlling cough. These drugs are widely used in proprietary cough mixtures because their sale is less strictly controlled than the narcotic antitussives, but in most cases their effectiveness is unproven by adequate clinical trials.

Many of these antitussive agents have been tested and found to be highly effective in suppressing chemically- or electrically-stimulated cough in experimental animals (see references 18 and 19, for example), and further studies in healthy human subjects have reaffirmed their effectiveness in controlling chemically-induced cough (see references 9 and 62, for example). Pathological cough is much less easy to study because it may arise from a number of different stimuli, it is under voluntary control and also subject to the placebo effect, and it is highly variable from day to day and may naturally disappear during the course of a drug trial. Nevertheless in the final analysis, the value of an antitussive should be judged primarily on its effectiveness in a properly conducted clinical trial, and very few of the non-narcotic antitussives pass this test, since all too often their stated efficacy is based on subjective assessments which are demonstrably unreliable.[71,91] Claims for the clinical efficacy of new antitussive drugs or of new concoctions of well-known preparations should therefore be studied critically by clinicians.

Dextromethorphan Dextromethorphan is a synthetic morphine derivative, *d*-3-methoxy-*N*-methyl-morphinan (Figure 2-1) which has been shown to be an effective centrally-acting antitussive agent without, however, any analgesic or addictive properties. It has been tested in a few controlled studies and found to be as effective as codeine in suppressing cough when given by mouth.[14,15,16] The usual adult dose of dextromethorphan hydrobromide is 15 to 30 mg every 4 to 6 hours, and for children one mg per kg body weight daily, divided into 3 or 4 doses. It is well-absorbed when given by mouth and forms a constituent of many proprietary cough medicines. Toxic symptoms of dizziness, headache, nausea, and vomiting have been described following single doses of 60 mg or more, but side-effects are infrequent with the usual oral dose and it has little if any liability to produce dependence of the morphine type.[43] Like other morphine derivatives, dextromethorphan should be used with caution in patients undergoing treatment with monoamine-oxidase inhibitors since the combination may lead to central nervous system depression and death.[66]

Other Non-narcotic Antitussive Agents A large number of other drugs have been advocated as antitussive agents and many of them are included in proprietary cough preparations and mixtures. For most of these drugs the paucity of good controlled clinical trials means that their effectiveness as specific cough suppressant agents remains uncertain, although no doubt many of the marketed preparations have a useful placebo effect and some, such as the antihistamines, have a contributory sedative action.

Noscapine is a non-narcotic, non-addictive alkaloid from the benzylisoquinoline fraction of opium. It has been shown to suppress experimentally-induced cough in man and animals and to produce subjective improvement in pathological cough,[70] but good controlled studies are lacking. A phenothiazine, *pipazethate* has been shown to protect experimental animals and man against cough produced by chemical stimulation,[62] but its value as an antitussive is not supported by a controlled study in patients with chronic lung disease.[85] *Levopropoxyphene napsylate* has shown evidence of a cough suppressant effect in experimental trials, but a good objective assessment of its effect in patients with various chronic lung conditions showed that it was ineffective.[91]

Two chemically-related agents with atropine-like effects and some local anaesthetic action, *caramiphen* and *carbetapentane,* are thought to have slight central antitussive action in experimental animals,[19,77] but there is no satisfactory evidence to show that they suppress pathological cough. *Benzonatate* is another local anaesthetic said to be clinically effective, although quoted evidence[8] seems disappointing. Recently the topical application of *lidocaine* (lignocaine) has been used to suppress intractable cough in a limited uncontrolled clinical trial,[41] and further studies are needed to confirm the usefulness of this procedure.

Antihistamines are included in many cough suppressant mixtures, although the mechanism of their antitussive action is not clear. Besides their antihistaminic action they have atropine-like, local anaesthetic and central sedative effects, but there is little evidence to suggest that their antitussive action is in any way specific. Cough is quite commonly a major symptom of asthma, especially in children, and its cause may be overlooked if wheeziness is minimal. It responds well to bronchodilator agents once the true aetiology is recognised.

EXPECTORANTS

Many physicians and patients believe that expectorant cough medicines are beneficial but it is very difficult to be certain whether the drugs which are given to "mobilise sputum" and promote expectoration are of value only as placebos, or whether they have a real effect on ventilatory function which provides symptomatic relief. Presumably the aim of treatment with an expectorant drug is to make it easier for the patient to rid his airways of obstructive secretions so that the distribution of ventilation is improved, the effort of breathing is minimised, and the irritation of excessive fluid in the airways more readily relieved by coughing. The objective criteria of effective treatment would therefore include (1) a decrease in the stickiness of the secretions coughed up, (2) an increase in the rate of mucus clearance, and (3) physiological evidence of improved ventilation. Admittedly the clearance of a large quantity of sputum appears to give satisfaction to some patients with chronic productive cough, but the benefit is purely subjective and it is arguable whether an increase simply in the *volume* of sputum coughed up is a measure of an effective agent, unless as an initial temporary phenomenon, since the hallmark of a useful expectorant must surely be to clear away excessive bronchial fluid rather than to promote its secretion.

Considered objectively, few if any of the numerous expectorant cough medicines available today can be said confidently to meet these three criteria of effective treatment. It is therefore advisable to prescribe such preparations with a measure of scepticism and to avoid their prolonged use if no benefit is achieved.

Traditional Expectorants

The number of drugs that have traditionally been used as expectorants comprises a surprisingly long list, of which the better known among them are guaiphanesin, ammonium salts, potassium iodide, terpin hydrate-related compounds, and ipecacuanha. Most of these agents have an emetic action due to vagal stimulation, and it has been suggested that subemetic doses of emetics cause expectoration rather than vomiting. There is very little evidence that any of them is effective, although they are included in innumerable preparations, both proprietary and non-proprietary.

Guaiphenesin is glyceryl guaiacolate, the glyceryl ether of guaiacol. It is said to be found in the sputum after oral administration, and there is a little evidence to suggest that it increases the rate of mucociliary clearance in chronic bronchitic patients.[82] However, there is no evidence to indicate that it reduces sputum viscosity[12] or that it is more effective than a placebo in increasing sputum volume or improving ventilatory function.[38]

Ammonium salts are used in small doses as ingredients of cough mixtures, but it is doubtful whether their irritant action on the gastric mucosa contributes to any expectorant action. *Potassium iodide* is actively removed from the blood stream by certain secretory tissues including the mucous glands of the tracheobronchial tree which are directly stimulated by the drug. The evidence that iodides affect sputum production or viscosity in asthmatics is inadequate,[30] and the toxicity of iodides in causing goitre, hypothyroidism, acneiform skin eruptions, and a variety of other adverse effects is of such magnitude that the drug is better avoided altogether.[21]

Terpin hydrate is said to increase bronchial secretion and assist expectoration, but the evidence is largely subjective.[78] The combination of terpin hydrate with cough suppressant drugs such as codeine and dextromethorphan in numerous proprietary and non-proprietary preparations has no logical basis except to provide a pleasant-tasting vehicle for the specific agents. *Ipecacuanha* is widely known for its emetic action and is traditionally used as an expectorant in small doses in various preparations, some of which combine antitussive and expectorant drugs. Objective evidence of its value is lacking and, as with many traditional cough medicines, definitive studies are needed to demonstrate to the critical physician that there are sound reasons for prescribing it at all.

Detergents

Detergents have been used in aerosol form for many years, with the objective of wetting sticky sputum and facilitating its expectoration.[79] Detergents are included in such formulations as Alevaire, which contains the nonionic deter-

gent tyloxapol, and Turgemist, which contains sodium 2-ethylhexyl-
sulphonate, an ionic detergent. Although detergents may increase aerosol
deposition in the bronchial tree by stabilising aqueous droplets,[87] the value
of this treatment in hydrating bronchial secretions is questionable since the
amount of water actually delivered to the airways by inhaled aerosol is so
small.[4] Studies by Palmer[58] suggested that a detergent aerosol was no more
effective than water in facilitating sputum expectoration, and although a later
double-blind investigation by Paez and Miller[57] demonstrated an increase in the
volume and dry weight of sputum following administration of tyloxapol as
compared with distilled water, the subjective improvement observed by the
patients was not significant and no changes were detected in the physical
findings or in measurements of lung function. It seems therefore that the value
of detergent-containing aerosols in the promotion of expectoration by patients
with chronic obstructive lung disease has not been established by the studies
which have so far been reported.

Mucolytic Agents

Since the rheological properties and the degree of cross-linking of bronchial
mucus are important factors in mucociliary transport, the effect of mucolytic
agents, particularly those which break disulphide bonds, have been widely
investigated. There is no doubt that several of these drugs are effective in
liquefying sputum *in vitro*, but it is usually difficult to establish whether the
patient obtains any significant benefit.

Sulphydryl Compounds   N-acetylcysteine has been shown *in vitro* to reduce
the viscosity of mucoprotein solutions[72] and to liquefy mucoid and purulent
bronchial secretions.[40] It can be administered either as a 5, 10, or 20 percent
solution by direct instillation of 1–2 ml into the bronchial tree through a
bronchoscope or tracheostomy, or as an aerosol by nebulisation of 2–5 ml of a
10 or 20 percent solution. Liquefaction of sputum is sometimes rapid after
intrabronchial instillation of acetylcysteine, and care must be taken to remove
the liquefied secretion promptly by suction.[51] Acetylcysteine attacks rubber
equipment and it is degraded by certain metals.
    The drug has an unpleasant smell and occasionally causes broncho-
spasm,[7,63] and for this reason it is commonly administered in conjunction with
a bronchodilator.[47] It is a difficult drug to use with an ultrasonic nebuliser
because it causes severe irritation and cough, and it inactivates a number of
antibiotics.[49] It should not therefore be combined with antibiotic aerosols, although it does not interfere with systemic antibiotic therapy.
    Objective measurements of the clinical usefulness of acetylcysteine in
treating patients with chronic obstructive lung disease have proved disappoint-

ing in that physical findings and spirometric measurements were not improved by the mucolytic agent, either in single dose studies[2] or in long-term trials of the drug combined with a bronchodilator.[38,47] Individual case reports suggest that it is sometimes of value in relieving mucoid impaction of the bronchi,[42] but it has never achieved wide acceptance for bronchial lavage, probably because saline solution is equally effective and is less likely to cause the immediate impairment of gas exchange which has been observed after acetylcysteine installation.[17] Clinical application of this drug has never fulfilled the promise suggested by its *in vitro* pharmacological properties, but it is the agent of choice when liquefaction of thick secretions *in situ* is contemplated.

Recent experimental work has shown that acetylcysteine can be measured in lung tissue and bronchial mucus several hours after oral administration,[67] but long-term studies of the effect of 600 mg of acetylcysteine daily by mouth in patients with chronic bronchitis failed to show objective evidence of improvement, although the frequency of exacerbations was said to be less in the treated group.[34]

Sodium 2-mercaptoethanesulphonate (Mistabron) is a mucolytic agent with a free sulphydryl group, similar structurally to N-acetylcysteine. The drug is not available at present in the United States. It is commonly administered as a 10 or 20 percent solution from a nebuliser, and although less unpleasant to take than acetylcysteine it is also liable to produce bronchospasm. In a clinical trial involving patients with chronic bronchitis on long-term treatment with this drug, its main effect was to cause thinning of the sputum[38]; but in another study, no objective benefit was apparent from measurements of pulmonary function or from clinical observations on a similar group of patients.[76]

S-Carboxymethylcysteine (Mucodyne) is a thiol derivative but it differs from N-acetyl-cysteine and mercaptoethanesulphonate in having no free sulphydryl group. It is unsuitable for aerosol therapy because of its poor solubility, but it is said to have mucolytic properties after oral administration. It is not available in the United States but is marketed in Britain where some investigations of its clinical efficacy have been carried out. One study on stable chronic bronchitic patients suggested that carboxymethylcysteine reduced sputum viscosity and increased sputum volume over a 10-day period of administration when compared to a placebo, and measurements of FEV_1 showed a small advantage to the treated group at the end of 1 month.[28] In contrast, a smaller study on a similar group of patients failed to show an increase in mucociliary clearance or ventilatory capacity after oral carboxymethylcysteine,[81] and it is clear that further studies are needed to justify the use of this drug in the routine treatment of chronic productive cough.

Bromhexine Hydrochloride   Bromhexine hydrochloride (Bisolvon) is a synthetic derivative of vasicine, which is the active principle of a plant, *Adhatoda vasica,* used in India as an antitussive and expectorant.[1] The drug is said to increase lysosomal activity in bronchial mucus and to increase the secretion of enzymes which can hydrolyse the mucopolysaccharide fibril structure of mucus.

Bromhexine is given by mouth in a dosage of 48 mg daily in three divided doses and may be increased to 72 mg daily if no clear response occurs. No serious adverse effects have been described, but the makers advise caution in its use in patients with peptic ulceration.

The results of some clinical studies show that bromhexine can alter the flow properties of sputum obtained from patients with chronic bronchitis,[20,36] but the evidence for clinical benefit or improvement in pulmonary function is conflicting (see reference 25) and studies of its effect on mucociliary clearance in chronic bronchitics show barely any advantage over a placebo.[80] Bromhexine also appears to be ineffective in hastening recovery from severe asthma.[68] It is still not clear whether the drug eases expectoration, but it would perhaps be reasonable to try bromhexine in patients who had difficulty in coughing up mucoid sputum, although its routine use for treating chronic bronchitics is not yet justified.[11]

L-arginine   Buffered L-arginine, which has mucolytic properties by virtue of its ability to break hydrogen bonds and chelate with calcium, has been proposed as a mucolytic aerosol in the treatment of cystic fibrosis. One report suggested that its use was accompanied by improved pulmonary function,[75] and it is also mentioned favourably in a review by Miller.[55]

Enzymes as Mucolytic Agents

The use of enzymes such as deoxyribonuclease, trypsin, and chymotrypsin instilled or inhaled into the bronchial tree has been advocated in the past for the mobilisation of tenacious bronchial secretions, but these agents are no more effective than *N*-acetylcysteine and are more liable to cause adverse reactions due to hypersensitivity to the foreign protein. At present they can only be said to have an occasional place in the treatment of respiratory tract obstruction.

Deoxyribonuclease   Deoxyribonuclease (Dornase) is a purified enzyme obtained from beef pancreas, and is used to liquefy purulent secretions which contain significant amounts of DNA. It may be administered as an aerosol in a dose of 50,000 to 100,000 units in 2 ml of normal saline or in 10 percent propylene glycol up to 3 times daily, but should not be continued for more than a few days because of the risk of developing hypersensitivity to beef protein. It may also be instilled directly into the tracheobronchial tree. It is used to reduce the viscosity of bronchial secretions and there is some objective evidence to suggest that it may be helpful in the treatment of cystic fibrosis,[50] but in general the use of this expensive and potentially toxic drug should be confined to those individuals in whom other forms of therapy have failed to relieve life-threatening bronchial obstruction which is attributable to purulent secretions.

Since DNA in sputum directly inhibits proteolytic enzyme activity, the addition of dornase encourages proteolysis, and this is the action which is probably largely responsible for the drug's effect in liquefying sputum. However proteolysis by naturally-occurring proteases is the cause of emphysema in individuals with alpha$_1$-antitrypsin deficiency,[29] and enzyme therapy should not therefore be used without prior assessment of the patient's serum alpha$_1$-antitrypsin level.[51]

Trypsin   Trypsin in aerosol form appears to be effective in treating individual cases of pulmonary alveolar proteinosis, although it is difficult to evaluate the drug independently because a variety of different forms of treatment are usually administered, together or in succession, and spontaneous remissions are common in the natural course of this rare disease.[24] Two recent case reports describe quite dramatic clinical and physiological improvement in patients with pulmonary alveolar proteinosis during treatment with trypsin aerosol[65,44] administered in divided dosage to a total of 100,000–200,000 units daily over a period varying from several weeks to 6 months. Because adverse effects such as cough, fever, soreness of the mouth and pharynx, hoarseness, and hypersensitivity reactions are common, it has been suggested that treatment should be initiated with small doses (25,000 units twice daily) and increased gradually according to the patient's tolerance. Clinical improvement can occur within 7 days or may not be seen for several weeks.

CLINICAL CONSIDERATIONS

Cough is a common symptom of many short-lived and trivial respiratory infections which lead to a few days' annoyance and inconvenience before resolving naturally. Most families have a favourite medicine which is administered on such occasions, and the universal need for such simple remedies is no doubt responsible for the innumerable proprietary preparations which are available over the counter. Many of these preparations are mixtures of drugs with different properties, often apparently conflicting; it is not uncommon for an agent with traditionally expectorant properties to be combined with a cough suppressant drug in the same preparation. Probably these medicines owe much of their value to their placebo effect, and if such a preparation is called for it is advisable to provide one which is palatable with a low risk of side-effects and no potential for causing dependence if it should be misused. Approved preparations which fulfill these criteria are Dextromethorphan Hydrobromide syrup N.F., Terpin Hydrate and Dextromethorphan Hydrobromide Elixir N.F., and Simple Linctus B.P.C.

More potent remedies are needed when the cough is persistent, exhausting, or painful and in these circumstances it is essential to reach a conclusion about the cause of the cough before a reasonable decision can be made about treatment. Once a diagnosis has been made it becomes possible to determine whether symptomatic treatment is needed and to make the choice between a cough suppressant and an expectorant drug.

Suppression of cough is indicated when it is exhausting or painful and of limited duration in terms of the natural history of the underlying disease. For example, it is entirely appropriate to prescribe codeine to control irritating nocturnal cough for a patient with acute tracheobronchitis whose illness will subside within a few days, or a methadone-containing preparation for a patient with persistent and perhaps painful cough due to inoperable bronchial neoplasm with a prognosis of several months. It would not be reasonable to advise either codeine or methadone to suppress the cough of a patient with chronic obstructive lung disease, not only because there is a risk of dependence if the patient were to use these drugs regularly, nor because they cause central nervous system depression and may precipitate respiratory failure, but also because the cough has a useful function in maintaining airway patency by expelling excessive secretions. In practice it is usually possible to limit the use of cough suppressant drugs to a period of a few days while an underlying inflammatory condition such as pneumonia resolves in response to specific chemotherapy; but there should be no hesitation in using effective opiate antitussives for longer periods to relieve distressing cough in cases of pulmonary malignancy.

The use of expectorants is controversial because their efficacy is disputed. For patients whose airways are obstructed by mucus it would be beneficial if the raising of excessive secretions could be eased so that the frequency and effort of coughing might be diminished. During exacerbations of chronic obstructive lung disease, whether due to bronchial asthma, chronic bronchitis, bronchiectasis, or cystic fibrosis, the most effective measures for treating the illness are specific chemotherapy to control infection, adequate hydration to promote mucociliary clearance of sputum, bronchodilators, regular physical therapy and if necessary appropriate supportive therapy (such as oxygen administration or assisted ventilation) to maintain cardiopulmonary function during the period of acute illness. In certain rare instances it may be helpful to instill or inhale a liquefying agent such as acetylcysteine into the tracheobronchial tree in order to mobilise viscid secretions, but for bronchial lavage many physicians would prefer simply to use normal saline. Humidification of inspired gas is essential if respiration is maintained via a tracheostomy or endotracheal tube, but in patients breathing normally the administration of nebulised solutions seems unlikely to have a very significant effect on bronchial secretions, since it appears that very little of the inspired aerosol is deposited in the tracheobronchial tree.[90] Some adverse effect on pulmonary function has been observed in patients with chronic bronchitis after inhaling ultrasonic saline aerosol, suggesting that the inhaled droplets may stimulate bronchoconstriction and aggravate ventilation-perfusion imbalance.[61] There is considerable variation in the views of different practitioners as to the value of nebulised aerosols in treating obstructive bronchial disease, particularly cystic fibrosis, but it is probably true to say that there is greater enthusiasm for this form of therapy in the United States than in Britain or elsewhere.

For patients with chronic obstructive lung disease who are in a stable phase, the most important remedies for chronic productive cough are the avoidance of environmental pollutants—especially smoking (it is astonishing how frequently such patients persist in smoking cigarettes)—regular physical therapy to get rid of excessive secretions,[45] and bronchodilators. There is insuffient evidence from good controlled clinical trials to justify the routine use of oral agents which are marketed for their expectorant properties, such as carboxymethylcysteine or bromhexine hydrochloride, although it may be reasonable to make a critical trial of such preparations in the case of those infrequent patients who appear to have real difficulty in raising sputum.

It is not always realised that cough is sometimes the only symptom of bronchial asthma.[22,53] This seems to be especially the case among asthmatic children whose parents often complain that the symptoms are particularly troublesome in the middle of the night, undoubtedly because of the well-known circadian variation in bronchial calibre which leads to maximal bronchoconstriction in the early hours of the morning, sometimes known as "morning dipping."[84] This symptom may be precipitated by a minor upper respiratory infection, and if asthma is suspected the usual clinical and physiological investigations should be carried out to establish the presence of atopy and evidence for reversible bronchoconstriction. This type of cough responds satisfactorily to measures usually given for mild asthma, such as cromolyn sodium (disodium cromoglycate) and bronchodilating agents.

REFERENCES

1. Amin AH, Mehta DR: A bronchodilator alkaloid (vasicinone) from *Adhatoda vasica* Nees. Nature 184: 1317, 1959.
2. Anderson G: A clinical trial of a mucolytic agent—acetyl cysteine—in chronic bronchitis. Bri J Dis Chest 60: 101–103, 1966.

3. ANDERSON IB, LUNDQVIST GR, PROCTOR DF: Human nasal mucosal function under four controlled humidities. Am Rev Resp Dis 106: 438–449, 1972.
4. ASMUNDSSON T, JOHNSON RF, KILBURN KH, GOODRICH JK: Efficiency of nebulisers for depositing saline in human lungs. Am Rev Resp Dis 108: 506–512, 1973.
5. BANG BG, BANG FB: Effect of water deprivation on nasal mucous flow. Proc Soc Exp Biol Med 196: 516–521, 1961.
6. BENNETT WM: Drug prescribing in renal failure. Drugs 17: 111–123, 1979.
7. BERNSTEIN LI, AUSDENMORE RW: Iatrogenic bronchospasm occurring during clinical trials of a new mucolytic agent, acetylcysteine. Dis Chest 46: 469–473, 1964.
8. BICKERMAN HA: The newer antitussive agents. Med Clin North Am 45: 805–821, 1961.
9. BICKERMAN HA, GERMAN E, COHEN BM, ITKIN SE; The cough response of healthy human subjects stimulated by citric acid aerosol. Part 2: evaluation of antitussive agents. Am J Med Sci 234: 191–206, 1957.
10. BICKERMAN HA, ITKIN SE: Further studies on the evaluation of antitussive agents employing experimentally induced cough in human subjects. Clin Pharmacol Ther 1: 180–191, 1960.
11. BRITISH THORACIC AND TUBERCULOSIS ASSOCIATION: A controlled trial of the effects of bromhexine on the symptoms of out-patients with chronic bronchitis. Br J Dis Chest 67: 49–60, 1973.
12. BÜRGI H: Changes in the fibre system and viscosity of the sputum of bronchitis during treatment with bromhexine and guaiphenesin (guaiacol glyceryl ether). Scand J Resp Dis (Supplement 90): 81–95, 1974.
13. CALESNICK B, CHRISTENSEN JA: Latency of cough response as a measure of antitussive agents. Clin Pharmacol Ther 8: 374–380, 1967.
14. CALESNICK B, CHRISTENSEN JA, MUNCH JC: Antitussive action of L-propoxyphene in citric acid-induced cough response. Am J Med Sci 242: 560–564, 1961.
15. CASS LJ, FREDERICK WS: Evaluation of a new antitussive agent. N Engl J Med 249: 132–136, 1953.
16. CASS LJ, FREDERICK WS, ANDOSCA JB: Qualitative comparison of dextromethorphan hydrobromide and codeine. Am J Med Sci 227: 291–296, 1954.
17. CEZEAUX G, TELFORD J, HARRISON G, KEATS AS: Bronchial lavage in cystic fibrosis. JAMA 199: 15–18, 1967.
18. CHAKRAVARTY NK, MATALLANA A, JENSEN R, BORISON HL: Central effects of antitussive drugs on cough and respiration. J Pharmacol Exp Ther 117: 127–135, 1956.
19. CHOU DT, WANG SC: Studies on the localisation of central cough mechanisms: site of action of antitussive drugs. J Pharmacol Exp Ther 194: 499–505, 1975.
20. COBBINS DM, ELLIOTT FM, REBUCK AS: The mucolytic agent bromhexine (Bisolvon) in chronic lung disease. A double-blind crossover trial. Aust NZ Med 1: 137–140, 1971.
21. COMMITTEE ON DRUGS OF THE AMERICAN ACADEMY OF PEDIATRICS: Adverse reactions to iodide therapy of asthma and other pulmonary diseases. Pediatrics 57: 272–274, 1976.
22. CORRAO WM, BRAMAN SS, IRWIN RS: Chronic cough as the sole presenting manifestation of bronchial asthma. N Engl J Med 300: 633–637, 1979.
23. CORSSEN G, ALLEN CR: Acetylcholine: its significance in controlling ciliary activity of human respiratory epithelium in vitro. J Appl Physiol 14: 901–904, 1959.

24. DAVIDSON JM, MACLEOD WM: Pulmonary alveolar proteinosis. Br J Dis Chest 63: 13–28, 1969.

25. DRUG AND THERAPEUTICS BULLETIN: Bisolvon and bisolvomycin up to date. Drug Ther Bull 9: 91–92, 1971.

26. EBBIGHAUSEN WOR, MOWAT J, VESTERGAARD P: Mass fragmentation detection of normorphine in urine of man after codeine intake. J Pharm Sci 62: 146–148, 1973.

27. EDDY NB, FRIEBEL H, HAHN KJ, HALBACH H: Codeine and its alternates for pain and cough relief. 4. Potential alternates for cough relief. Bull WHO 40: 639–719, 1969.

28. EDWARDS GF, STEEL AE, SCOTT JK, JORDAN JW: S-carboxymethyl-cysteine in the fluidification of sputum and treatment of chronic airway obstruction. Chest 70: 506–513, 1976.

29. ERIKSSON S: Studies in alpha 1-antitrypsin deficiency. Acta Med Scand 177 (Supplement 432): 1965.

30. FALLIERS CJ, MCCANN WP, CHAI H, ELLIS EF, YAZDI N: Controlled study of iodotherapy for childhood asthma. J Allergy Clin Immunol 38: 183–192, 1966.

31. GIORDANO A, SHIH CK, HOLSCLAW DS, KHAN MA, LITT M: Mucus clearance: in vivo canine tracheal vs in vitro bullfrog palate studies. J Appl Physiol 42: 761–766, 1977.

32. GOLDSTEIN A, ARONOW L, KALMAN SM: The narcotic analgesics. in Principles of Drug Action Ed 2, p 33–36. New York: Wiley, 1974.

33. GOSSELIN GE: Physiological regulators of ciliary motion. Am Rev Resp Dis 93 (Symposium): 41–59, 1966.

34. GRASSI C, MORANDINI GC: A controlled trial of intermittent oral acetylcysteine in the long-term treatment of chronic bronchitis. Eur J Clin Pharmacol 9: 393–396, 1976.

35. GREEN MG: Alveolobronchiolar transport mechanisms. Arch Intern Med 131: 109–114, 1973.

36. HAMILTON WFD, PALMER KNV, GENT M: Expectorant action of bromhexine in chronic obstructive bronchitis. Br Med J 3: 260–261, 1970.

37. HIRSCH JA, TOKAYER JL, ROBINSON MJ, SACKNER MA: Effects of dry air and subsequent humidification on tracheal mucous velocity in dogs. J Appl Physiol 39: 242–246, 1975.

38. HIRSCH SR, VIERNES PF, KORY RC: Clinical and physiological evaluation of mucolytic agents nebulised with isoproterenol: 10% N-acetylcysteine versus 10% 2-mercaptoethane sulphonate. Thorax 25: 737–743, 1970.

39. HIRSCH SR, VIERNES PF, KORY RC: The expectorant effect of glyceryl guaiacolate in patients with chronic bronchitis. A controlled in vitro and in vivo study. Chest 63: 9–14, 1973.

40. HIRSCH SR, ZASTROW JE, KORY RC: Sputum liquefying agents: A comparative in vitro evaluation. J Lab Clin Med 74: 346–353, 1969.

41. HOWARD P, CAYTON RM, BRENNAN SM, ANDERSON PB: Lignocaine aerosol and persistent cough. Br J Dis Chest 71: 19–24, 1977.

42. IRWIN RS, THOMAS HM: Mucoid impaction of the bronchus. Diagnosis and treatment. Am Rev Resp Dis 108: 955–959, 1973.

43. ISBELL H, FRASER HF: Actions and addiction liabilities of Dromoran derivatives in man. J Pharmacol Exp Ther 107: 524–530, 1953.

44. JAY SJ: Pulmonary alveolar proteinosis. Successful treatment with aerosolized trypsin. Am J Med 66: 348–354, 1979.

45. JONES NL: Physical therapy—present state of the art. Am Rev Resp Dis 110: in Proceedings of the Conference on the Scientific Basis of Respiratory Therapy, p 132–136, 1974.

46. KING M, GILBOA A, MEYER FA, SILBERBERG A: On the transport of mucus and its rheological simulants in ciliated systems. Am Rev Resp Dis 110: 740–745, 1974.

47. KORY RC, HIRSCH SR, GIRALDO J: Nebulisation of N-acetylcysteine combined with a bronchodilator in patients with chronic bronchitis. Dis Chest 54: 504–509, 1968.

48. LAIDLAW J, REID AE, SHERLOCK S: Morphine tolerance in hepatic cirrhosis. Gastroenterology 40: 389–396, 1961.

49. LAWSON D, SAGGERS BA: NAC and antibiotics in cystic fibrosis. Br Med J 1: 317, 1965.

50. LIEBERMAN J. Dornase aerosol effect on sputum viscosity in cases of cystic fibrosis. JAMA 205, 312–313, 1968.

51. LIEBERMAN J: The appropriate use of mucolytic agents. Am J Med 49: 1–4, 1970.

52. London DR, Milne MD: Dangers of monoamine oxidase inhibitors. Br Med J 2: 1752, 1962.

53. McFADDEN ER: Exertional dyspnoea and cough as preludes to acute attacks of bronchial asthma. N Engl J Med 292: 555–559, 1975.

54. McHORSE TS, WILKINSON GR, JOHNSON RF, SCHENKER S: Effect of acute viral hepatitis in man on the disposition and elimination of meperidine. Gastroenterology 68: 775–780, 1975.

55. MILLER WF: Aerosol therapy in acute and chronic respiratory disease. Arch Intern Med 131: 148–155, 1973.

56. MULINOS MG, NAIR KGS, EPSTEIN IG: Clinical investigation of antitussive properties of pholcodine. NY State J Med 62: 2373–2377, 1962.

57. PAEZ PN, MILLER WF: Surface active agents in sputum evacuation: a blind comparison with normal saline solution and distilled water. Chest 60: 312–317, 1971.

58. PALMER KNV: Effect of an aerosol detergent in chronic bronchitis. Lancet 1: 611–613, 1957.

59. PARKS CR, ALDEN ER, STANDAERT TA, WOODRUM DE, GRAHAM B, HODSON WA: The effect of water nebulisation on cough transport of pulmonary mucus in the mouth-breathing dog. Am Rev Resp Dis 108: 513–519, 1973.

60. PAVIA D, THOMSON ML, CLARKE SW: Enhanced clearance of secretions from the human lung after the administration of hypertonic saline aerosol. Am Rev Resp Dis 117: 199–203, 1978.

61. PFLUG AE, CHENEY FW, BUTLER J: The effect of ultrasonic aerosol on pulmonary mechanics and arterial blood gases in patient with chronic bronchitis. Am Rev Resp Dis 101: 710–714, 1970.

62. PRIME FJ: The assessment of antitussive drugs in man. Br Med J 1: 1149–1151, 1961.

63. RAO S, WILSON DB, BROOKS RC, SPROULE BJ: Acute effects of nebulisation of N-acetylcysteine on pulmonary mechanics and gas exchange. Am Rev Resp Dis 102: 17–22, 1970.

64. REID :L Measurement of the bronchial mucous gland layer: A diagnostic yardstick in chronic bronchitis. Thorax 15: 132–141, 1960.

65. RIKER JB, WOLINSKY H: Trypsin aerosol treatment of pulmonary alveolar proteinosis. Am Rev Resp Dis 108: 108–113, 1973.

66. RIVERS N, HORNER B: Possible lethal reaction between Nardil and dextromethorphan. Can Med Assoc J 103: 85, 1970.

67. RODENSTEIN D, DECOSTER A, GAZZANIGA A: Pharmacokinetics of oral acetylcysteine: absorption, binding and metabolism in patients with respiratory disorders. Clin Pharmacokinet 3: 247–254, 1978.

68. RUDOLF M, RIORDAN JF, GRANT BJB, MABERLY DJ, SAUNDERS KB: Bromhexine in severe asthma. Br J Dis Chest 72: 307–312, 1978.

69. SADÉ J, ELIEZER N, SILBERBERG A, NEVO AC: The role of mucus in transport by cilia. Am Rev Resp Dis 102: 48–52, 1970.

70. SEGAL MS, GOLDSTEIN MM, ATTINGER EO: The use of Noscapine (Narcotine) as an antitussive agent. Dis Chest 32: 305–309, 1957.

71. SEVELIUS H, McCOY JF, COLMORE JP: Dose response to codeine in patients with chronic cough. Clinical Pharmacol Ther 12: 449–455, 1971.

72. SHEFFNER AL: The reduction *in vitro* in viscosity of mucoprotein solutions by a new mucolytic agent, N-acetyl-L-cysteine. Ann NY Acad Sci 106: 298–310, 1963.

73. SHIH CK, LITT M, KHAN A, WOLF DP: Effect of nondialyzable solids concentration and viscoelasticity on ciliary transport of tracheal mucus. Am Rev Resp Dis 115: 989–995, 1977.

74. SNELL ES, ARMITAGE P: Clinical comparison of diamorphine and pholcodine as cough suppressants by a new method of sequential analysis. Lancet 1: 860–862, 1957.

75. SOLOMONS CC, COTTON EK, DUBOIS R, PINNEY M: The use of buffered L-arginine in the treatment of cystic fibrosis. Pediatrics 47: 384–390, 1971.

76. STEEN SN, ZIMENT I, FREEMAN ARIT, THOMAS JS: Evaluation of a new mucolytic drug. Clin Pharmacol Ther 16: 58–62, 1974.

77. STEFKO PL, DENZEL J, HICKEY L: Experimental investigation of nine antitussive drugs. J Pharm Sci 50: 216–221, 1961.

78. SUMNER ED: Formulations in terpin hydrate preparations. J Am Pharm Assoc 8: 250–254, 1968.

79. TAINTER ML, NACHOD FC, BIRD JG: Alevaire as a mucolytic agent. N Engl J Med 253: 764–767, 1968.

80. THOMSON ML, PAVIA D, GREGG I, STARK JE: Bromhexine and mucociliary clearance in chronic bronchitis. Br J Dis Chest 68: 21–27, 1974.

81. THOMSON ML, PAVIA D, JONES CJ, McQUISTON TAC: No demonstrable effect of S-carboxymethylcysteine on clearance of secretion from the human lung. Thorax 30: 669–673, 1975.

82. THOMSON ML, PAVIA D, McNICOL MW: A preliminary study of the effect of guaiphenesin on mucociliary clearance from the human lung. Thorax 28: 742–747, 1973.

83. TOREMALM NG: The daily amount of tracheo-bronchial secretions in man. Acta Oto-Laryngol (Suppl) 158: 43–53, 1960.

84. TURNER-WARWICK M: On observing patterns of airflow obstruction in chronic asthma. Br J Dis Chest 71: 73–86, 1977.

85. VAKIL BJ, MEHTA AJ, PRAJAPAT KD: Trial of pipazethate as an antitussive. Clin Pharmacol Ther 7: 515–519, 1966.

86. VAN AS A: Pulmonary airway clearance mechanisms: A reappraisal. Am Rev Resp Dis 115: 721–726, 1977.

87. WALKENHORST W, DAUTREBANDE L: New studies on aerosols. 13. Experimental observations on various factors influencing weight, number, flowrate and size distribution of aerosol particles. Arch Int Pharmacodyn Ther 150: 264–294, 1964.

88. WHO TECHNICAL REPORT: Opiates and their alternates for pain and cough relief. WHO Tech Rep Ser 495: 5–19, 1972.

89. WIDDICOMBE JG: Respiratory reflexes from the trachea and bronchi of the cat. J Physiol 123: 55–69, 1954.

90. WOLFSDORF J, SWIFT DL, AVERY ME: Mist therapy reconsidered: an evaluation of the respiratory deposition of labelled water aerosols produced by jet and ultrasonic nebulisers. Pediatrics 43: 799–808, 1969.

91. WOOLF CR, ROSENBERG A: Objective assessment of cough suppressants under clinical conditions using a tape recorder system. Thorax 19: 125–130, 1964.

3

Introduction
to the
Use of Antimicrobial
Chemotherapy

Modern antibacterial chemotherapy began in the 1930s when sulphonilamide first came to be used systemically to treat bacterial infections, and it expanded dramatically in 1941 with the advent of penicillin, which opened the way to the discovery of a host of antibiotic and synthetic chemotherapeutic agents. These drugs have changed the whole aspect of medical practice, nowhere more strikingly than in the field of respiratory medicine where they have transformed the morbidity and mortality of childhood infections and have improved the prospects for successful treatment in nearly every sort of pulmonary disease. Nevertheless it is widely recognised that antimicrobial chemotherapy is often used unnecessarily and ineffectively both in hospital and in office practice, causing serious morbidity from adverse reactions, increasing the pool of antibiotic-resistant bacteria, and wasting a great deal of money. Since respiratory infections constitute the major reason for antibiotic administration, especially in general practice,[7] it is appropriate that a discussion about the use of antimicrobials in the field of respiratory medicine should be preceded by a cautionary comment on their current misuse.

A number of surveys on the use of antibiotics in hospitals have shown that the proportion of cases in which antibiotic administration was considered to be either not indicated or inappropriate in terms of drug or dosage was astonishingly high—between 52 and 66 percent[12,37,57]—while in general practice antibiotics, although widely used, have been shown to be of no value in the treatment of the minor upper respiratory illnesses of children.[25,67] And yet adverse reactions to all antimicrobials have been demonstrated in nearly 5 percent of hospital inpatients[10] and to an even greater extent (7 percent) of those treated with ampicillin[59]—one of the most widely used of current antibiotics. Clearly, some share of the morbidity of antimicrobial therapy must fall to those patients who are treated unnecessarily, and some of whom may even die.[55]

Uncritical use of antimicrobial drugs enlarges the pool of resistant micro-organisms by (1) increasing the likelihood of suboptimal regimens of antibiotic therapy, (2) favouring the elimination of sensitive bacteria in normal human microbial flora and allowing resistant organisms to flourish, and (3) increasing the opportunities for acquired resistance through transfer from other bacteria. It is also well recognised that selective pressure exerted by antimicrobial agents encourages the development of nosocomial (that is, hospital acquired) infections with resistant bacteria.[49,52] For these reasons the risks of prophylactic antibiotic therapy have been increasingly emphasised and its benefits widely questioned, particularly in surgery where the criteria for antibiotic prophylaxis are extremely variable.[60,69,73] In the field of respiratory medicine prophylactic chemotherapy should be confined to the prevention of tuberculosis in certain susceptible subjects (see Chapter 6) with isoniazid, and the treatment of susceptible whooping cough contacts with a 5-day course of erythromycin.

Growing doubts about the usefulness of much of the antimicrobial chemotherapy doled out in homes and hospitals have naturally given rise to observations about the cost of a form of treatment which is often ineffective and may sometimes do positive harm. Suffice it to say that in 1976 the total cost for antimicrobial agents at 19 hospitals in the United States amounted to over $2.1 million, nearly 30 percent of the pharmacy drug costs at these hospitals,[16] while a figure of $1.55 billion was forecast for the wholesale cost of anti-infective agents to be supplied in the United States in 1979.[36]

These reflections emphasise the fact that antibacterial chemotherapy has implications which extend beyond the individual patient to the well-being of other members of the community who will suffer the consequences of infection with resistant bacterial populations.[56] More than with other drugs, a decision to use an antimicrobial agent should not be taken lightly but with due consideration for its possible wider effects. Sometimes the drug is not really necessary.

FACTORS DETERMINING THE RESPONSE TO ANTIMICROBIAL CHEMOTHERAPY

Just as pharmacological agents act by combining with receptors in the target tissue to bring about an alteration in biochemical processes which change the rate of a reaction, so chemotherapeutic antimicrobial agents act by binding to receptor sites in the cells of micro-organisms and interfering with their metabolism, causing cell death in the case of bactericidal agents or inhibiting bacterial replication in the case of bacteriostatic drugs. This effect can only occur if a sufficient concentration of the drug reaches the site of infection, and it is likely to be short-lived if the patient suffers adverse effects and the drug has to be withdrawn. Thus the pharmacologic factors which influence the response to any drug, described in the opening chapter of this book, apply equally to antimicrobial agents, but because of the dynamic nature of the interaction between the host organism and microbial penetration, several additional factors need to be taken into account when antimicrobial chemotherapy is being considered.

Host Determinants

The Immune Response   The inflammatory reactions which relate to the immune response and the mechanical barriers of the skin and mucous membranes constitute the normal defence mechanisms of the body to infection and are effective enough to deal with the vast majority of infections encountered day by day. Chemotherapy is needed to tip the balance in favour of the infected person when the virulence of the infecting organism or the weakness of the host's responses threaten to cause death or lasting tissue damage. Lack of normal immune and inflammatory reactivity imposes a severe and often lethal handicap in an environment where infective micro-organisms are unavoidable, as manifested by the shortened life span of children affected by inherited abnormalities of immunity, for example, chronic familial granulomatosis[34] or the increased liability to infection of patients receiving immune-suppressant drugs.[76] In this context the infection is often known as "opportunistic" and may result from micro-organisms which are traditionally pathogenic or from those which are usually considered to be of low pathogenicity, such as fungi or atypical mycobacteria[63] (Table 3-1).

Since the efficacy of antimicrobial drugs depends to a very large extent upon the integrity of host defence mechanisms, it is of some importance that the physician take notice of any concurrent disease or treatment which might prejudice the outcome of antimicrobial chemotherapy and might encourage him to consider (1) the possibility of infection by organisms which are usually of low pathogenicity, (2) the use of bactericidal in preference to bacteriostatic drugs, and (3) the use of serotherapy as an adjunct to chemotherapy in patients whose immune mechanisms are compromised.[22,38] Some of the conditions which are most characteristically associated with an impaired immunological response are listed in Table 3-2.

Table 3-1 / Opportunistic Infections

Traditionally Pathogenic Organisms Occurring With Abnormal Frequency in the Compromised Host	Traditionally Pathogenic Organisms Causing Abnormally Severe Disease in the Compromised Host	Organisms that Rarely Cause Disease Except in the Compromised Host
Bacteria: *Mycobacterium tuberculosis*, Gram-positive cocci, Gram-negative bacteria	Viruses: Measles, Varicella } causing chronic disease Enteroviral infection spreading to CNS	Viruses: Cytomegalovirus, BCG, Vaccinia Bacteria: *Nocardia asteroides*, atypical mycobacteria, *Listeria monocytogenes*
Fungi: *Cryptococcus neoformans*, *Candida albicans*	Bacteria: *Mycoplasma pneumoniae*, in sickle-cell disease	Fungi: *Mucor mercedo* (in diabetic acidosis) Protozoa: *Pneumocystis carinii*

Table 3-2 / Some Conditions or Diseases Associated With an Impaired Immunologic Response

Mechanism of Impairment	Examples	References
Inherited immune deficiency	Sex-linked agammaglobulinaemia	8, 54
	Swiss-type agammaglobulinaemia (hereditary thymic aplasia)	54
Acquired immune deficiency	Multiple myeloma, macroglobulinaemia	19
	Chronic lymphatic leukaemia	61
	Malignant lymphoma	21
Inherited pmn leucocyte deficiency	Chronic granulomatous disease	34
	Chediak-Higashi syndrome	13
	Lazy-leucocyte disease	44
Acquired pmn leucocyte deficiency	Acute or chronic granulocytopenia (as in drug allergy)	3, 31
	Acute leukaemia	6
Consequences of radiotherapy, immune suppressant and cytotoxic drugs, and corticosteroids	Organ transplantation	29
	Chemotherapy for malignancy	27
	Long-term, high-dose corticosteroids	24, 68
Unknown or multiple factors	Malnutrition	5, 58, 65
	Protein-losing states, (such as nephrotic syndrome)	66
	Metabolic disorders, (such as diabetes mellitus, uraemia, iron deficiency in mucocutaneous candidiasis)	17, 35, 46, 75
	Sickle-cell disease	1, 62

Superinfection   Among the factors which play a part in determining the host's resistance to infective disease are the normal bacterial flora of such areas as the skin, the oropharynx, the vagina, the genital and perineal areas, the external auditory meatus, the conjunctivae, and the gastrointestinal tract. Apart from a role simply as occupants of the area competing for essential nutrients in the same way that a well-stocked flower bed discourages the growth of weeds, the harmless resident bacteria also produce compounds which inhibit the growth of other organisms (for example, colicins produced by enteric bacilli which kill sensitive bacteria in specific ways), or which alter the chemical environment, making it unfavourable for some bacteria (for example, the maintenance of an acid pH in the adult vagina by lactobacillus).

This type of ecological balance is easily upset by broad-spectrum or combination antimicrobial chemotherapy which may suppress the growth of harmless members of the normal microbial flora and encourage potential pathogens which are inherently insensitive or which develop resistance to the chemotherapeutic regimen causing, for example, second pulmonary infections with Gram-negative organisms following therapy for primary bacterial pneumonia.[26,71] Antibiotic-associated colitis[48] is another instance of secondary infection due to antibiotic therapy with a number of drugs (lincomycin, clindamycin, ampicillin, tetracycline, penicillin G, trimethoprim-sulphamethoxazole, cephalosporins, chloramphenicol, and metronidazole have all been incriminated); therapy with these drugs can lead to the multiplication of a toxin-producing clostridium, *C. difficile*, which causes diffuse mucosal changes in the colon with protracted, copious diarrhoea often referred to as pseudomembranous colitis.[70]

In some circumstances the liability to superinfection may be increased by host factors which alter the microbiological flora in favour of potential pathogens. For example, although Gram-negative enteric bacilli such as *Klebsiella*-Enterobacter species and *Pseudomonas* do not normally colonise the upper respiratory tract of healthy individuals, they may do so in the elderly,[72] in alcoholics,[23] and in hospitalised patients,[33] possibly because of impaired oropharyngeal clearance mechanisms. This alteration in pharyngeal flora may represent an important step in the pathogenesis of Gram-negative pneumonias.

Local Factors   Local factors which are unfavourable to the resolution of an infection may be responsible for the failure of antimicrobial chemotherapy. The commonest example in respiratory medicine is probably bronchial obstruction due to tumour or to a foreign body which prevents drainage of secretions from the distal part of the lung and allows a focus of infection to develop. Tissue necrosis and suppuration may reduce the response to chemotherapy because local antibiotic concentrations are low due to the poor vascular supply, and phagocytic function may be impaired because of hypoxia and inadequate nutrition. It is important to recognise the presence of an abscess or the localisation of pus in the pleural cavity or other tissue space, since the infection is unlikely to resolve without surgical drainage.

Occasionally the presence of a foreign body may be overlooked as the cause of persisting infection; this may occur with suture material, and it is sometimes forgotten that urinary tract infection is a common consequence of urethral catheterisation for longer than 48 hours.

Bacterial Determinants

Intrinsic Resistance   Obviously some antimicrobial agents are ineffective against micro-organisms which lack the specific receptor site with which the drug interacts—for example, the antituberculosis drug isoniazid is effective against mycobacteria by inhibiting the synthesis of mycolytic acids which are constituents of mycobacterial cell membranes; but ineffective against other bacteria which do not make use of that synthetic pathway and are therefore inherently insensitive to isoniazid. Alternatively, the target for drug action may be present but relatively inaccessible to the inhibiting chemical agent. For example, the penicillins and cephalosporins owe their bactericidal effect to the inhibition of a transpeptidation step in the cross-linking of peptidoglycan polymers to synthesise cell walls, but the narrow-spectrum penicillins (for example, penicillin G) have difficulty in penetrating the restrictive lipopolysaccharide-containing outer membrane of the Gram-negative organisms and do not reach the target site in sufficient concentration to have an inhibitory effect.[15] Modification of the molecule to yield broader spectrum semi-synthetic penicillins such as ampicillin and carbenicillin increases the ability of the drug molecule to penetrate the external cell membrane of Gram-negative organisms.

Micro-organisms can also avoid the inhibitory effect of chemotherapeutic agents to which they are inherently sensitive if the chemical environment is able to provide a physical or chemical factor which invalidates the drug action. For example, bacteria growing in a sufficiently high osmotic environment may be able to convert to a form (protoplast or L form) which lacks a cell wall, enabling the organism to resist the effect of antibacterial agents which act by preventing cell wall synthesis.[39] An alternative mechanism is illustrated by the sulphonamides which act by competitively inhibiting the bacterial synthesis of folic acid, an essential step in the biosynthesis of purine, thymine, serine, and methionine. Availability of these synthetic end-products in the environment renders the micro-organism independent of the folic acid synthetic pathway and therefore unaffected by the presence of sulphonamides—a situation which may arise in infections involving extensive tissue breakdown (for example, a lung abscess[20]).

Acquired Drug Resistance   Bacterial populations, particularly large ones, are liable to contain small numbers of organisms which have developed antibiotic resistance by spontaneous mutation. This may occur either as a *large-step mutation* in which, for example, the genetic change results in an alteration in the receptor site for the drug, which is no longer bound and therefore no longer exerts its effect; or as a *multiple-step mutation* whereby progressive, small mutations reduce the affinity of the organism for the drug in a stepwise fashion so that increasing levels of the drug are required to achieve a therapeutic effect. Administration of the antibiotic to a patient infected with such a bacterial population will exert a selective pressure by preventing the growth of the sensitive organisms while favoring the resistant strain, which ultimately becomes dominant. Thus, after an initial beneficial clinical response to the antibiotic, the patient suffers a relapse as the infection becomes refractory to treatment. This explains why the use of two effective drugs is mandatory in the treatment of tuberculosis since the emergence of resistant strains of bacilli is otherwise rapid. It is equally logical to use combination chemotherapy in other types of infection although, with certain exceptions, it is usually possible to obtain adequate control by the use of a single agent in sufficient dosage without the additional risk of using a second drug.

The other way in which antibiotic resistance develops in a bacterial population is by transfer of resistant properties from one strain of bacteria to another through the transmission of the gene coding for drug resistance. This is located on a ring-shaped extrachromasomal piece of DNA called an *R plasmid*, which can carry genetic information for determining resistance to one antibiotic or to several different antibiotics at the same time. It can be transferred (1) through *transduction* by means of a bacteriophage which carries over a piece of the genome (that is, the genetic data bank) of the resistant cell—the means by which staphylococci and streptococci transfer resistance (Figure 3-1); (2) through *transformation*, whereby resistant genes formed by another bacterium are incorporated from the environment into a bacterial cell; and (3) through *conjugation,* which permits the transfer of resistance from one bacterium to another by direct contact. Transfer of multiple drug resistance occurs principally in the enteric bacteria by the process of conjugation, which involves the replication of the R plasmid in the resistant bacterium and transfer of genetic material to the non-resistant strain (Figure 3-2).[30] R plasmids occur widely among the enterobacteria both in humans[45] and in animal populations, their proliferation being favoured by the extensive use of antibiotics. Since they may contain information for determining resistance to a number of antibiotics simultaneously, they may be responsible for the sudden development of multiple drug resistance in a previously sensitive organism. Non-pathogenic coliform organisms can serve as a reservoir of resistance which can be transmitted to pathogens, and the likelihood of infection due to multi-resistant pathogens is greatest in hospitals where the pool of resistant coliforms is continually restimulated by the wide variety of antibiotics used and the frequent courses of treatment. The use of antibiotics in animal feed-stuffs may make an additional contribution to the pool of resistant organisms since it has been shown that drug resistance in animal bacterial flora can be transferred to the resident flora of man.

The mutations which lead to drug resistance are modifications in biochemical mechanisms, such as the deletion or alteration of an enzyme or some other cell component. The major mechanisms of resistance by microorganisms to antibiotics include the following:

1. Alteration in drug uptake by the bacterial cell, leading to a reduction in its intracellular concentration. This is the predominant mechanism of tetracycline resistance.
2. Increased destruction of the drug by inactivating enzymes produced by the mutant (resistant) bacteria. The principle method by which bacteria

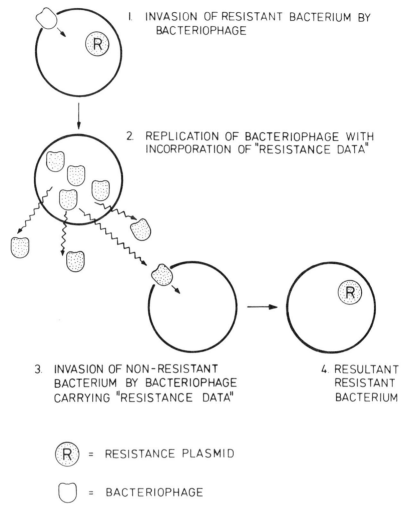

1. INVASION OF RESISTANT BACTERIUM BY BACTERIOPHAGE

2. REPLICATION OF BACTERIOPHAGE WITH INCORPORATION OF "RESISTANCE DATA"

3. INVASION OF NON-RESISTANT BACTERIUM BY BACTERIOPHAGE CARRYING "RESISTANCE DATA"

4. RESULTANT RESISTANT BACTERIUM

(R) = RESISTANCE PLASMID

⬭ = BACTERIOPHAGE

Figure 3-1 *Schematic diagram of resistance transfer by transduction.*

become resistant to the penicillins is by the production of beta-lactamase which cleaves the beta-lactam ring of penicillin and destroys antibacterial activity. Similar mechanisms are important in the development of resistance to cephalosporins, the aminoglycosides, and chloramphenicol.

3. Diminished conversion of the drug to its active metabolite. The conversion of flucytosine to 5-fluouracil is an absolute requirement for the

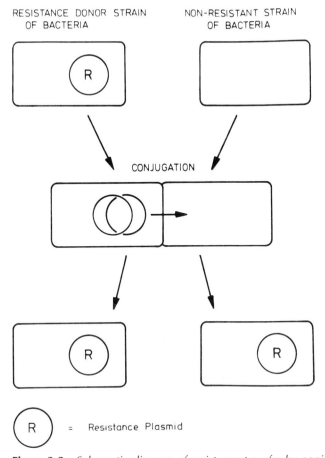

RESISTANCE DONOR STRAIN
OF BACTERIA

NON-RESISTANT STRAIN
OF BACTERIA

CONJUGATION

R   =   Resistance Plasmid

Figure 3-2   *Schematic diagram of resistance transfer by conjugation.*

drug to be effective. Fungal resistance to flucytosine is conferred by a mutation which abolishes the activity of cytosine deaminase, the enzyme responsible for this step.

4. Increased conversion of the drug to an antagonist metabolite. This mechanism has been observed rarely in staphylococci resistant to sulphonamide, due to the production by mutant cells of an excessive amount of para-aminobenzoic acid which competitively antagonises the inhibitory effect of the drug.

5. Decreased affinity of the receptors for the drug. Resistance to sulphonamides, rifampicin, erythromycin, trimethoprim, and streptomycin has been demonstrated in bacteria by this mechanism.

Combinations of Chemotherapeutic Agents

As a general principle it is advisable to use a single antimicrobial drug with a narrow spectrum of activity which is effective against the organisms causing the infection but does not upset the normal bacterial flora. In the treatment of respiratory infections it is sometimes impossible to meet these criteria because (1) the organism is known to become resistant very quickly if a single drug is used, (2) effective therapy is urgently needed before the exact nature of the infecting organism and its sensitivities can be ascertained, or (3) the infection is a mixed one with bacteria of differing antibiotic sensitivities.

Prevention of Resistance   The rapid development of resistance to a single chemotherapeutic agent is characteristic of the mycobacteria which in any case demand rather prolonged treatment with the currently available drugs to achieve eradication of the infection. The average frequency of occurrence of a resistant mutant for a particular drug in the case of a particular organism is one per 10–50 million bacteria, but if two antimicrobial drugs are used the chance that an organism will be resistant to both drugs is 1 in 10^{-14} or less, a probability which is most unlikely to be encountered in normal infections. The use of two drugs concurrently in the treatment of tuberculosis is therefore necessary but effective, provided that the infecting strain of mycobacteria is sensitive to both.

Although *Mycobacterium tuberculosis* is the classic example, there are other micro-organisms which develop resistance rapidly to certain antibiotics if used singly. For example, *Klebsiella* species develop resistance to streptomycin, and staphylococci develop resistance to fusidic acid or rifampin.[7] If it is necessary to use one such antibiotic for the treatment of these infections, especially if the infection is a chronic one which is likely to require prolonged chemotherapy, it would be appropriate to combine it with another effective agent, giving both in full dosage.

Severe Undiagnosed Infection   The use of combination chemotherapy is also acceptable for the treatment of desperately ill patients, for example, those with severe pneumonia or septicaemia, whose need for urgent effective treatment overrides the desirability for initial microbiological guidance in the choice of chemotherapy. In such situations it is best to use high-dosage combinations of bactericidal agents given parenterally which will provide a broad spectrum of chemotherapy to cover the micro-organisms considered on clinical or epidemiological grounds the most likely to be responsible for the infection. For example, a combination of flucloxacillin and ampicillin is used in the case of a severe pneumonia, with the possible addition of gentamicin if a Gram-negative organism is believed to be a likely pathogen. A highly important practical point is that specimens for microbiological examination should be obtained from all likely sources (sputum, blood, pleural exudate, etc.) before the first dose of chemotherapy is given, so that reliable bacteriological information is available in the shortest possible time for guiding future management.

Mixed Infections   Combinations of antibiotics may be necessary in the treatment of mixed infections. Although more than one organism may sometimes be cultured from the sputum most respiratory tract infections are due at any one time to a single predominant species which is responsible for that particular illness, and the treatment directed toward the eradication of that organism is usually curative. The exceptions occur in chronic recurring infections such as chronic bronchitis and bronchiectasis, in cystic fibrosis when organisms such as staphylococci and Gram-negative bacteria commonly coexist,[42] and in aspiration pneumonias or lung abscess which often result from a mixed infection with a variety of aerobic and anaerobic micro-organisms.[2] In these conditions the choice of antimicrobial therapy depends heavily on culture of the infecting organisms prior to therapy, and transtracheal aspiration may be necessary for a reliable diagnosis if anaerobic infection is suspected.[53]

Synergism and Antagonism Between Antimicrobial Agents   An enhanced antibacterial effect may be obtained through synergism between two chemotherapeutic agents, for example, between trimethoprim and sulphamethoxazole which when combined form the potent bacterial agent known in Britain as co-trimoxazole.[32] Carbenicillin and gentamycin synergy has been demonstrated against *Pseudomonas aeruginosa*,[64] and penicillins and aminoglycosides are combined for their synergistic action in enterococcal endocarditis.[41]

The disadvantages of combination chemotherapy lie not only in an increased risk of toxic side-effects or drug interactions from a multiplicity of drugs, or a greater liability to superinfection with resistant organisms because of the broader spectrum of combined therapy, but also in the possibility of antagonism between the antimicrobial effects of two or more chemotherapeutic agents. Antimicrobial agents have an effect in the patient which is either bactericidal or bacteriostatic (Table 3-3). Bacteriostatic drugs inhibit bacterial replication but do not kill the organisms, which are destroyed *in vivo* by the immunological and other defence mechanisms of the host; in contrast, bactericidal drugs kill and lyse micro-organisms. There is some laboratory and clinical evidence that combinations of bacteriostatic and bactericidal agents are less effective than treatment with one drug alone: for example, mortality due to pneumococcal meningitis was greater in patients treated with a combination of penicillin plus chlortetracycline than in those treated with penicillin alone.[40] Antagonism between penicillin and chloramphenicol has been observed in experimental canine pneumococcal meningitis[74] and in streptococcal endocar-

Table 3-3 / Bactericidal and Bacteriostatic Antimicrobial Agents

Primarily bactericidal	Penicillins
	Cephalosporins
	Aminoglycosides
	Polymyxins
	Trimethoprim-sulphamethoxazole
Primarily bacteriostatic	Tetracyclines
	Chloramphenicol
	Erythromycin
	Lincomycins

ditis in rabbits,[11] but favourable results with this combination have been recorded in the treatment of clinical pneumococcal pneumonia.[18] The conflict between experimental and most clinical evidence of antagonism between penicillins on the one hand and chloramphenicol or tetracyclines on the other may be related to differences in the relative concentrations of the drugs in different anatomical situations, or possibly to the timing of their administration in relation to one another. Similar uncertainty exists about the significance of *in vitro* antagonism between aminoglycosides and chloramphenicol or tetracycline, and between aminoglycosides and lincomycins, the available clinical evidence appearing to refute the pessimistic prognostications of the laboratory data. The evidence is reviewed and tabulated by Rahal,[50] whose practical recommendations tend to oppose the combinations of chloramphenicol or tetracyclines with penicillins or with aminoglycosides, except in the special cases of brucellosis and plague.[9,51]

RATIONAL CHOICE OF ANTIMICROBIAL AGENTS FOR RESPIRATORY INFECTIONS

Treatment of any infection must be based if possible on an accurate microbiological diagnosis which determines the infecting organism and its sensitivities. Before starting therapy, therefore, the physician has a first priority to obtain specimens for culture, including throat swab, sputum, transtracheal aspirate, pleural aspirate, or blood as the clinical situation warrants, and to send them to the laboratory without delay. Gram and Ziehl-Neilsen staining may provide morphological information about the infecting organism and plates should be set up for anaerobic or fungal cultures if these types of infection are anticipated. If possible antibiotics should not be prescribed without guidance from these investigations, but it is often necessary to start therapy for acute respiratory infections on the basis of a clinical diagnosis of the most likely causative organism.[14] It is easier for the clinician to make a rational choice of antibiotic if he is aware of current local infections and sensitivity patterns, and if he has a particular organism in mind before starting treatment.

Although the choice of antibiotic is primarily determined by the identity of the infecting organism, whether known or suspected, there is usually a short list of drugs available which are all active against the infection to a greater or lesser extent. The antibiotic of choice is usually the one which comes nearest to the concept of the "ideal drug," that is, one which has the following qualities[47]:

1. High activity against the micro-organism in question but preferably with a narrow spectrum of action, since this reduces the risks of super-infection and bacterial resistance.
2. Suitable pharmacological characteristics which result in adequate drug levels in the infected tissues for a convenient length of time.
3. Minimal side-effects with a low incidence of adverse reactions.
4. Preferably bactericidal action rather than bacteriostatic, making it effective in patients with impaired defence mechanisms.
5. Low cost.

Many antibiotics are far from ideal and some which have the most suitable spectrum of activity are also the most likely to cause toxic side-effects. It is therefore necessary for the clinician to weigh the relative importance of activity and toxicity of the various alternative antimicrobial drugs in each case with special attention to age, possible pregnancy, a history of hypersensitivity reactions, the presence of underlying disease, and the state of hepatic and renal function.

For many antimicrobial drugs there is a narrow margin of effectiveness between suboptimal dosage and toxicity so that factors which alter the drug's absorption or elimination are especially important. This applies not only to the aminoglycosides and vancomycin which are all ototoxic and nephrotoxic to some extent, but also to the tetracyclines which may affect hepatic as well as renal function in pregnancy; it also applies to ethambutol, which may cause optic neuritis, and to 5-fluorocytosine, which can seriously depress the bone marrow. These serious side-effects may be irreversible and special care must be taken to avoid them: an enquiry into renal and hepatic function is a natural precaution in the assessment of any patient for antibiotic treatment so that any constraints are recognised from the outset. They may result in the exclusion of certain drugs of choice because there is an unreasonable risk of toxicity, or in modification of dosage of the chosen drug based on the age of the patient, as in the routine use of streptomycin, or based on some measure of renal function as applied to gentamicin dosage.

The determination of blood antibiotic levels is a valuable aid to dose adjustment with these drugs in avoiding excessive accumulation or inadequate dosage.[28] If dosage modification is necessary it can be achieved either by reducing the size of each dose or by increasing the interval between doses, and tables are available which indicate the appropriate method and scale of dosage reduction at various levels of renal failure for different antibiotics.[4] Dosage can then be monitored by measurements of the peak plasma concentration in blood obtained at the appropriate interval after administration, and of the trough concentration shortly before the next dose is due (times and levels of peak concentrations for different antibiotics are listed in references 28 and 43). Such assays may provide an early indication of excessive or inadequate dosage, although the ultimate determinant is the clinical response of the patient to therapy.

The essential steps which should be taken to ensure a reasonable chance of successful antimicrobial therapy can be summarised formally as follows:

1. Diagnosis of the pathogen based on microbiological or clinical criteria.
2. Selection of a short list of alternative antimicrobial agents with the appropriate spectrum of activity.
3. Review of the patient's individual clinical features to identify factors which might influence the choice of therapy.
4. Selection of the most suitable drug.
5. Choice of administration route most likely to produce adequate drug levels at the site of infection.
6. Surveillance of therapy to ensure adherence to the prescribed drug regimen.
7. Where indicated, monitoring of dosage by serial determinations of plasma drug concentration.

REFERENCES

1. BARRETT-CONNOR E: Bacterial infection and sickle cell anaemia. An analysis of 250 infections in 166 patients and a review of the literature. Medicine 50: 97–112, 1971.
2. BARTLETT JG, GORBACH SL, FINEGOLD JM: The bacteriology of aspiration pneumonia. Am J Med 56: 202–207, 1974.
3. BENNETT N McK: Drug induced agranulocytosis and septicaemia. Med J Aust 2: 575–577, 1963.
4. BENNETT WM, SINGER I, GOLPER T, FEIG P, COGGINS CJ: Guidelines for drug therapy in renal failure. Ann Intern Med 86: 754–783, 1977.
5. BISTRIAN BR, SHERMAN M, BLACKBURN GL, MARSHALL R, SHAW C: Cellular immunity in adult marasmus. Arch Intern Med 137: 1408–1411, 1977.

6. BODEY GF, RODRIGUEZ V, CHANG HY, NARBONI G: Fever and infection in leukaemic patients. Cancer 41: 1610–1622, 1978.
7. BRITISH MEDICAL JOURNAL: Antibiotics and respiratory illness. Br Med J 2: 1, 1974.
8. BRUTON OC: Agammaglobulinaemia. Pediatrics 9: 722–728, 1952.
9. BUCHANAN TM, FABER LC, FELDMAN RA: Brucellosis in the United States, 1960–1972. An abattoir-associated disease. Part 1. Clinical features and therapy. Medicine 53: 403–413, 1974.
10. CALDWELL JR, CLUFF LE: Adverse reactions to antimicrobial agents. JAMA 230: 77–80, 1974.
11. CARRIZOSA J, KOBASA WD, KAYE D: Antagonism between chloramphenicol and penicillin in streptococcal endocarditis in rabbits. J Lab Clin Med 85: 307–311, 1975.
12. CASTLE M, WILFERT CM, CATE TR, OSTERHOUT S: Antibiotic use at Duke University Medical Center. JAMA 237: 2819–2822, 1977.
13. CLARK RA, KIMBALL HR: Defective granulocyte chemotaxis in the Chediak-Higashi Syndrome. J Clin Invest 50: 2645–2652, 1971.
14. COLE RB: Problems in the diagnosis and treatment of pneumonia. Practitioner 223: 765–770, 1979.
15. COSTERTON JW, INGRAM JM, CHENG KJ: Structure and function of the cell envelope of Gram-negative bacteria. Bacteriol Rev 38: 87–110, 1974.
16. CRAIG WA, UMAN SJ, SHAW WR, RAMGOPAL V, EAGAN LL, LEOPOLD ET: Hospital use of antimicrobial drugs. Survey at 19 hospitals and results of antimicrobial control program. Ann Intern Med 89: 793–5, 1978.
17. DANIELS JC, SAKAI H, REMMERS AR, SARLES HE, FISH JC, COBB EK, LEVIN WC, RITZMANN SE: *In vitro* reactivity of human lymphocytes in chronic uraemia: analysis and interpretation. Clin Exp Immunol 8: 213–227, 1971.
18. DAVIS WM: Successful treatment of pneumococcal pneumonia with combination of chloramphenicol and penicillin. Am J Med Sci 227: 391–397, 1954.
19. FAHEY JL, SCOGGINS R, UTZ JP, SZWED CF: Infection, antibody response and gamma globulin components in multiple myeloma and macroglobulinaemia. Am J Med 35: 698–707, 1963.
20. FEINGOLD DS: Antimicrobial chemotherapeutic agents; the nature of their action and selective toxicity. N Engl J Med 269: 900–907 and 957–964, 1963.
21. FELD R, BODEY GP Infections in patients with malignant lymphoma treated with combination chemotherapy. Cancer 39: 1018–1025, 1977.
22. FELLER I, PIERSON C: *Pseudomonas* vaccine and hyperimmune plasma for burned patients. Arch Surg 97: 225–229, 1968.
23. FUXENCH-LOPEZ Z, RAMIREZ-RONDA CH: Pharyngeal flora in ambulatory alcoholic patients. Prevalence of Gram-negative bacilli. Arch Intern Med 138: 1815–1816, 1978.
24. GINZLER E, DIAMOND H, KAPLAN D, WEINER M, SCHLESINGER M, SELEZNICK M: Computer analysis of factors influencing frequency of infection in systemic lupus erythematosus. Arthritis Rheum 21: 37–44, 1978.
25. GORDON M, LOVELL S, DUGDALE AE: The value of antibiotics in minor respiratory illness in children. Med J Aust 1: 304–306, 1974.
26. GRAYBILL JR, MARSHALL LW, CHARACHE P, WALLACE CK, MELVIN VB: Nosocomial

pneumonia. A continuing major problem. Am Rev Resp Dis 108: 1130–1140, 1973.

27. Hersh EM, Freirech EJ: Host defence mechanisms and their modification by cancer chemotherapy. in H Busch (ed), Methods in Cancer Research, Vol 4. p. 355, New York: Academic Press, 1968.

28. Hewitt WL, McHenry MC: Blood level determinations of antimicrobial drugs. Some clinical considerations. Med Clin North Am 62: 1119–1140, 1978.

29. Hill RB, Dahrling BE, Starzl TE, Rifkind D: Death after transplantation. An analysis of sixty cases. Am J Med 42: 327–334, 1967.

30. Holloway BW, Asche LV: Mechanisms and clinical implications of antibiotic resistance in bacteria. Drugs 14: 283–290, 1977.

31. Howard MW, Strauss RG, Johnston RB: Infections in patients with neutropenia. Am J Dis Child 131: 788–790, 1977.

32. Hughes DTD: Use of combinations of trimethoprim and sulphamethoxazole in the treatment of chest infections. J Infect Dis 128: (Suppl) S701–S705, 1973.

33. Johanson WG, Pierce AK, Sanford JP: Changing pharyngeal bacterial flora of hospitalised patients. Emergence of Gram-negative bacilli. N Eng J Med 281: 1137–1140, 1969.

34. Johnston RB, McMurry JS: Chronic familial granulomatosis. Report of five cases and review of the literature. Am J Dis Child 114: 370–378, 1967.

35. Kass EH: Hormones and host resistance to infection. Bacteriol Rev 24: 177–185, 1960.

36. Kunin CM: Antibiotic accountability. N Engl J Med 301: 380–381, 1979.

37. Kunin CM, Topasi T, Craig WA: Use of antibiotics. A brief exposition of the problem and some tentative solutions. Ann Intern Med 79: 555–560, 1973.

38. Lancet: Pneumococcal vaccines. Lancet 1: 131–132, 1978.

39. Lederberg J: Bacterial protoplasts induced by penicillin. Proc Nat Acad Sci USA 42: 574–577, 1956.

40. Lepper MH, Dowling HF: Treatment of pneumococcic meningitis with penicillin compared with penicillin plus aureomycin. Arch Intern Med 88: 489–494, 1951.

41. Mandell GL, Kaye D, Levison ME, Hook EW: Enterococcal endocarditis. An analysis of 38 patients observed at the New York Hospital—Cornell Medical Center. Arch Intern Med 125: 258–264, 1970.

42. May JR, Herrick NC, Thompson D: Bacterial infection in cystic fibrosis. Arch Dis Child 47: 908–913, 1972.

43. McHenry MC, Gavan TL, Selection and use of antimicrobial drugs. Progr Clin Pathol 6: 205–266, 1975.

44. Miller ME, Oski FA, Harris MB: Lazy-leucocyte syndrome. A new disorder of neutrophil function. Lancet 1: 665–669, 1971.

45. Moorhouse EC: Transferable drug resistance in enterobacteria isolated from unborn infants. Br Med J 2: 405–407, 1969.

46. Perillie PE, Nolan JP, Finch SC: Studies of the resistance to infection in diabetes mellitus: local exudative cellular response. J Lab Clin Med 59: 1008–1015, 1962.

47. Petersdorf RG, Featherstone H: New antimicrobial drugs and their value in the treatment of respiratory infections. Am Rev Resp Dis 117: 1–3, 1978.

48. PITTMANN FE: Antibiotic-associated colitis—An update. Adverse Drug Reaction Bulletin 75: 268–271, 1979.

49. PRICE DJE, SLEIGH JD: Control of infection due to Klebsiella aerogenes in a neuro-surgical unit by withdrawal of all antibiotics. Lancet 2: 1213–1215, 1970.

50. RAHAL JJ: Antibiotic combinations: the clinical relevance of synergy and antagon-sim. Medicine 57: 179–195, 1978.

51. REED WP, PAMER DL, WILLIAMS RC, KISCH AL: Bubonic plague in the southwestern United States. A review of recent experience. Medicine 49: 465–486, 1970.

52. RIDLEY M, BARRIE D, LYNN R, STEAD KC: Antibiotic resistant Staphylococcus aureus and hospital antibiotic policies. Lancet 1: 230–233, 1970.

53. RIES K, LEVISON ME, KAYE D: Transtracheal aspiration in pulmonary infection. Arch Intern Med 133: 453–458, 1974.

54. ROSEN FS, JANEWAY CA: The gamma globulins III. The antibody deficiency syn-dromes. N Engl J Med 275: 709–715 and 769–775, 1966.

55. ROSENTHAL A; Follow-up study of fatal penicillin reactions. JAMA 167: 1118–1121, 1958.

56. SACK RB: Prophylactic antibiotics? The individual versus the commonity. N Engl J Med 300: 1107–8, 1979.

57. SCHECKLER WE, BENNETT JV: Antibiotic usage in seven community hospitals. JAMA 213: 264–267, 1970.

58. SETH V, CHANDRA RK: Opsonic activity, phagocytosis, and bacterial capacity of polymorphs in undernutrition. Arch Dis Child 47: 282–284, 1972.

59. SHAPIRO S, SLONE D, SISKIND V, LEWIS GP, JICK H: Drug rash with ampicillin and other penicillins. Lancet 2: 969–972, 1969.

60. SHAPIRO M, TOWNSEND TR, ROSNER B, KASS EH: Use of antimicrobial drugs in general hospitals. N Engl J Med 301: 351–355, 1979.

61. SHAW RK, SZWED C, BOGGS DR, FAHEY JL, FREI E, MORRISON E, UTZ JP: Infection and immunity in chronic lymphocytic leukaemia. Arch Intern Med 106: 467–478, 1960.

62. SHULMAN S, BARTLETT J, CLYDE WA, AYOUB EM: The unusual severity of mycoplas-mal pneumonia in children with sickle-cell disease. N Engl J Med 287: 164–167, 1972.

63. SMITH H: Opportunistic infection. Br Med J 2: 107–110, 1973.

64. SMITH CB, WILFERT JN, DANS PE, KURRUS TA, FINLAND M: In vitro activity of carbenicillin and results of treatment of infections due to *Pseudomonas* with carbe-nicillin singly and in combination with gentamicin. J Infect Dis 122 (Suppl): S14–S25, 1970.

65. SMYTHE PM, SCHONLAND M, BRERETON-STILES GG, COOVADIA HM, CRACE HJ, LOENING WEK, MAFOYANE A, PARENT MA, VOS GH: Thymolymphatic deficiency and depression of cell-mediated immunity in protein-calorie malnutrition. Lancet 2: 939–943, 1971.

66. SOOTHILL J: Immune deficiency states. in Gell PGH, Coombes RRA, Lachman PJ (eds) Clinical Aspects of Immunology, Ch 23 Oxford: Blackwell, 1975.

67. SOYKA LF, ROBINSON DS, LACHANT N, MONACO J: The misuse of antibiotics for treatment of upper respiratory tract infections in children. Pediatrics 55: 552–556, 1975.

68. Staples PJ, Gerding DN, Decker JL, Gordon RS: Incidence of infection in systemic lupus erythematosus. Arthritis Rheum 17: 1–10, 1974.

69. Study Group on the Use of Antimicrobial Drugs: Prophylactic antimicrobial drug therapy at five London teaching hospitals. Lancet 1: 1351–1353, 1977.

70. Tedesco F, Markham R, Gurwith M, Christie D, Bartlett JG: Oral vancomycin for antibiotic-associated pseudomembranous colitis. Lancet 2: 226–228, 1978.

71. Tillotson JR, Finland M: Bacterial colonisation of the respiratory tract complicating antibiotic treatment of pneumonia. J Infect Dis 119: 597–624, 1969.

72. Valenti WM, Trudell RG, Bentley DW: Factors predisposing to oropharyngeal colonisation with Gram-negative bacilli in the aged. N Engl J Med 298: 1108–1111, 1978.

73. Veterans Administration Ad Hoc Interdisciplinary Advisory Committee on Antimicrobial Drug Usage Prophylaxis in Surgery. JAMA 237: 1003–1008, 1977.

74. Wallace JF, Smith RH, Garcia M, Petersdorf RG: Studies on the pathogenesis of meningitis. 4. Antagonism between penicillin and chloramphenicol in experimental pneumococcal meningitis. J Lab Clin Med 70: 408–418, 1967.

75. Wells RS, Higgs JM, Macdonald A, Valdimarsson H, Holt PJL: Familial chronic mucocutaneous candidiasis. Journal of Medical Genetics 9: 302–310, 1972.

76. Whitecar JF, Luna M, Bodey GP: Pseudomonas bacteremia in patients with malignant diseases. Am J Med Sci 260: 216–223, 1970.

77. Wright GLT, Harper J: Fusidic acid and lincomycin therapy in staphylococcal infections in cystic fibrosis. Lancet 1: 9–14, 1970.

4

Antimicrobial Agents I

The list of antimicrobial agents seems to grow longer almost daily and it would be impossible to review their applications and characteristics in detail without turning this book into a catalogue and thus destroying its original purpose of providing a practical guide for the respiratory physician. I have therefore chosen to discuss only those drugs which are currently widely used in respiratory medicine, basing the discussion partly on personal experience in their use and also on my own assessment of published reports and reviews. Information about new chemotherapeutic agents can be obtained from regular critical reviews such as those published in *Drugs* (Australia), the *Drug and Therapeutic Bulletin* (Britain), or from *The Medical Letter* and from *Rational Drug Therapy* (United States). The comprehensive review entitled *The Use of Antibiotics*[54] has been regularly updated and it provides a wealth of information about the pharmacology and clinical applications of a wide range of antimicrobial drugs. The drugs which I have chosen to discuss in this and the following chapters are those included in Table 4-1.

PENICILLINS

General Properties

Penicillin was developed from the mould *Penicillium notatum*, which was observed by Fleming in 1928 to inhibit bacterial growth in laboratory cultures. These observations were developed by Florey and his associates with the isolation of a crude preparation of penicillin which was shown to have a useful

Table 4-1 / Micro-organisms Causing Respiratory Infections: Appropriate Drug Therapy[54,68,102]

Micro-organism	Initial Chemotherapy	Alternative Chemotherapeutic Agents
Aerobic micro-organisms		
Gram-positive cocci		
Streptococcus pyogenes	Penicillin G or V	Erythromycin; a cephalosporin
Streptococcus pneumoniae	Penicillin G	Erythromycin; a cephalosporin
Staphylococcus aureus (penicillin G-sensitive)	Penicillin G	A cephalosporin; clindamycin, erythromycin
Staphylococcus aureus (penicillin G-resistant)	Isoxazolyl penicillin	Methicillin; nafcillin; a cephalosporin
Staphylococcus aureus ("methicillin-resistant")	Depends on in vitro sensitivities	Vancomycin; kanamycin; sodium fusidate; gentamicin
Gram-negative bacilli		
Escherichia coli	Gentamicin	Ampicillin; a cephalosporin, a tetracycline
Klebsiella pneumoniae	Gentamicin	A cephalosporin, a tetracycline
Proteus species	Gentamicin	Tobramycin; kanamycin
Salmonella typhi	Chloramphenicol	Ampicillin; trimethoprim-sulphamethoxazole
Haemophilus influenzae	Ampicillin	A tetracycline; trimethoprim-sulphamethoxazole
Bordetella pertussis	Erythromycin	
Yersinia pestis	Streptomycin	A tetracycline
Brucella species	Streptomycin	A tetracycline
Pseudomonas aeruginosa	Tobramycin	Carbenicillin
Chlamydia psittaci	A tetracycline	Erythromycin
Coxiella burneti	A tetracycline	Erythromycin
Mycoplasma pneumoniae	A tetracycline	Erythromycin
Legionella pneumophila	Erythromycin	A tetracycline; rifampin
Anaerobic micro-organisms		
Gram-positive cocci		
Peptococcus, peptostreptococcus	Penicillin G	Clindamycin; metronidazole; chloramphenicol
Gram-negative bacilli		
Bacteroides fragilis	Clindamycin	Metronidazole; chloramphenicol
Bacteroides melaninogenicus	Penicillin G	Clindamycin; metronidazole; chloramphenicol
Fusobacterium	Penicillin G	Clindamycin; metronidazole; chloramphenicol

If possible, in vitro sensitivity tests should always be done to determine the most suitable antimicrobial agent for treating a particular infection. The choices shown in this table indicate the drugs most likely to be successful in treating infection due to a particular micro-organism, taking due account of drug toxicities.

therapeutic effect against bacterial infections in humans.[16] Manufacture of penicillin in large quantities is now carried out from mutant strains of *Penicillium* which have been developed and selected for high yield. The semi-synthetic penicillins are obtained by incorporating specific precursors in the cultures of the mould, by chemical modification of natural penicillin or, more effectively, by synthesis from 6-amino penicillanic acid, which is a product of the enzymatic hydrolysis of penicillin. In the original search for penicillin in the 1940s a number of natural penicillins were identified with differing properties which were designated alphabetically. Penicillin G or benzylpenicillin proved superior to the others and is the prototype with which more specialised penicillins are compared.

Structure   The chemical structure of penicillin G is shown in Figure 4-1 which also depicts the changes in the side chain responsible for the characteristic properties of some widely-used semi-synthetic penicillins. Penicillin G is inactivated by penicillinase (beta-lactamase) which splits the beta-lactam ring of the penicillin molecule to form inactive penicilloic acid, a step which is prevented by the synthetic side-chain alterations of methicillin and the isoxazolyl penicillins.

Mode of Action   The penicillins act by blocking the formation of cross-links between units of the bacterial cell wall which maintain its rigid structure. These cross-links consist of peptide bonds between peptidoglycan strands which are the basic repeating units or "building blocks" of the cell wall. The cross-linking process is carried out by a transpeptidase enzyme which is inhibited by penicillins and cephalosporins, probably by binding between the antibiotic and the enzyme at its substrate binding site and thus preventing it from carrying out its transpeptidation function.[97] Although this inhibitory action prevents cell-wall synthesis it does not in itself explain the cell lysis and death which result; this is probably due to the continuous action of cell-wall autolytic enzymes which exert a prevailing destructive effect on the bacterial cell walls in the absence of biosynthesis, causing weaknesses which allow protrusion and rupture of the cell membrane.[88,90]

Resistance   The usual basis of the development of bacterial resistance to penicillin is the production of penicillinase. For example, resistance to penicillin G by this mechanism developed rather rapidly among strains of *Staphylococcus aureus* within a few years of its introduction, and now many strains are resistant even outside hospitals.[10] Group A streptococci have remained sensitive, but recently strains of pneumococci relatively or completely resistant to penicillin have been detected, and multiple-resistant strains have emerged in South Africa.[4,48]

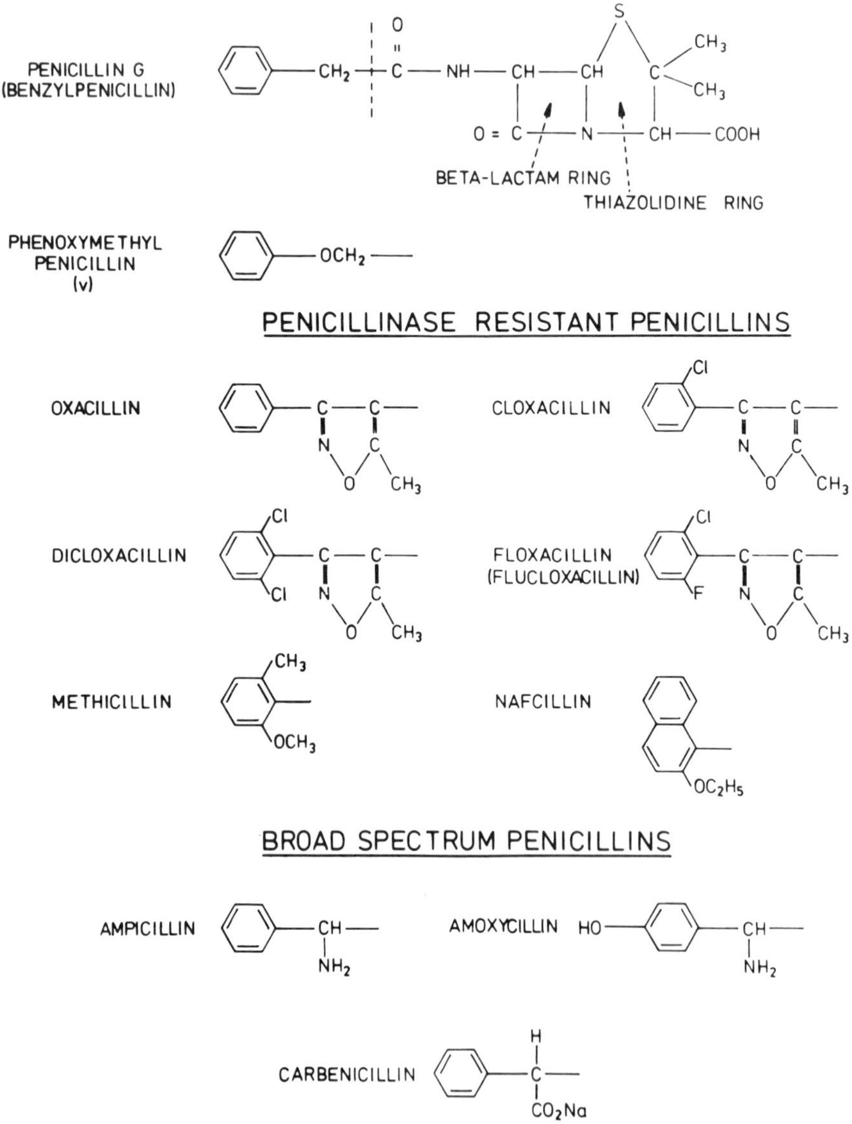

Figure 4-1 *Chemical structure of selected penicillins. Side-chain alterations are responsible for variations in the antimicrobial properties of different penicillins.*

Staphylococci also show another form of resistance known as "tolerance" in which they appear to lack the normal autolytic enzyme activity which is responsible for cell destruction following bacterial cell wall damage initiated by penicillin.[12] As a result the antibiotic loses its bactericidal effect although it continues to inhibit the organism. Tolerance of this type applies to all penicillins, to cephalosporins, and usually to vancomycin, but does not apply to gentamycin, rifampin, or cycloserine.

Staphylococci have also been able to adapt to penicillinase-resistant penicillins such as methicillin, and they are referred to as "methicillin-resistant" strains which have occurred sporadically in North America and Europe, nearly always in a hospital environment. The mechanism of this resistance is unknown.[6,76]

Penicillin Allergy   Hypersensitivity reactions to penicillins are responsible for a high proportion of allergic drug reactions, the main antigenic determinant being the penicilloyl derivative which acts as a haptene in combining with protein to form the antigen. Hypersensitivity is usually common to all penicillins, and cross-sensitivity also occurs with the cephalosporins but only in 5 to 10 percent of patients.[22] The most serious forms of penicillin allergy are anaphylactic shock, urticarial reactions, and angioneurotic oedema, serum sickness, fever, various skin rashes, immune haemolytic anaemia, and thrombocytopenia.[59]

The most important measure in avoiding allergic reactions to penicillins is to seek a history of previous reactions before administering the first dose. There appears to be little or no correlation between penicillin hypersensitivity and a previous or family history of atopy,[37,44] and atopic patients should not be denied penicillin if it is otherwise indicated. Parenteral injections are more likely to induce an allergic reaction, and oral administration is to be preferred outside hospital where emergency measures for the treatment of acute anaphylaxis are less readily available. Practical and effective screening tests for identifying penicillin-hypersensitive individuals are still unsatisfactory, although a multivalent antigen for skin testing is available, penicilloyl-polylysine (PPL), which has some value in predicting reactors. However, negative responders to PPL may still react severely to other "minor" antigenic determinants of penicillin for which there is currently no commercially available skin testing preparation, although a "minor determinant mixture" has been described.[58] Combined skin testing with PPL and the minor determinant mixture is said to be helpful in screening patients with a possible history of penicillin allergy, because if both are negative the likelihood of an immediate penicillin reaction is extremely small.[1] However, skin testing carries the risk of precipitating the reaction one is seeking to avoid and should not be carried out without the immediate availability of epinephrine for injection, appropriate airway support, and the necessary trained personnel. There is as yet no satisfactory single *in vitro* test for Type I allergies.

If the use of penicillin is considered to be absolutely essential in a penicillin-sensitive individual, hyposensitisation can be attempted—although it is hazardous and not always successful. Parker[75] begins with an oral dose of 1,000 units, doubling it every 20 or 30 minutes up to a dose of approximately 50,000 units. Thereafter he begins with 1,000 units subcutaneously or intradermally, doubling the dose until comparable oral and parenteral doses of penicillin are reached, whereupon full therapeutic doses are administered parenterally and the oral dose is discontinued. Hyposensitisation may also be achieved more slowly using an extended programme of gradually increasing dosage over a period of days or weeks. Emergency medications and resuscitative equipment should be available for immediate use throughout any attempt at hyposensitisation.

Penicillin G (Benzylpenicillin)

Penicillin G has a narrow range of activity against Gram-positive aerobic and anaerobic bacteria and against a few Gram-negative species, some anaerobic bacilli (but not *Bacteroides fragilis*), and the *Neisseria* species.

Clinical Pharmacology   Only about one-third of the oral dose of penicillin G is absorbed from the gastrointestinal tract. It is unstable in acid solution and absorption is unreliable, probably because of variation in the degree of acid inactivation. It is therefore customarily administered parenterally by intramuscular or intravenous injection. Immediate high serum levels are obtained after rapid intravenous injection of crystalline penicillin G, with a rapid decrease in the first hour followed by a slower decline. Intermittent intravenous dosage of 2 or 3 million units (1 million units is equal to 600 mg) administered every 2 or 3 hours produces a mean concentration of approximately 20 µg/ml. After intramuscular injection of 1 million units a serum level of 6–8 µg/ml is reached within 30 minutes. Diffusion into most tissues and serous spaces is rapid, particularly in the presence of inflammation, but it is poor into abscess cavities and avascular areas and is negligible into uninflamed bone or CSF, except when the meninges are inflamed. Penicillin G is rapidly excreted by glomerular filtration and renal tubular secretion, which results in about 75 percent of an injected dose being excreted within 6 hours, largely as the active drug. Probenecid competes with penicillin for its proximal tubular excretory pathway and can be used to increase the serum concentration. A small amount of penicillin is excreted in the bile, and the remainder is inactivated in the liver to penicilloic acid.

Preparations and Dosage Crystalline penicillin G is available for intramuscular or intravenous administration, either as the sodium or the potassium salt in vials of dry powder containing 0.2 to 20 million units each. The usual dose is 0.5 to 3 million units (300 mg to 1.8 g) every 4 to 6 hours, but it is seldom necessary to exceed 12 million units (7.2 g) daily. Penicillin is inactivated if mixed in solution prior to injection with some other drugs, including hydrocortisone, lincomycin, and kanamycin; if intravenous administration is indicated, penicillin should be given by intermittent bolus injection because it is inactivated within a few hours in alkaline carbohydrate solutions and because the major product of such inactivation, penicilloic acid, is antigenic. Benzathine and procaine salts of penicillin G are available for intramuscular injection to provide lower but prolonged blood levels, but if an oral penicillin preparation is required phenoxymethylpenicillin (penicillin V) should be used, because absorption is more reliable.

Toxic Effects Hypersensitivity reactions are more likely to occur if the penicillin solution has not been freshly prepared. Haemolysis and a positive Coomb's test may occur during prolonged penicillin treatment and interstitial nephritis with eosinophilia and fever is a rare complication. Very high levels of penicillin in the CSF may cause fits and coma due to a direct irritative effect on the central nervous system, and it is most likely to occur in patients with impaired renal function who are treated with high dosage. One million units of the potassium salt of crystalline penicillin G contains 1.5 mEq of potassium ion, while the same dose of the sodium salt contains 1.7 mEq of sodium ion: complications can arise if massive doses are given in patients with cardiac or renal failure.

Clinical Practice Parenteral penicillin G is the antibiotic of choice in the treatment of unclassified pneumonia arising outside hospital (because *Streptococcus pneumoniae* is the most likely infecting micro-organism), or in the treatment of hospital-acquired pneumonia shown to be due to penicillin-sensitive streptococcal or staphylococcal infections (Table 4-2). The treatment of streptococcal pharyngitis is sometimes initiated with a single dose of penicillin G followed by oral penicillin V, or alternatively a single dose of long-acting benzathine penicillin or combined benzathine and procaine penicillins can be used.[9,81] The possibility of an acute allergic reaction should be borne in mind and appropriate precautions should be taken. Penicillin G is also the drug of choice in the initial treatment of suspected anaerobic lung infections and in the therapy of actinomycosis.

Table 4-2 / Major Clinical Indications for Penicillin G and V in Respiratory Infections

Priority	Indication
Drug of choice	Streptococcal pharyngitis
	Undiagnosed pneumonia arising outside the hospital
	Pneumonia due to penicillin-sensitive streptococci or staphylococci
	Anaerobic chest infections (excluding those caused by *Bacteroides fragilis*)
	Actinomycosis

Penicillin V (Phenoxymethylpenicillin)

Penicillin V (Figure 4-1) is a natural penicillin prepared by adding phenoxyacetic acid to the fermentation medium of the culture. The range of activity is similar to that of penicillin G, but it is somewhat less active, and its major advantage is that it is more stable in acid solution and therefore better absorbed from the gastrointestinal tract. It is administered by mouth as the potassium salt—Penicillin V Potassium, U.S.P. or penicillin V B.P.—in various formulations of tablets, capsules, granules, suspensions, and the like. Penicillin V is given every 6 hours and the usual dosage in children is 125 mg (1 to 5 years) and 250 mg (6 to 12 years); and in adults 250–500 mg. Peak serum levels are improved if the drug is taken an hour before meals.

The pharmacology, mode of action, and toxicity of penicillin V are otherwise similar to those of penicillin G. The main uses of penicillin V in the respiratory field is for the treatment of streptococcal pharyngitis and for the convalescent phase of pneumonia due to sensitive pneumococcal infection.

Isoxazolyl Penicillins

This group of semi-synthetic penicillins comprises oxacillin, cloxacillin, dicloxacillin, and flucloxacillin (Figure 4-1). Since these drugs are stable in acid medium, they are reliably absorbed by mouth and have the important property of resistance to penicillinase, which gives them their primary role in the treatment of penicillinase-producing staphylococcal infection. They are all somewhat less active than penicillin G against bacteria which are sensitive to it. Because of cross-resistance between methicillin and other penicillinase-resistant penicillins the so-called "methicillin-resistant" staphylococci are also resistant to the isoxazolyl penicillins, although this resistance is relative rather than absolute.[62]

Clinical Pharmacology   After oral administration the isoxazolyl penicillins attain a peak serum level in ½–1 hour and maintain significant levels for 4 to 6 hours, the serum concentration reached by oxacillin being approximately half that of the other three drugs in the same dosage because of differences in absorption and rate of excretion. Higher concentrations are achieved with all four compounds when given parenterally, compared with the oral route. They diffuse widely into body tissues, serous cavities, and into inflamed bones and joints. Although the isoxazolyl penicillins are over 90 percent bound to serum proteins, it is uncertain what effect this may have on their therapeutic activity; protein-binding may increase the duration of action by maintaining a reservoir of the drug which is released as the free portion is metabolised or excreted; on the other hand, protein-binding lowers the peak drug concentration achieved at the site of drug action.[53] In spite of this uncertainty adequate serum concentrations and a satisfactory therapeutic effect can be readily achieved with these compounds. Like penicillin G they are largely excreted unchanged by renal glomerular filtration, tubular secretion, and to a slight extent by the biliary tract. Some inactivation occurs in the liver, more so in the case of oxacillin than in the others. Cystic fibrosis patients eliminate dicloxacillin and possibly other isoxazolyl penicillins much more rapidly than do normal persons because of an increased capacity for renal tubular secretion,[50] resulting in the need for increased dosage and monitoring of serum antibiotic levels to ensure adequate therapeutic concentrations.

Preparations and Dosage   For adults, the usual oral dose of the isoxazolyl penicillins is 200–500 mg every 6 hours, given about 1 hour before meals in order to improve absorption. The dose can be doubled or even further increased in severe infections, and probenecid can be used concurrently to increase the serum concentration. Oxacillin, cloxacillin, and dicloxacillin are available in the United States, while in Britain the preparations of choice are cloxacillin and flucloxacillin. The preferred drugs for oral administration are dicloxacillin and flucloxacillin because they are both well absorbed and produce prolonged effective serum concentrations.[95]

All four isoxazolyl penicillins give similar peak serum concentrations after a single intramuscular injection. The usual adult dose for severe infections is 1 g intravenously every 4 to 6 hours, but lower doses are sufficient for less serious infections and can be given intramuscularly. In the United States the only parenteral preparation available is Oxacillin Sodium for Injection, U.S.P., in 250 mg, 500 mg, and 1 g vials. In Britain Cloxacillin Injection B.P. and Flucloxacillin Injection B.P. are available in 250 mg and 500 mg vials.

Table 4-3 / Major Clinical Indications for Penicillinase-resistant Penicillins in Respiratory Infections

Priority	Indication
Drug of choice	Pneumonia known to be, or suspected of being due to staphylococci resistant to penicillin G

Toxic Effects   These penicillins cause hypersensitivity reactions in penicillin allergic patients and may cause nausea and diarrhoea after oral administration. Oxacillin is mildly hepatotoxic as shown by abnormal liver function tests which resolve when the drug is discontinued; raised SGOT levels have been observed in patients on cloxacillin.[11] Convulsions may occur in patients with high serum levels of isoxazolyl penicillins because of excessive dosage or reduced excretion due to impaired renal function. Neutropenia can occur and reversible agranulocytosis has been reported.[104]

Clinical Practice   The only indication for the isoxazolyl penicillins is in the treatment of staphylococcal infections known to be or suspected to be resistant to penicillin G. For example, their use is indicated in the initial treatment of severe undiagnosed pneumonia, especially that acquired in hospital or during an influenza epidemic. It should be borne in mind that these penicillins are less effective than penicillin G except in penicillin-G-resistant infections (Table 4-3).

Other Penicillinase-resistant Penicillins

Methicillin   Methicillin (Figure 4-1) was the first of the penicillinase-resistant penicillins to be discovered. It is one of the most stable and active in the presence of staphylococcal penicillinase, but it is unsuitable for oral adminis-tration because it is unstable in an acid medium. The pharmacokinetics and toxicity are similar to the other penicillins, but methicillin seems to be more liable to cause interstitial nephritis.[32] Methicillin Injection is given in a dose of 1 g every 4 hours intramuscularly, or as a bolus injection intravenously.

Because of its greater tendency to cause nephritis, its unsuitability for oral administration, and its rapid excretion, methicillin is being discarded by many clinicians in favour of the isoxazolyl penicillins.

Nafcillin   Nafcillin (Figure 4-1) is comparable to methicillin in its stability to staphylococcal penicillinase, and it has had considerable clinical use in North

America. Its spectrum of activity is wider than the isoxazolyl penicillins, in that it is effective against some strains of pneumococci and haemolytic streptococci. The pharmacokinetics and toxicity are similar to those of the other penicillins, but it has better penetration of the CSF than other penicillins and is therefore considered by some to be the drug of choice in treating staphylococcal meningitis. Nafcillin Sodium U.S.P. is available for oral and parenteral use, but because gastrointestinal absorption of the drug is unreliable, its use by mouth should be avoided.

Ampicillin and Amoxycillin

These two closely-related penicillins (Figure 4-1) have a similar antibacterial spectrum which is broader than that of the penicillins so far considered. Besides their activity against Gram-positive organisms, which is only slightly inferior to that of penicillin G in respect of most streptococci and better than penicillin G against *Streptococcus faecalis,* ampicillin and amoxycillin are effective against some of the Gram-negative enteric bacteria such as *Escherichia coli, Proteus mirabilis,* and most *Salmonella* and *Shigella* species. Most staphylococci are resistant but *Haemophilus influenzae* is usually susceptible to these two antibiotics, although some increase in resistant strains has been reported since 1974.[45] Like penicillin G, some Gram-negative anaerobic bacilli are sensitive to ampicillin and amoxycillin, although this is not true of *Bacteroides fragilis.*

Clinical Pharmacology Both ampicillin and amoxycillin are acid stable and well-absorbed by mouth, but amoxycillin has the advantage of considerably better absorption which is less affected by food in the stomach.[72] Peak serum levels for both drugs are reached about 2 hours after an oral dose, and they can be detected in the serum for about 6 hours, although effective concentrations of amoxycillin are detectable for rather longer. Ampicillin and amoxycillin diffuse widely throughout body tissues: amoxycillin penetrates better into bronchial secretions, but in purulent sputum there is little difference between the two drugs.[67] Both are excreted in a manner similar to the other penicillins.

Preparations and Dosage Both drugs are available for oral administration as capsules or as liquid preparations. The usual adult dose of ampicillin in the treatment of mild to moderate lower respiratory infections, such as an acute exacerbation of chronic bronchitis, is 500 mg 6-hourly; and for amoxycillin it is 250 mg 8-hourly, but these dosage regimens can be doubled if the infection is severe. For serious chest infections it is best to administer ampicillin parenterally in divided doses of 1–2 g every 6 hours.

Table 4-4 / Major Clinical Indications for Amoxycillin and Ampicillin In Respiratory Infections

Priority	Indications
Drug of choice	In patients with chronic obstructive lung disease who develop pneumonia or acute exacerbations of bronchitis
Possible alternative	Bronchopulmonary infection due to Salmonella typhi, Escherichia coli or Proteus species

Toxicity Ampicillin and amoxycillin are liable to cause the same sort of hypersensitivity and toxic effects as the natural penicillins, and because cross-allergenicity can occur, their use is contraindicated in penicillin-sensitive individuals. Both drugs are particularly likely to cause maculopapular eruptions in 3 to 5 percent of patients treated,[5,13] and these reactions are thought to be specific to ampicillin and amoxycillin rather than a characteristic of a general penicillin sensitivity. Rashes are particularly common in patients with glandular fever who are given either drug, and the use of these antibiotics for treating acute pharyngitis is therefore inappropriate. Nausea and diarrhoea are encountered with both drugs,[39] and pseudomembranous colitis has been reported.

Clinical Practice The main indication for ampicillin and amoxycillin (Table 4-4) is in the initial treatment of respiratory infections in patients with chronic obstructive lung disease who develop pneumonia or an acute exacerbation of chronic bronchitis which is likely to be due either to *Streptococcus pneumoniae* or *Haemophilus influenzae*. In my experience, the only practical advantage of amoxycillin over ampicillin is that oral administration can be limited to 3 doses per day.

Carbenicillin

The most valuable characteristic of this semi-synthetic penicillin (Figure 4-1) and its esters, carbenicillin indanyl sodium and carfecillin, is their activity against *Pseudomonas aeruginosa,* and to a lesser extent against *Proteus* species and other Gram-negative bacteria.[42] *Klebsiella* species are nearly always resistant. Ticarcillin, a derivative of carbenicillin with slightly greater anti-*Pseudomonas* activity, offers no significant clinical advantage. Carbenicillin is acid labile and must be given by injection, but indanyl carbenicillin and carfecillin are absorbed after oral administration and are then broken down *in vivo* to produce carbenicillin; however, they are unsuitable for the treatment of

Table 4-5 / Major Clinical Indication for Carbenicillin In Respiratory Infections

Priority	Indication
Drug of choice	In combination with gentamicin or tobramycin in treating severe bronchopulmonary infections due to *Pseudomonas aeruginosa*

systemic infections because adequate serum levels are not attained; the main indication for their use is the oral treatment of urinary tract infections. After an intramuscular injection of 1 g of carbenicillin, a peak serum level of 25 µg/ml is reached in 1 hour and falls to 4 µg/ml after 6 hours. To achieve serum levels of greater than 100 µg/ml in the treatment of *Pseudomonas* septicaemia, 20–30 g daily must be given intravenously. The drug is distributed in body tissues similarly to penicillin G and excreted mainly by the kidneys. Carbenicillin is available for parenteral injection as the disodium salt in sterile vials containing 1–10 g doses, and it is usually administered intravenously in an adult daily dose of 30 g. Higher blood levels can be achieved by giving probenecid concurrently.

The side-effects and toxicity of carbenicillin parallel those of the other penicillins; neurotoxicity may be a problem because of the very high dosage which is commonly necessary, and the high sodium content of the preparation (4.7 mEq/g) can lead to hypernatraemia and hypokalaemia, particularly if renal function is impaired.[43] The drug should be reserved for the treatment of serious infections and septicaemia due to *Pseudomonas aeruginosa*[82] (Table 4-5). Acute bronchial or pulmonary infections with *Pseudomonas aeruginosa* are uncommon, but they have a high mortality and require early systemic therapy with carbenicillin, while chronic suppurative infections sometimes occur in bronchiectasis, cystic fibrosis, and chronic lung abscess and are very difficult to eradicate even if an initial response to carbenicillin therapy is achieved.[14] To prevent the emergence of resistant strains, carbenicillin should be used in conjunction with gentamycin when treating *Pseudomonas* infections.

CEPHALOSPORINS

General Properties

The cephalosporins originate from a mould, *Cephalosporium acrimonium*. The most important of these drugs is cephalosporin C, from which many semi-synthetic derivatives have been developed by side-chain alterations. The 7-

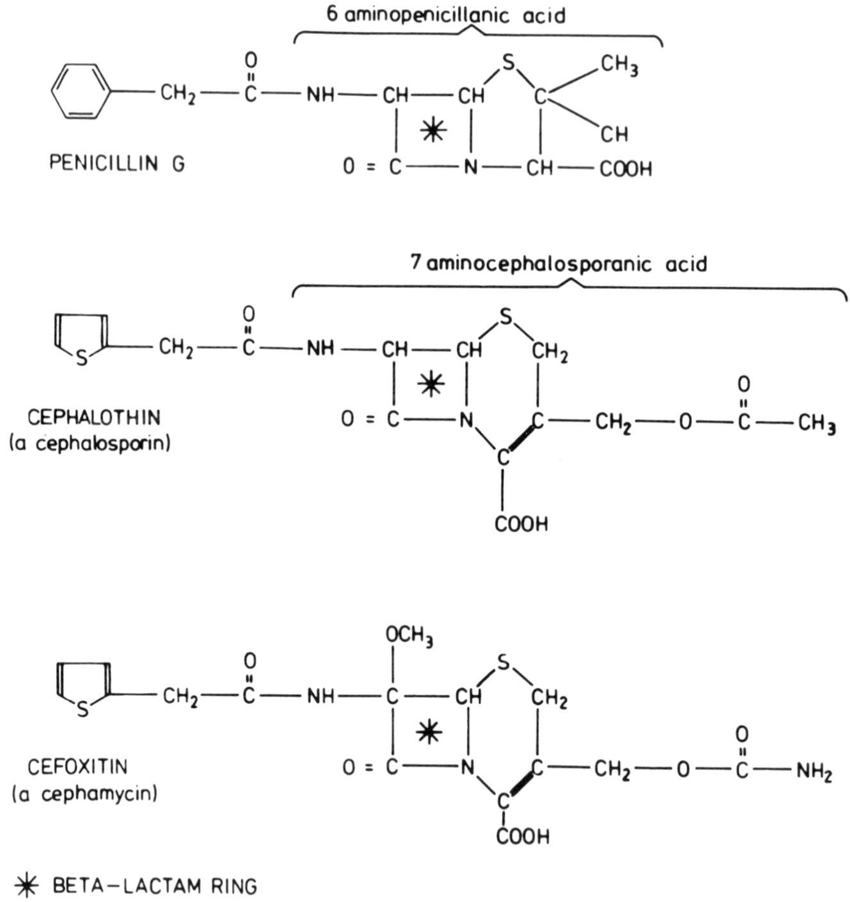

Figure 4-2 *Comparison of the structure of cephalosporins and cephamycins with penicillin, showing that these antibiotics all possess the characteristic beta-lactam ring.*

aminocephalosporanic acid nucleus bears a close resemblance to the 6-aminopenicillanic acid structure of the penicillins with the characteristic beta-lactam ring (Figure 4-2), which accounts for the similar bactericidal action of the cephalosporins in inhibiting bacterial cell wall synthesis. The cephamycins are also beta-lactam antibiotics derived from cephamycin C which is a naturally occurring substance produced by *Streptomyces lactamdurans.*

Spectrum of Activity   An important characteristic of the cephalosporins and cephamycins is their relatively broad spectrum of activity against many of the common pathogenic Gram-positive cocci and a variety of Gram-negative organisms. It may be argued that this broad spectrum enhances the usefulness in the initial treatment of unclassified pneumonia and other acute lung infections,[49] but in this respect the limitations of the cephalosporins have to be remembered, in particular their lack of activity against *Pseudomonas aeruginosa* and *Bacteroides fragilis,* both of which may be important pathogens in aspiration pneumonias or chronic suppurative lung infections; also worth noting is their relative lack of activity against *Haemophilus influenzae,* which is so common a pathogen in chronic obstructive lung disease. The cephalosporins are more active against penicillinase-producing staphylococci than the first generation penicillins such as penicillins G and V and ampicillin, but the antibiotics of choice against these organisms are methicillin or the isoxazolyl penicillins. In patients who are allergic to penicillin, however, the cephalosporins provide a useful alternative against *Streptococcus pneumoniae* and the other Gram-positive cocci, although cross-hypersensitivity to the cephalosporins occurs in 5 to 10 percent of penicillin-sensitive individuals.

Among the Gram-negative organisms, *Haemophilus influenzae* and *Bordetella pertussis* are rather resistant, but the former is sensitive to some of the newer cephalosporins; possibly the most useful attribute of the cephalosporins and cephamycins is their activity against *Klebsiella* species.

Clinical Pharmacology   Many cephalosporins and cephamycins are unstable in acid medium and have to be administered parenterally. Tissue distribution is similar to that of the penicillin but penetration into the sputum is said to be poor.[20] Protein binding varies considerably between different members of the group, but this factor seems to have little effect on their relative bacterial activity or toxicity. Elimination is primarily renal by a combination of glomerular filtration and tubular secretion, and excretion is retarded by concomitant probenecid administration in all except cephaloridine which is eliminated almost entirely by glomerular filtration. Dosage modification of these drugs is therefore necessary in patients with impaired renal function. The serum half-lives of the cephalosporins vary between 30 minutes and 2 hours.[71]

Toxicity   Nephrotoxicity is the most important adverse effect of the cephalosporins, occurring predominantly with cephaloridine which may cause acute tubular necrosis in high dosage, particularly when used in combination with potent tubular diuretics such as furosemide and ethacrynic acid.[25] Cephalothin may also impair renal function,[15] but nephrotoxicity is rarely encountered with the other cephalosporins or cefoxitin, and analysis of individual case reports suggests in some that additional factors may have contributed to the renal impairment.[41,100] Pain at intramuscular injection sites and thrombophlebitis due to intravenous administration are rather common complications. Skin rashes occur in about 2 percent of patients, and hypersensitivity reactions occur in a

Table 4-6 / A Summary of Selected Cephalosporins and a Cephyamycin

Name	Route of Administration	Adult Dose	Special Advantage or Disadvantages in Treating Respiratory Infections
Cephaloridine	I.M. or I.V.	0.5–1.0 gm every 6–8 hours (not more than 6 gm daily in all)	Very active against S. aureus, S. pneumoniae, S. viridans, and S. pyogenes, including penicillinase-producing strains, and therefore useful in penicillin-sensitive individuals. Effective in Gram-negative bacterial pneumonias due to E. coli, Proteus mirabilis, and Klebsiella aerogenes, but relatively ineffective against H. influenzae. Nephrotoxic in high dosage, in renal failure or combined with some diuretics (such as furosemide). Can only be administered parenterally.
Cephalothin	I.V. (I.M.)	0.5–1.0 gm every 4–6 hours	Similar spectrum of activity to cephaloridine; less nephrotoxic. Frequent doses are required because of short half-life. Intramuscular injection painful and intravenous route preferable with higher doses.
Cephalexin	Oral	250–500 mg four times daily	Well-absorbed orally but has inferior activity to cephaloridine and cephalothin and should not be relied on in treating pneumonia or bronchial infections. (It is highly concentrated in the urine and is most useful for urinary tract infections.)
Cephradine	Oral, I.M., or I.V.	0.5 gm every 6 hours	Well-absorbed orally, but like cephalexin it has less intrinsic antibacterial activity than cephaloridine or cephalothin and should not be relied on for serious respiratory infections.
Cefazolin	I.M. or I.V.	0.5 gm every 8 hours	Similar spectrum of activity to cephaloridine but achieves higher blood levels for a longer period; 75 percent protein bound. Not known to be nephrotoxic but eosinophilia and hypersensitivity reactions may be common.[86]
Cefamandole	I.M. or I.V.	0.5–2.0 gm every 4–6 hours	High activity against Enterobacteria, Staph. aureus and H. influenzae but less than cephalothin against Strep. pneumoniae and most streptococci. Little evidence of nephrotoxicity. May prove useful for Gram-negative pulmonary infections.[28,70]
Cefuroxime	I.M. or I.V.	0.5–2.0 gm every 8 hours	Highly active against H. influenzae[29] and active against many other Gram-negative aerobic bacilli but not Pseudomonas aeruginosa or most strains of faecal streptococci. Effective in lower respiratory tract infections.[21]
Cefoxitin	I.V. (I.M.)	1.0–2.0 gm every 6–8 hours	A cephamycin. High activity against Gram-negative bacilli including indole-positive Proteus, Ser. marcescens, E. coli and Klebsiella species but not Pseudomonas aeruginosa. Also effective against Bacteroides fragilis.[35] May prove useful for Gram-negative pneumonias.[34] Little evidence of nephrotoxicity. Intramuscular injection is very painful.

small proportion of penicillin-sensitive individuals. Like the penicillins the cephalosporins are relatively safe to use in pregnancy.

Choice of Cephalosporins

A synopsis of the major characteristics of selected cephalosporins and a cephamycin, cefoxitin, is given in Table 4-6. For an oral preparation there is little to choose between cephalexin and cephradine, but neither has much part to play in the treatment of respiratory infections except perhaps in the convalescent therapy of patients treated during the acute illness with a parenteral cephalosporin. They are less effective and more expensive than ampicillin for treating acute exacerbations of bronchitis. Cephazolin is among the best of the parenteral cephalosporins because of its long half-life of 1.5–2.0 hours and the relative absence of pain after intramuscular injection. It attains high levels in the blood, but the significance of this is uncertain because it is highly protein bound, and tissue concentrations at the site of infection may be low.[85]

The cephalosporins are "second-string" drugs in respiratory medicine, for use in certain special situations.[33] Despite their general lack of toxicity and their bactericidal action, they are somewhat less effective than the penicillins against the majority of Gram-positive bacteria and are considerably less active than the aminoglycosides against Gram-negative organisms. They are more costly and less effective than ampicillin, tetracycline, or trimethoprim-sulphamethoxazole for chronic bronchitis, and their main claim for consideration arises either when penicillins cannot be used because of hypersensitivity, or when combination therapy with gentamycin is desirable in the treatment of acute *Klebsiella* pneumonia (Table 4-7). The wider spectrum of activity of cefoxitin and the most recent cephalosporins may increase the value of this group of drugs in the treatment of Gram-negative pneumonias.

Table 4-7 / Major Clinical Indications for the Cephalosporins in Respiratory Infections

Priority	Indications
Drug of choice	In combination with gentamicin in treating severe pneumonia due to *Klebsiella pneumoniae*
Possible alternative	Bronchopulmonary gram-positive infections in penicillin-allergic individuals
	Pneumonia due to penicillinase-producing *Staphylococcus aureus*

AMINOGLYCOSIDES

General Properties

The aminoglycosides are a group of compounds which consist of amino sugars in glycosidic linkages. They are polycations and their polarity accounts for their common properties of poor oral absorption, limited diffusion into the cerebrospinal fluid, and rapid renal excretion. With the exception of the recently introduced semi-synthetic drugs amikacin and netilmicin, all the aminoglycosides were isolated from different species of *Streptomyces,* and all are chemically similar.

Mode of Action   These drugs prevent bacterial protein synthesis at initiation by binding to the 30S ribosomal subunits, and they also interfere with the fidelity of messenger translocation which leads to the incorporation of "wrong" amino acids into the newly synthesised bacterial proteins. Although presumably disadvantageous, these distortions of protein synthesis do not in themselves cause cell death and the fact that the aminoglycosides are bactericidal is still unexplained.[80] Resistance to these drugs develops readily, either by single step mutation which results in prevention of drug binding by the ribosome, or more commonly by the transmission of resistance by R plasmids which convey the facility for producing drug-metabolising enzymes and may confer resistance to several antibiotics at the same time.

Clinical Pharmacology   All the aminoglycosides are poorly absorbed from the gastrointestinal tract and are administered parenterally. Estimates of protein binding seem to depend on the experimental conditions, but for practical purposes these antibiotics appear not to be bound to serum proteins.[77] Diffusion into the pleural space is rather slow with streptomycin, but adequate levels are achieved with repeated doses; levels of gentamicin in the pleural, pericardial and ascitic fluids are about half those of plasma at the same time, and tobramycin seems to behave similarly. Kanamycin diffuses well into serous fluids, achieving concentrations equal to that in serum. Passage of the aminoglycosides into the CSF is negligible under normal conditions, and even in the presence of meningeal inflammation CSF levels are unreliable. Intrathecal streptomycin is now seldom used to treat tuberculous meningitis.

There is little metabolic inactivation of the aminoglycosides which are largely excreted unchanged by glomerular filtration. Adjustment of dosage is therefore necessary when renal function is poor, and a number of formulae, nomograms, and computer programmes have been devised to determine the appropriate dosage; monitoring of serum antibiotic levels is also necessary to ensure satisfactory control of therapy.

Toxicity   The aminoglycosides are rather toxic, and because the excretion pathway is by glomerular filtration impairment of renal function leads to their accumulation and an increased risk of adverse effects. An assessment of renal functional status is therefore essential before embarking on aminoglycoside therapy. The commonest types of adverse effect are described below:

1. Ototoxicity, affecting both vestibular and auditory function; some of the aminoglycosides, such as streptomycin or gentamicin, are liable to affect balance, while others such as kanamycin and amikacin mainly affect hearing. Ototoxicity is due to very high peak blood levels or to prolonged lower blood concentrations, and may be potentiated by the diuretics furosemide and ethacrynic acid.[69] Aminoglycosides should be used with particular care in elderly patients, who often have pre-existing loss of hearing, and serial audiometry may help to detect early changes in auditory acuity. Headache, nausea, and tinnitus are signs of early eighth nerve damage and should prompt immediate withdrawal of aminoglycoside therapy; some recovery of function may result but permanent hearing loss or vestibular deficiency is usual.
2. A curare-like effect causing neuromuscular blockade is attributed to suppression of acetylcholine release, and this effect is most marked in patients with myasthenia gravis or those who have received neuro-muscular blocking agents.[83]
3. Renal tubular damage manifested by protein, casts, and cells in the urine, and impaired renal function which may progress to acute renal failure. Streptomycin is the least nephrotoxic of the aminoglycosides and only occasionally causes a reversible decrease in renal function,[3] but the others all cause renal toxicity, which may include acute tubular necrosis. They should be used with caution in patients with depressed renal function. Some reports suggest that the combination of gentamicin with cephalothin leads to increased renal toxicity but this is not confirmed by recent data.[30]
4. Hypersensitivity reactions in the form of rashes and fever occur most often with streptomycin, but these and other forms of allergic reaction can occur rarely with any of the aminoglycosides.

Clinical Uses of the Aminoglycosides

Streptomycin   The role of streptomycin in the treatment of acute respiratory infections has gradually declined over the past twenty years partly because of the development of more active and less toxic antibiotics, but also because of therapeutic failures due to the rapid development of resistance to streptomycin during treatment and the emergence of many streptomycin-resistant bacterial

Table 4-8 / Major Clinical Indications for Streptomycin in Respiratory Infections

Priority	Indication
Drug of choice	Plague (with tetracycline)
	Brucella pneumonia (with tetracycline)
First alternative	To isoniazid, rifampin, and ethambutol in pulmonary tuberculosis

strains. The drug has been increasingly reserved for the treatment of tuberculosis, but here too it is gradually being displaced by rifampin and ethambutol. It is still used in the treatment of plague, tularaemia, and brucellosis[65,92] (Table 4-8).

An important consideration in its use is the danger of vestibular upset which is much increased when renal function is impaired. Young adults should receive 1 g intramuscularly daily in a single dose, but those over 40 years of age should only be given 0.75 g daily or 1 g on alternate days, 3 times per week. In children the dosage is 20–40 mg/kg body weight per day, but only 10–20 mg/kg per day in infants.[106] In renal failure the serum half-life of streptomycin may increase from 2.5 to 100 hours and in patients with a creatinine clearance of less than 10 ml/min, dosage adjustments can be made by administering the normal loading dose followed by half the normal dose every 3 or 4 days.[56] Streptomycin is removed by haemodialysis, and a suitable regime for patients on dialysis is 10 mg/kg body weight every 5 to 7 days.[99] When renal function is impaired dosage should be monitored by measuring the peak plasma streptomycin level 1 hour before administration, which should not exceed 40–50 μg/ml, while the prevailing plasma concentration prior to the next dose should not exceed 20 μg/ml.

The use of streptomycin in its main role, the treatment of tuberculosis, is described in the next chapter.

Gentamicin This drug has a wide range of actions against Gram-negative bacteria and staphylococci but not against streptococci or against clostridia and *Bacteroides* species. Gentamicin resistance among Enterobacteriaceae has been increasingly observed in hospital infections, and it is often associated with resistance to other antibiotics.

Gentamicin is not absorbed by mouth and is largely eliminated unchanged by glomerular filtration. It is normally administered intramuscularly, but it can also be given intravenously by bolus injection over 2 to 3 minutes

Table 4-9 / Major Clinical Indications for Gentamicin in Respiratory Infections

Priority	Indication
Drug of choice	Pneumonia due to gram-negative micro-organisms
	Aspiration pneumonia
Possible alternative	Pneumonia due to resistant staphylococci

in the same dosage.[54] The drug has a narrow therapeutic range with a high risk of ototoxicity which mainly affects vestibular function,[47] and it also bears a risk of nephrotoxicity. The recommended initial dosage for adults is 4–5 mg/kg body weight per day for patients with normal renal function and average weight given in 3 divided doses[66,73]; but higher starting doses are advocated for seriously ill patients, that is, 7–8 mg/kg per day.[87] Modification of the dosage schedule is necessary if renal function is abnormal, based either on blood urea levels[36] or derived more accurately by consideration of age, body weight, and serum creatinine level with the help of a nomogram.[17,66] Measurement of serum gentamicin levels is the most reliable method of therapeutic monitoring.[8] The dosage schedule should be adjusted to produce peak serum levels of approximately 6–10 µg/ml 1 hour after intramuscular injection, while the serum level just before the next dose should not exceed 2 µg/ml.[64] Children need relatively large doses of gentamicin to reach the same serum levels as adults.[26] Gentamicin is removed readily by conventional haemodialysis and adequate blood levels can be maintained by single doses of 1 mg/kg body weight after each dialysis; but the drug may accumulate if modern, short dialysis techniques are used.

The main clinical indications for the use of gentamicin in respiratory infections (Table 4-9) is in the treatment of life-threatening pneumonia which is likely to be due to aerobic Gram-negative bacteria, for example, in hospital-acquired aspiration pneumonia[61] and in the treatment of severe respiratory infections caused by sensitive aerobic Gram-negative organisms or by staphylococci which are resistant to the less toxic antibiotics customarily used. Penetration of aminoglycosides into bronchial secretions appears to be rather unpredictable, and this factor may be responsible in part for the poor response to therapy of some infections such as bronchiectasis and *Pseudomonas* bronchopneumonia treated with parenteral aminoglycoside therapy.[77]

Tobramycin   This aminoglycoside has a spectrum of action similar to that of gentamicin, with the advantage of greater activity against *Pseudomonas* species.[101] However, it is less active against the other Gram-negative bacteria. The adverse effects are similar to those of gentamicin and it is prescribed according to the same dosage recommendations. The only indication for its use in respiratory infections is in the treatment of severe bronchial or pulmonary disease due to *Pseudomonas aeruginosa,* for example, in cystic fibrosis.[63]

Kanamycin   The general properties of kanamycin are similar to those of the other aminoglycosides, and it has a comparable range of activity against Gram-negative bacteria, although it is not effective against *Pseudomonas* species. Its role in the treatment of Gram-negative infections has largely been taken over by gentamicin. Kanamycin has some activity also against mycobacteria, and before ethambutol and rifampin were available it was a possible reserve drug for the treatment of resistant tuberculosis.[51] However, it is more ototoxic and nephrotoxic than streptomycin, and it has now been all but discarded in anti-tuberculosis therapy.

Amikacin   This aminoglycoside is a semi-synthetic derivative of kanamycin and is active against *Staphylococcus aureus* and the same range of Gram-negative bacilli as the other drugs of the group. Its particular advantage is that it is frequently effective against many strains which fail to respond to gentamicin and tobramycin.[7] Amikacin is nephrotoxic and ototoxic, tending to cause deafness rather than vestibular damage. At present its use should be reserved for patients who have severe infections due to Gram-negative organisms which are resistant to gentamicin and tobramycin.[91]

TETRACYCLINES

This group of antibiotics plays an important role in the treatment of respiratory infections, particularly in the management of chronic bronchitis, in the treatment of mycoplasmal and other "atypical" pneumonias, and as alternative chemotherapeutic agents to the penicillins in the treatment of acute bacterial lung infections. There has been a gradual decline in their use in recent years because their side-effects have been more widely recognised and because tetracycline-resistant organisms have become increasingly prevalent, particularly in hospital. They are considered here as a group, followed by brief notes about the special characteristics of individual tetracyclines.

General Properties

The tetracyclines are all derived from *Streptomyces* species which were iso-lated by large-scale systematic screening of soil samples in the search for antibiotic-producing micro-organisms. They all have the same basic polycyclic structure.

Mode of Action and Resistance   At tissue levels obtainable with pharmacolog-ical dosage, the tetracyclines are bacteriostatic although they become bacte-ricidal at higher concentrations. Their mechanism of action is through interfer-ence with bacterial protein synthesis by binding reversibly to ribosomes and to messenger RNA. This action is not limited to bacteria, for tetracyclines also inhibit protein synthesis in mammalian cells; their selective effect as antibacte-rial agents is ascribed to preferential accumulation of the drug in bacterial cells due to an active process which is absent from mammalian cells. The develop-ment of resistance among the tetracyclines is due to decreased drug uptake by the bacterial cell, and there is usually complete cross-resistance to all the tetracyclines, the only exception being with minocycline and certain strains of *Staphylococcus aureus*. Most bacteria are slow to become resistant to the tetracyclines, but their extensive use over the years has led to fairly wide-spread resistance in hospitals among certain micro-organisms, for example, staphylococci,[89] pneumococcus,[78] and haemolytic streptococcus,[19] although this has been less of a drawback among the general population.[31,40] Transfer of tetracycline resistance among Enterobacteria and other Gram-negative or-ganisms is mediated by R plasmids and may be multiple against a num-ber of antibiotics, especially in hospitals. Resistance to tetracyclines among *Haemophilus influenzae* strains appears to be relatively uncommon in Britain.[45]

Spectrum of Activity   The tetracyclines have a very broad range of activity which includes most Gram-positive and Gram-negative organisms, although not *Proteus* species or *Pseudomonas aeruginosa,* but their usefulness as first-choice antibacterial agents is much diminished because of the prevalence of resistant strains. Their activity against a number of specific infections possibly gives the tetracyclines their most important role in respiratory medicine at the present time: against mycoplasmas, *Chlamydia psittaci, Legionella pneumo-phila,* and rickettsiae, and against less common infections such as *Brucella abortus* and *Yersinia pestis.*

Clinical Pharmacology[57]   Tetracyclines are absorbed from the stomach and all levels of the bowel, but absorption is incomplete and tends to be further reduced if there is food in the stomach and in the presence of chelating agents such as iron, calcium, magnesium, and aluminum. These antibiotics should therefore be administered in the fasting state, and concurrent ingestion of milk, antacids, or oral iron preparations should be avoided. They may also be administered intravenously in severe illness or in the presence of nausea and vomiting, but intramuscular injection is unsatisfactory because of local discomfort and poor absorption. Following absorption the tetracyclines are widely distributed and penetrate readily into joint and serous cavities but relatively slowly into the CSF, uninfluenced by meningeal inflammation. Protein binding varies between different preparations, being greatest with methacycline and minocycline (70–80 percent) and least with tetracycline and oxytetracycline (20–30 percent). Tetracyclines are concentrated temporarily in the liver and kidneys, but their incorporation into calcified tissue has an important long-term effect in causing the discolouration of developing teeth. This precludes their use in pregnant or lactating women (because of the untoward effect in the child) and in children under the age of seven years.

The primary route of excretion for most of the tetracyclines is by glomerular filtration, and the risk of toxicity is increased if renal function is impaired. The exception is doxycycline which is largely excreted by the liver. All are to some extent metabolised and excreted by the liver into the bile and thence into the bowel from which they are again partly reabsorbed. The half-lives of different tetracyclines cover a considerable range, from 6 to 9 hours for tetracycline to nearly 20 hours for doxycycline and minocycline.

Toxicity   Certain constraints are placed on the use of tetracyclines by the increased incidence of toxic side-effects in a number of conditions. These constraints include the following observances:

1. Avoidance of their use in children because of tooth discolouration (see above).
2. Avoidance of their use in pregnancy because of damage to foetal teeth and increased risk of maternal hepatic and renal damage.[55]
3. Special caution with their use in liver disease, avoiding parenteral administration of high dosage tetracyclines.
4. Extreme caution with their use in renal disease because of a direct toxic effect on the kidneys which is increased in the presence of pre-existing renal disease.[27,60] If tetracycline therapy is unavoidable in a patient with decreased renal function, doxycycline is the drug of choice, although it should be used with care.[74] Nephrogenic diabetes insipidus and renal failure is a particular complication of treatment with demeclocycline[93]; it is dose-dependent and reversible.

Tetracyclines have numerous other troublesome side-effects which include gastrointestinal irritation leading to nausea, epigastric discomfort, vomiting and diarrhoea; phototoxicity, occurring mainly with demeclocycline; bone marrow depression causing mild leucopenia or thrombocytopenia; hypersensitivity reactions which include urticaria, morbilliform rash and exfoliative dermatitis, angioneurotic oedema, asthma, and acute anaphylaxis; and reversible vestibular disturbances occurring only with minocycline. Because of their broad antibacterial spectrum tetracyclines are particularly liable to induce superinfections causing oral or vaginal candidiasis, colonisation of the respiratory tract with resistant Gram-negative micro-organisms, and occasional fulminating diarrhoea due to staphylococcal enterocolitis or pseudomembranous colitis.

The administration of outdated and degraded tetracycline can lead to a renal tubular acidosis syndrome which resolves when the drug is discontinued.

Drug Interactions The interference of antacid and iron preparations in the absorption of oral tetracycline has been mentioned above, and this should be avoided by careful spacing of the treatment regimen if concurrent administration is necessary. The disturbance of bowel flora by broad spectrum antimicrobials such as the tetracyclines may reduce bacterial synthesis of vitamin K in the gut and potentiate the activity of anticoagulant drugs such as warfarin, but it is probable that this interaction is clinically important only when there is also dietary deficiency of vitamin K.[2]

Clinically important antagonism has been shown to occur when penicillins and tetracyclines are used together in the treatment of pneumococcal meningitis, and this combination is contraindicated in Gram-positive penicillin sensitive infections.[84]

Clinical Uses

The tetracyclines are valuable for the treatment of primary atypical pneumonias due to *Mycoplasma pneumoniae, Chlamydia psittaci,* and *Coxiella burneti,* and they are the drugs of choice in these infections (Table 4-10). They are also effective against *Legionella pneumophila,* although erythromycin seems to be favoured more highly at the present.[52,98] In combination with streptomycin, tetracyclines constitute the preferred treatment in severe brucella infections and in bubonic plague. They are also widely used in treating acute exacerbations of chronic bronchitis, particularly those arising outside the hospital environment where resistant strains of *Haemophilus influenzae* are less prevalent, and they may be useful in long-term low dosage for controlling infection in the severe bronchitic with frequent winter exacerbations,[46] although this practice is controversial.[94,96]

Table 4-10 / **Major Clinical Indications for the Tetracyclines in Respiratory Infections**

Priority	Indication
Drug of choice	Pneumonia due to *Mycoplasma pneumoniae*, *Chlamydia psittaci*, and *Coxiella burneti*
Possible alternative	Acute exacerbations of chronic bronchitis occurring outside the hospital

Tetracycline, Oxytetracycline, and Chlortetracycline   There is little difference among these three antibiotic "variants" on which to base a choice, but there is considerable variation in cost from one proprietary preparation to the next. The oral preparations are available in capsule or tablet form in dosages ranging from 50–500 mg, the usual oral dose in adults being 250–500 mg 4 times daily. If given intravenously the total daily dose is normally 0.5–1.0 g administered in two equal 12-hourly doses by infusion. Thrombophlebitis of the infusion site is a common complication.

Demeclocycline and Methacycline   Both of these drugs have half-lives longer than those discussed above, and they are given by mouth in rather lower adult dosage of 150 mg 4 times daily or 300 mg 2 times daily. Demeclocycline has a special use in the treatment of patients with inappropriate secretion of antidiuretic hormone (ADH) which is associated most commonly with bronchial carcinoma.[18,24] It has also been used for treating sodium and water retention due to congestive cardiac failure resistant to other forms of therapy[107] and to cirrhosis of the liver.[23] However, continued use leads to elevation of serum urea and creatinine levels with impairment of renal function, although these changes are reversed when treatment is stopped.[79] Renal function should be kept under careful review when using demeclocycline, and the dosage should be reduced when function is impaired.

Doxycycline   Doxycycline is more active than tetracycline and is not excreted by the kidneys to the same extent as the others so that it accumulates to a much lesser degree and is the preferred alternative in patients with renal failure. The half-life after oral administration is from 18 to 22 hours, and the adult oral dose is a single one of 200 mg on the first day followed by 100 mg per day thereafter. Unlike the other tetracyclines the absorption of doxycycline is not seriously impaired by the presence of food in the upper gastrointestinal tract.[103] An intravenous preparation is also available.

Minocycline   Minocycline is more active than the other tetracyclines against *Staphylococcus pyogenes* and is also more likely to be effective against strains of Gram-positive cocci and Gram-negative bacteria which are resistant to the other tetracyclines. Like doxycycline it is slowly excreted and can be given in a single daily dose, the usual adult dose being 200 mg on the first day followed by a maintenance of 100 mg every 12 hours. However it suffers from the serious defect of causing vestibular toxicity leading to nausea, vomiting, dizziness, and ataxia in 50–90 percent of subjects.[38,105] These symptoms subside within 48 hours when the drug is discontinued.

References

1. ADKINSON NF, THOMSON WL, MADDREY WC, LICHTENSTEIN LM: Routine use of penicillin skin testing on an inpatient service. N Engl J Med 285: 22–24, 1971.
2. ANSELL JE, KUMAR R, DEYKIN D: The spectrum of vitamin K deficiency. JAMA 238: 40–42, 1977.
3. APPEL GB, NEU HC: The neprotoxicity of antimicrobial agents. N Engl J Med 296: 663–670, 722–728, 784–787, 1977.
4. APPELBAUM PC, SCRAGG JN, BOWEN AJ, BHAMJEE A, HALLET AF, COOPER RC: Streptococcus pneumoniae resistant to penicillin and chloramphenicol. Lancet 2: 995–997, 1977.
5. ARNDT KA, JICK H: Rates of cutaneous reactions to drugs. A report from the Boston Collaborative Drug Surveillance Program. JAMA 235: 918–923, 1976.
6. BARRETT FF, MCGEHEE RF, FINLAND M: Methicillin-resistant Staphylococcus aureus at Boston City Hospital. N Engl J Med 279: 441–448, 1968.
7. BARTLETT JG: Amikacin treatment of pulmonary infections involving gentamicin-resistant Gram-negative bacilli. Am J Med 62: 945–948, 1977.
8. BARZA M, LAVERMANN M: Why monitor serum levels of gentamicin? Clin Pharmacokinet 3: 202–215, 1978.
9. BASS JW, CRAST FW, KNOWLES CR, ONUFER CN: Streptococcal pharyngitis in children. A comparison of four treatment schedules with intramuscular penicillin G benzathine. JAMA 235: 1112–1116, 1976.
10. BENGTSSON S, FORSGREN A, MELLBIN T: Penicillinase production in community strains of Staphylococcus aureus. Scand J Infect Dis 9: 23–25, 1977.
11. BERGER M, POTTER DE: Pitfall in diagnosis of viral hepatitis on haemodialysis unit. Lancet 2: 95–96, 1977.
12. BRITISH MEDICAL JOURNAL: New light on pencillin. Br Med J 1: 986–987, 1977.
13. BROGDEN RN, SPEIGHT TM, AVERY GS: Amoxycillin: a review of its antibacterial and pharmacokinetic properties and therapeutic use. Drugs 9: 88–140, 1975.
14. BURNS MW: Significance of Pseudomonas aeruginosa in sputum. Br Med J 3: 382–383, 1973.
15. BURTON JR, LICHTENSTEIN NS, COLVIN RB, HYSLOP NE: Acute renal failure during cephalothin therapy. JAMA 229: 679–682, 1974.

16. Chain E, Florey HW, Gardner AD, Heatley NG, Jennings MA, Orr-Ewing J, Sanders AG: Penicillin as a chemotherapeutic agent. Lancet 2: 226–228, 1940.
17. Chan RA, Benner EJ, Hoeprich PD: Gentamicin therapy in renal failure: a nomogram for dosage. Ann Intern Med 76: 773–778, 1972.
18. Cherrill DA, Stote RM, Birge JR, Singer I: Demeclocycline treatment in the syndrome of inappropriate antidiuretic hormone secretion. Ann Intern Med 83: 654–656, 1975.
19. Dadswell JV: Survey of the incidence of tetracycline-resistant haemolytic streptococci between 1958 and 1965. J Clin Pathol 20: 641–642, 1967.
20. Daikos GK, Kosmidis J, Stathakis C, Anyfantis A, Plakoutsis T, Papathanassiou B: Bioavailability of cefuroxime in various sites including bile, sputum and bone. Proc R Soc Med 70 (Suppl 9): 38–41, 1977.
21. Daikos GK, Kosmidis JC, Stathakis Ch, Giamarellou H: Cefuroime: antimicrobial activity, human pharmacokinetics and therapeutic efficacy. J Antimicrob Chemother 3: 555–562, 1977.
22. Dash CH: Penicillin allergy and the cephalosporins. J Antimicrob Chemother (Suppl 1): 107–118, 1975.
23. De Troyer A, Pilloy W, Broeckaert I, Demanet JC: Demeclocycline treatment of water retention in cirrhosis. Ann Intern Med 85: 336–337, 1976.
24. De Troyer A: Demeclocycline treatment for syndrome of inappropriate antidiuretic hormone secretion. JAMA 237: 2723–2726, 1977.
25. Dodds MG, Foord RD: Enhancement by potent diuretics of renal tubular necrosis induced by cephaloridine. Br J Pharmacol 40: 227–236, 1970.
26. Echeverria P, Siber GR, Paisley J, Smith AL, Smith DH, Jaffe N: Age-dependent dose response to gentamicin. J Pediatr 87: 805–808, 1975.
27. Edwards OM, Huskisson EC, Taylor RT: Azotaemia aggravated by tetracycline. Br Med J 1: 26–27, 1970.
28. Eykyn S, Jenkins C, King A, Phillips I: Antibacterial activity of cefamandole, a new cephalosporin antibiotic, compared with that of cephaloridine, cephalothin, and cephalexin. Antimicrob Agents Chemother 3: 657–661, 1973.
29. Eykyn SA, Jenkins C, King A, Phillips I: Antibacterial activity of cefuroxime, a new cephalosporin antibiotic, compared with that of cephaloridine, cephalothin and cefamandole. Antimicrob Agents Chemother 9: 690–695, 1976.
30. Fanning WL, Gump D, Jick H: Gentamicin-and cephalothin-associated rises in blood urea nitrogen. Antimicrob Agents Chemother 10: 80–82, 1976.
31. Finland M: Twenty-fifth anniversary of the discovery of Aureomycin: the place of the tetracyclines in antimicrobial therapy. Clin Pharmacol Ther 15: 3–8, 1974.
32. Galpin JE, Shinaberger JH, Stanley TM, Blumenkrantz MJ, Bayer AS, Friedman GS, Montogomerie JZ, Guze LB, Coburn JW, Glassock RJ: Acute interstitial nephritis due to methicillin. Am J Med 65: 756–765, 1978.
33. Garrod LP: Choice among penicillins and cephalosporins. Br Med J 3: 96–100, 1974.
34. Geddes AM, Schnurr LP, Ball AP, McGhie D, Brookes GR, Wise R, Andrews J: Cefoxitin: a hospital study. Br Med J 1: 1126–1128, 1977.
35. Geddes AM, Wilcox RML: Treatment of abdominal sepsis with cefoxitin. in Current Chemotherapy: Proceedings of the 10th International Congress of Che-

motherapy, Siegenthaler W, Luthy R (eds). Zurich, Switzerland, 1977, p. 299–300. Washington: American Society for Microbiology, 1978.

36. GINGELL JC, WATERWORTH PM: Dose of gentamicin in patients with normal renal function and renal impairment. Br Med J 2: 19–22, 1968.

37. GREEN GR, ROSENBLUM A: Report of the Penicillin Study Group-American Academy of Allergy. J Allergy Clin Immunol 48: 331–343, 1971.

38. GUMP DW, ASHIKAGA T, FINK TJ, RADIN AM: Side effects of minocycline: different dosage regimens. Antimicrob Agents Chemother 12: 642–646, 1977.

39. GURWITH MJ, RABIN HR, LOVE K, CO-OPERATIVE ANTIBIOTIC DIARRHEA STUDY GROUP: Diarrhea associated with clindamycin and ampicillin therapy: preliminary results of a co-operative study. J Infect Dis 135 (Suppl): S104–S110, 1977.

40. HASSAM ZA, SHAW EJ, SHOOTER RA, CARO DB: Changes in antibiotic sensitivity in strains of Staphylococcus aureus, 1952–78. Br Med J 2: 536–537, 1978.

41. HESELTINE PNR, BUSCH DF, MEYER RD, FINEGOLD SM: Cefoxitin: clinical evaluation in thirty-eight patients. Antimicrob Agents Chemother 11: 427–434, 1977.

42. HEWITT WL, WINTER RE: The current status of parenteral carbenicillin. J Infect Dis 127 (Suppl): S120–S129, 1973.

43. HOFFBRAND BI, STEWART JDM: Carbenicillin and hypokalaemia. Br Med J 4: 746, 1970.

44. HOROWITZ L: Atopy as a factor in penicillin reactions. N Engl J Med 292: 1243–1244, 1975.

45. HOWARD AJ, HINCE CJ, WILLIAMS JD: Antibiotic resistance in Streptococcus pneumoniae and Haemophilus influenzae. Report of a study group on bacterial resistance. Br Med J 1: 1657–1660, 1978.

46. HUGHES D: Chemoprophylaxis in chronic bronchitis. J Antimicrob Chemother 2: 320–322, 1976.

47. JACKSON GG, ARCIERI G: Ototoxicity of gentamicin in man: a survey and controlled analysis of clinical experience in the United States. J Infect Dis 124 (Suppl): S130–S137, 1971.

48. JACOBS MR, KOORNHOF HJ, ROBINS-BROWNE RM, STEVENSON CM, VERMAAK ZA, FREIMAN I, MILLER GB, WITCOMB MA, ISAACSON M, WARD JL, AUSTRIAN R: Emergence of multiply resistant pneumococci. N Engl J Med 299: 735–740, 1978.

49. JENKINSON SG, GEORGE RB, LIGHT RW, GIRARD WM: Cefazolin vs Penicillin. Treatment of uncomplicated pneumococcal pneumonia. JAMA 241: 2815–2817, 1979.

50. JUSKO WJ, MOSOVICH LL, GERBRACHT LM, MATTAR ME, YAFFE SJ: Enhanced renal excretion of dicloxacillin in patients with cystic fibrosis. Pediatrics 56: 1038–1044, 1975.

51. KASS I: Kanamycin in the therapy of pulmonary tuberculosis in the United States. Ann NY Acad Sci 132: 892–900, 1966.

52. KIRBY BD, SNYDER KM, MEYER RD, FINEGOLD SM: Legionnaires' disease: clinical features of twenty-four cases. Ann Intern Med 89: 297–309, 1978.

53. KOCH-WESER J, SELLERS EM: Binding of drugs to serum albumin. N Engl J Med 294: 311–316, 1976.

54. KUCERS A, BENNETT NM: The Use of Antibiotics, 3rd Ed. London: Heinemann, 1979.

55. KUNELIS CT, PETERS JL, EDMONDSON HA: Fatty liver of pregnancy and its relationship to tetracycline therapy. Am J Med 38: 359–377, 1965.
56. KUNIN CM: A guide to use of antibiotics in patients with renal disease. Ann Intern Med 67: 151–158, 1967.
57. KUNIN CM, FINLAND M: Clinical pharmacology of the tetracycline antibiotics. Clin Pharmacol Ther 2: 51–69, 1961.
58. LEVINE BB, ZOLOV DM: Prediction of penicillin allergy by immunological tests. J Allergy 43: 231–244, 1969.
59. LEVINE BB, REDMOND AP, VOSS HE, ZOLOV DM: Prediction of penicillin allergy by immunological tests. Ann NY Acad Sci 145: 298–318, 1967.
60. LEW HT, FRENCH SW: Tetracycline toxicity and nonoliguric acute renal failure. Arch Intern Med 118: 123–128, 1966.
61. LORBER B, SWENSON RM: Bacteriology of aspiration pneumonia. Ann Intern Med 81: 329–331, 1974.
62. LOWBURY EJL, LILLY AA, KIDSON A: "Methicillin-resistant" Staphylococcus aureus: reassessment by controlled trials in burns unit. Br Med J 1: 1054–1056, 1977.
63. McCRAE WM, RAEBURN JA, HANSON EJ: Tobramycin therapy of infections due to *Pseudomonas aeruginosa* in patients with cystic fibrosis: effect of dosage and concentration of antibiotic in sputum. J Infect Dis 134 (Suppl): S191–S193, 1976.
64. McGHIE D, HUTCHISON JGP, GEDDES AM: Serum gentamicin. Lancet 2: 1463–1464, 1974.
65. MARTIN WJ: The present status of streptomycin in antimicrobial therapy. Med Clin North Am 54: 1161–1172, 1970.
66. MAWER GE, AHMAD R, DOBBS SM, McGOUGH JG, LUCAS CB, TOOTH JA: Prescribing aids for gentamicin. Br J Clin Pharmacol 1: 45–50, 1974.
67. MAY JR, INGOLD A: Amoxicillin in the treatment of infections of the lower respiratory tract. J Infect Dis (Suppl) 129: S189–S193, 1974.
68. MEDICAL LETTER: The choice of antimicrobial drugs. Med Lett Drugs Ther 18: 9–16, 1976.
69. MERIWETHER WD, MANGI RJ, SERPICK AS: Deafness following standard intravenous dose of ethacrynic acid. JAMA 216: 795–798, 1971.
70. MINOR MR, SANDE MA, DILWORTH JA, MANDELL GL: Cefamandole treatment of pulmonary infection caused by Gram-negative rods. J Antimicrob Chemother 2: 49–53, 1976.
71. MOELLERING RC, SWARTZ MN: The newer cephalosporins. N Engl J Med 294: 24–28, 1976.
72. NEU HC: Antimicrobial activity and human pharmacology of amoxicillin. J Infect Dis (Suppl) 129: S123–S131, 1974.
73. NOONE P, PARSONS TMC, PATTISON JR, SLACK RCB, GARFIELD-DAVIES D, HUGHES K: Experience in monitoring gentamicin therapy during treatment of serious Gram-negative sepsis. Br Med J 1: 477–481, 1974.
74. ORR LH, RUDISILL E, BRODKIN R, HAMILTON RW: Exacerbation of renal failure associated with doxycycline. Arch Intern Med 138: 793–794, 1978.
75. PARKER CW: Practical aspects of diagnosis and treatment of patients who are hypersensitive to drugs. in International Encyclopaedia of Pharmacology and Therpeutics, Section 75: Hypersensitivity to Drugs, Vol 1. Samter M, Parker CW (eds). pp. 367–394. Oxford: Pergamon Press, 1972.

76. PARKER MT, HEWITT JH: Methicillin resistance in Staphylococcus aureus. Lancet 1: 800–804, 1970.
77. PECHERE JC, DUGAL R: Clinical pharmacokinetics of aminoglycoside antibiotics. Clin Pharmacokinet 4: 170–199, 1979.
78. PERCIVAL A, ARMSTRONG EC, TURNER GC: Increased incidence of tetracycline-resistant pneumococci in Liverpool in 1968. Lancet 1: 998–1000, 1969.
79. PERKS WH, WALTERS EH, TAMS IP, PROWSE K: Demeclocycline in the treatment of the syndrome of inappropriate secretion of antidiuretic hormone. Thorax 34: 324–327, 1979.
80. PESTKA S: Inhibitors of ribosome functions. Ann Rev Microbiol 25: 487–562, 1971.
81. PETER G, SMITH AL: Group A streptococcal infections of the skin and pharynx. N Engl J Med 297: 311–317, 365–370, 1977.
82. PINES A, RAAFAT H, SIDDIQUI GM, GREENFIELD JSB: Treatment of severe pseudomonas infections of the bronchi. Br Med J 1: 663–665, 1970.
83. PITTINGER C, ADAMSON R: Antibiotic blockade of neuromuscular function. Ann Rev Pharmacol 12: 169–184, 1972.
84. RAHAL JJ: Antibiotic combinations: the clinical relevance of synergy and antagonism. Medicine 57: 179–195, 1978.
85. REGAMEY C, GORDON RC, KIRBY WMM: Cefazolin vs Cephalothin and Cephaloridine. Arch Intern Med 133: 407–410, 1974.
86. RIES K, LEVISON ME, KAYE D: Clinical and in vitro evaluation of cefazolin, a new cephalosporin antibiotic. Antimicrob Agents Chemother 3: 168–174, 1973.
87. RIFF, LJ AND JACKSON GG: Pharmacology of gentamicin in man. J Infect Dis 124 (Suppl): S98–S105, 1971.
88. ROGERS HJ, FORSBERG CW: Role of antolysins in the killing of bacteria by some bactericidal antibiotics. J Bacteriol 108: 1235–1243, 1971.
89. SABATH LD: Current concepts: Drug resistance of bacteria. N Engl J Med 280: 91–94, 1969.
90. SABATH LD, WHEELER N, LAVARDIERE M, BLAZEVIC D, WILKINSON BJ: A new type of penicillin resistance of Staphylococcus aureus. Lancet 1: 443–446, 1977.
91. SCHIFFMAN DO: Evaluation of amikacin sulfate (amikin). A new aminoglycoside antibiotic. JAMA 238: 1547–1550, 1977.
92. SIMON HJ: Streptomycin, kanamycin, neomycin and paromomycin. Pediatr Clin North Am 15: 73–83, 1968.
93. SINGER I, ROTENBERG D, Demeclocycline-induced nephrogenic diabetes insipidus. In vivo and in vitro studies. Ann Intern Med 79: 679–683, 1973.
94. STOTT NCH, WEST RR: Randomised controlled trial of antibiotics in patients with cough and purulent sputum. Br Med J 2: 556–559, 1976.
95. SUTHERLAND R, CROYDON EAP, ROLINSON GN: Flucloxacillin, a new isoxazolyl penicillin, compared with oxacillin, cloxacillin and dicloxacillin. Br Med J 4: 455–460, 1970.
96. TAGER I, SPEIZER FE: Role of infection in chronic bronchitis. N Engl J Med 292: 563–571, 1975.
97. TIPPER DJ, STROMINGER JL: Biosynthesis of the peptidoglycan of bacterial cell walls: inhibition of cross-linking by penicillins and cephalosporins. J Biol Chem 243: 3169–3179, 1968.

98. TSAI TF, FINN DR, PLIKAYTIS BD, MCCAULEY W, MARTIN SM, FRASER DW: Legionnaires' disease: clinical features of the epidemic in Philadelphia. Ann Intern Med 90: 509–517, 1979.

99. USUDA Y, SEKINE O: Chemotherapy of tuberculosis in patients on dialysis. in Current Chemotherapy: Proceedings of the 10th International Congress of Chemotherapy, Vol 1. Siegenthaler W, Luthy R (eds). pp. 241–243, Washington: American Society for Microbiology, 1978.

100. VERMA S, KEFF E: Cephalexin-related nephropathy. JAMA 234: 618–619, 1975.

101. WATERWORTH PM: The *in vitro* sensitivity of tobramycin compared with that of other aminoglycosides. J Clin Pathol 25: 979–983, 1972.

102. WEINSTEIN L: Antimicrobial agents. General considerations. in The Pharmacological Basis of Therapeutics, 5th Ed. Goodman LS, Gilman A, (eds). Ch. 55, pp. 1090–1112. New York: Macmillan, 1975.

103. WELLING PG, KOCH PA, LAU CC, CRAIG WA, Bioavailability of tetracycline and doxycycline in fasted and non-fasted subjects. Antimicrob Agents Chemother 11: 462–469, 1977.

104. WESTERMAN EL, BRADSHAW MW, WILLIAMS TW: Agranulocytosis during therapy with orally administered cloxacillin. Am J Clin Pathol 69: 559–560, 1978.

105. WILLIAMS DN, LAUGHLIN LW, LEE YH: Minocycline: possible vestibular side-effects. Lancet 2: 744–746, 1974.

106. YAFFE SJ, BACH N: Pediatric pharmacology. Postgrad Med 40: 193–201, 1966.

107. ZEGERS DE BEYL D, NAEIJE R, DE TROYER A: Demeclocycline treatment of water retention in congestive cardiac failure. Br Med J 1: 760, 1978.

5
Antimicrobial Agents II

The drugs briefly described in this chapter are for the most part used less frequently in the treatment of respiratory infections than those already described in the preceding chapter, mainly because they are less effective or more toxic. This division is quite arbitrary, however, and the two chapters should be considered in continuity.

VANCOMYCIN

Like the penicillins and cephalosporins vancomycin is a bactericidal antibiotic which exerts its therapeutic effect by interfering with bacterial cell wall synthesis although by a mechanism different from that discussed above: vancomycin inhibits the formation of the peptidoglycan polymer "building blocks" which constitute the basic structure of the wall.[102] The drug has two uses which may be important to the respiratory physician—the treatment of serious "methicillin-resistant" staphylococcal infections and the control of antibiotic associated colitis (pseudomembranous colitis) due to bowel superinfection with *Clostridium difficile* during the course of broad-spectrum antibiotic therapy.

Vancomycin is a natural antibiotic originating from a soil actinomycete, *Streptomyces orientalis,* and is prepared as a water soluble white powder, vancomycin hydrochloride. It is active mainly against Gram-positive cocci, and a synergistic effect can be obtained with aminoglycosides against *Streptococcus faecalis*[129] and with rifampicin against *Staphylococcus aureus.*[121] The drug is poorly absorbed by mouth and for systemic infections it is administered

Table 5-1 / Major Clinical Indications for Vancomycin in Respiratory Infections

Priority	Indication
Reserve drug	Severe "methicillin resistant" staphylococcal bronchopulmonary infections

intravenously, the usual adult dose being 0.5–1.0 g daily in 2 to 4 doses. For oral administration in the treatment of antibiotic associated colitis the dose is 500 mg 4 times daily.[117]

Vancomycin diffuses readily into most tissues and into serous cavities. It is largely excreted by the kidneys, more than 80 percent of the dose being recovered in the urine within 24 hours. The serum half-life is 6 hours. Vancomycin is ototoxic[105] and possibly nephrotoxic, although the latter has recently been questioned.[3] Deafness is related to high serum levels and may persist or progress even when the drug is withdrawn; great care is therefore necessary in treating patients with renal impairment since accumulation will occur unless adjustments to dosage are made with the aim of maintaining the serum vancomycin level in the range of 2.5–25 μg/ml.[42,76] Allergic reactions including skin rashes, fever, and anaphylactic shock have been described.

Vancomycin is a reserve drug for treating severe resistant staphylococcal infections[12] (Table 5-1). It is a drug of choice for the treatment of antibiotic-associated colitis, and for this purpose it appears to be relatively non-toxic because gastrointestinal absorption is minimal.

CHLORAMPHENICOL

Chloramphenicol is a broad-spectrum bacteriostatic antibiotic, but its usefulness is restricted because of the risk of aplastic anaemia. It was originally isolated from a soil actinomycete, *Streptomyces venezuelae*, and has subsequently been synthesised chemically. It is effective against a wide range of Gram-negative bacteria including salmonellae and shigellae, but transferable chloramphenicol-resistance mediated by R plasmids occurs quite widely among the Enterobacteriaceae and many other organisms. Resistant strains of *Haemophilus influenzae* are rare.[56] Chloramphenicol is also effective against anaerobic Gram-negative organisms, including *Bacteroides fragilis*. It is active against many Gram-positive organisms including penicillase-producing *Staphylococcus aureus*, and against mycoplasmas and rickettsiae.

General Properties

Mode of Action   Chloramphenicol acts by preventing bacterial protein synthesis, specifically by binding to 30S ribosomal subunits and inhibiting peptide bond formation. The ribosomal binding of chloramphenicol is reversible and dilution of a chloramphenicol-treated culture *in vitro* allows it to begin growing again. Although the action of chloramphenicol is selective for bacterial ribosomes this selectivity is not complete, and in mammalian cells the small amount of protein synthesis which is undertaken by mitochondria is also inhibited by the drug; the toxicity of chloramphenicol toward the bone marrow may be related to this effect.[44,79]

Clinical Pharmacology   Absorption from the gastrointestinal tract is rapid and peak levels are reached in the plasma in about 2 hours. The half-life of the drug is 1.6–3.3 hours, and adequate therapeutic levels can be maintained by 6- or 8-hourly dosage regimens. Chloramphenicol passes readily into body fluid spaces and into the cerebrospinal fluid. It is largely conjugated in the liver by glucuronyl transferase and the inactive glucuronide is excreted by glomerular filtration.

Preparations and Administration   For oral administration chloramphenicol is available in capsules (50, 100, and 250 mg) or as an oral suspension containing chloramphenicol palmitate equivalent to 150 mg chloramphenicol base in 5 ml; or for parenteral administration, chloramphenicol sodium succinate injection in 1 g vials. For adults the usual dosage is 1 g every 6 to 8 hours and for children over 1 month of age, 50 mg/kg body weight per day in 4 divided doses; below this age, 25 mg/kg body weight is given daily in 4 doses.

Toxic Effects   Chloramphenicol has two sorts of toxic effect on the bone marrow[132]:

1. Anaemia, with or without thrombocytopenia and/or leucopenia, due to toxic bone marrow depression which is reversible and probably attributable to inhibition of mitochrondrial protein synthesis in haemopoietic cells.[133] It is dose related and associated with a decreased uptake of iron by normoblasts, leading to diminished reticulocyte count, high serum iron, and a fall in haemoglobin. The condition appears during the course of therapy and recovery is the rule after chloramphenicol has been discontinued.
2. Aplastic anaemia, which is probably idiosyncratic, due possibly to a genetically-determined defect in bone marrow cells[37]; it is not dose-

related and often occurs after the cessation of prolonged therapy or following more than one course of the drug. The incidence in one study was estimated as 1 in 11,500 with a mortality of 1 in 18,500,[52] and similar rates have been recorded in different parts of the world.

The other toxic effects of chloramphenicol include the "grey syndrome," a severe illness in neonates consisting of vomiting, diarrhoea, cyanosis, and abdominal distension within the first 4 days of therapy, due to failure of chloramphenicol metabolism and excretion. Hypersensitivity reactions causing skin rashes, fever, and angioneurotic oedema are fairly uncommon complications. Superinfections are apt to occur during chloramphenicol therapy and may cause oropharyngeal candidiasis or pseudomembranous colitis.

Clinical Use

The toxicity of chloramphenicol toward the bone marrow precludes its use except in three situations: (1) typhoid fever, (2) *Haemophilus influenzae* meningitis or epiglottitis, and (3) severe infections for which other less toxic antibiotics cannot be used and chloramphenicol is the better alternative (Table 5-2). Its use in respiratory medicine should therefore be a rare event, arising only in the treatment of pneumonia secondary to *Salmonella typhi* infections, in Gram-negative lung infections, particularly due to *Klebsiella pneumoniae* for which cephalosporins and aminoglycosides are excluded because of bacterial resistance or drug allergy, or *Bacteroides fragilis* infections when clindamycin cannot be used. Chloramphenicol should never be used casually for minor

Table 5-2 / Major Clinical Indications for Chloramphenicol in Respiratory Infections

Priority	Indication
Drug of choice	Pneumonia secondary to *Salmonella typhi* infection
Possible alternative	Gram-negative bronchopulmonary infections, particularly due to *Klebsiella pneumoniae*, for which less toxic antibiotics are excluded by hypersensitivity or resistance
	Anaerobic infections due to *Bacteroides fragilis*

upper respiratory infections or in cases for which another antibiotic would do as well, but is appears that a good many doctors are still insufficiently aware of its dangers.[46,103]

CLINDAMYCIN

Clindamycin is a derivative of lincomycin, which is a naturally occurring antibiotic isolated from *Streptomyces lincolnensis*. Both are bacteriostatic antibiotics which, like chloramphenicol and the tetracyclines, act by binding to bacterial ribosomes and inhibiting protein synthesis. Clindamycin is a more useful drug than lincomycin because it is more active, particularly against staphylococci, and it is better absorbed from the gastrointestinal tract. It is effective against most aerobic and anaerobic Gram-positive bacteria, but nearly all Gram-negative aerobes are resistant to it. However the *Bacteroides* species including *B. fragilis* are usually sensitive.

Effective plasma levels of clindamycin are achieved after oral administration which is unaffected by food in the stomach. The drug is widely distributed in the tissues including bone but does not enter the CSF to a significant extent. It is 90 percent protein bound. The majority of the drug is inactivated in the liver to conjugates which are excreted in the urine and bile; only 10 percent is excreted unchanged in the urine, and no dosage adjustment is indicated in patients with chronic renal disease.[16] Because of the extensive hepatic metabolism, however, some modification of dosage is necessary in patients with seriously impaired hepatic function.

Clindamycin is usually administered by mouth in an adult dose of 150–200 mg every 6 hours, and in children the usual dose is 8–16 mg/kg body

---

Table 5-3 / Major Clinical Indications for Clindamycin in Respiratory Infections

Priority	Indication
Drug of choice	Anaerobic chest infections due to *Bacteroides fragilis*
Possible alternative	To penicillins for bronchopulmonary gram-positive infections in penicillin-allergic individuals
	To isoxazolyl penicillins in resistant staphylococcal pneumonia

weight per day in 3 or 4 divided doses. It can also be given parenterally in 2 to 4 divided doses totalling 600 mg to 2.4 g per day for adults, depending on the severity of the infection, and in children 10–40 mg/kg per day in 3 or 4 doses. Intramuscular injection may cause local irritation, and allergic reactions have been observed occasionally. Nausea, vomiting, and abdominal cramps are sometimes troublesome, but a more important side-effect is pseudomembranous colitis due to the toxin produced by superinfection with *Clostridium difficile*.[48] Oral vancomycin appears effective in controlling the infection.

Clindamycin is most likely to be needed (Table 5-3) in the treatment of anaerobic bronchopulmonary infection or lung abscess due to *Bacteroides fragilis*, which is the most commonly encountered anaerobe.[45] It also has a place in the treatment of penicillin-resistant or "methicillin-resistant" staphylococcal pneumonia,[109] and in treating streptococcal or staphylococcal infections in patients who are allergic to the penicillins.[77]

ERYTHROMYCIN

Erythromycin is one of a group of antibiotics known as macrolides which have a chemical structure consisting of a large lactone ring to which sugars are attached. It was originally isolated from *Streptomyces erythreus* and acts by binding selectively to bacterial ribosomes causing inhibition of protein synthesis.

General Properties

Spectrum of Activity   *In vitro* erythromycin is bacteriostatic in low concentrations and bactericidal in high concentrations. Its spectrum of activity embraces most Gram-positive bacteria including many anaerobes, some Gram-negative bacteria including *Haemophilus influenzae* and *Bordetella pertussis,* but not the Enterobacteriaceae or *Pseudomonas* species; it also includes a number of organisms which cause important respiratory infections, such as mycoplasmas, chlamydiae, rickettsiae, *Legionella pneumophila,* and some of the atypical mycobacteria such as *M. kansasii.* Resistance to erythromycin is uncommon among streptococci and pneumococci, but resistant staphylococcal strains are encountered, especially in hospitals. The drug can be used freely outside hospital with little risk of meeting resistance,[72] but in a hospital environment sensitivity testing of staphylococci is necessary.[51]

Clinical Pharmacology   Although erythromycin base is well absorbed from the upper small intestine, it is destroyed by gastric acid. It is therefore administered either in capsules with an acid-resistant coating or in the form of a derivative, such as erythromycin stearate or estolate, which is more acid stable than the parent substance. Diffusion of erythromycin into most body spaces occurs readily, and effective penetration of the cerebrospinal fluid takes place when the meninges are inflamed. A small proportion of the drug is excreted unchanged in the urine, but the major portion is concentrated in the liver and either excreted in the bile or inactivated. Dosage adjustment is unnecessary in renal failure.

Administration Erythromycin is usually administered by mouth in an adult dose of 250–500 mg every 6 hours, depending on the severity of the infection. The oral dose in children is 30–50 mg/kg body weight per day in four divided doses. For parenteral therapy, erythromycin gluceptate, lactobionate, and ethylsuccinate are available, the usual adult dose being 500 mg 6-hourly by intravenous injection; intramuscular injection is also possible but painful, and it may cause sterile abscesses.

Toxicity Erythromycin is a relatively safe drug with few side effects, although it does cause mild nausea, vomiting, and diarrhoea in some patients. Erythromycin estolate is hepatotoxic, causing jaundice about 10 to 14 days after starting treatment, which is sometimes associated with abdominal pain, fever, pruritus, and a rash. The jaundice is mainly cholestatic in character and subsides rapidly when the drug is withdrawn.[23,119] Liver toxicity does not occur with the other erythromycin derivatives. Ototoxicity causing tinnitus and transient deafness has been described in a few patients, possibly associated with excessively high serum levels of the drug.[88,126]

Clinical Uses

The major indication for erythromycin (Table 5-4) is in the treatment of Gram-positive infections such as pneumococcal pneumonia in patients who are allergic to penicillins, and it is the antibiotic of choice in the treatment of legionnaire's disease.[120] Erythromycin is an effective alternative to tetracyclines in the treatment of atypical pneumonias due to mycoplasmal, rickettsial, or chlamydial infections. It prevents the development of whooping cough in susceptible individuals if given as soon as possible after exposure,[2] and it may also reduce the severity of the illness if given early in its course; however, it has no influence once the paroxysmal stage is reached.[11]

TRIMETHOPRIM-SULFAMETHOXAZOLE (COTRIMOXAZOLE)

This combined preparation of trimethoprim and sulfamethoxazole[130] was devised to take advantage of the synergism between sulphonamides and

Table 5-4 / Major Clinical Indications for Erythromycin in Respiratory Infections

Priority	Indication
Drug of choice	Legionnaire's disease
	Prevention of whooping cough, or treatment in the early stages
First alternative	To penicillins for upper respiratory or bronchopulmonary Gram-positive infections in penicillin-allergic individuals
	To tetracyclines for pneumonia due to *Mycoplasma pneumoniae*, *Coxiella burneti*, or *Chlamydia psittaci*

trimethoprim, which results from the inhibitory effect of the two drugs on different enzymes in the same biosynthetic pathway. Folic acid (Figure 5-1) is necessary for the growth of bacterial and mammalian cells because in its reduced form, tetrahydrofolic acid, it acts as a coenzyme in certain one-carbon transfer reactions which are essential for RNA, DNA, and protein synthesis. Mammalian cells and some bacteria depend upon an external supply of dihydrofolic acid, but other micro-organisms manufacture their own supply and are vulnerable if this production line is interrupted by the competition of sulphonamides for para-aminobenzoic acid. A further stage in the process is the reduction of dihydrofolic acid to tetrahydrofolic acid by the enzyme dihydrofolate

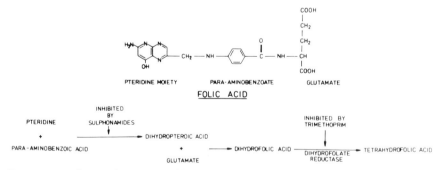

Figure 5-1 *Chemical structure of folic acid and sites of action of sulphonamides and trimethoprim in inhibiting the folate synthetic pathway.*

reductase. This reaction takes place both in mammalian and bacterial cells but is blocked by trimethoprim, which has at least 10,000 times more inhibitory effect on the bacterial than on the mammalian enzyme. Figure 5-1 illustrates the successive reactions which lead to the production of the essential coenzymes and indicates the site of action of sulphonamides and trimethoprim at different stages in the process.[26,53]

General Properties

Spectrum of Activity Trimethoprim-sulfamethoxazole has a wide spectrum of action against Gram-positive and Gram-negative micro-organisms. Of particular importance to the respiratory physician is its activity against *Streptococcus pneumoniae,* most *Streptococci* and many *Staphylococci, Haemophilus influenzae,* and most *Klebsiella* strains. It is also highly effective against *Pneumocystis carinii.*

Clinical Pharmacology The combination is rapidly and almost completely absorbed from the gastrointestinal tract, the serum half-lives of trimethoprim and sulfamethoxazole being 14.5 and 11 hours respectively, a difference which does not significantly affect the ratio of the two drugs in the blood. The combined preparation consists of sulfamethoxazole 400 mg and trimethoprim 80 mg, a ratio of 5:1; after absorption of this formulation and distribution in body tissues the plasma ratio of the two drugs in the free state is approximately 18:1 which is the optimum for antibacterial synergy.[66] Both drugs are widely distributed throughout all body tissues and variations in this ratio will occur in different tissues according to the distribution properties of each drug, but synergy occurs over a wide range of ratios and the antibacterial effect is not seriously impaired. Penetration into sputum produces therapeutically effective levels of both drugs.[57] The two agents are metabolised in the liver and excreted primarily by glomerular filtration, although sulfamethoxazole is also excreted to a lesser extent by renal tubular secretion. In renal failure the renal clearance of both drugs is diminished and dosage adjustment is necessary in end-stage renal disease (glomerular filtration rate less than 10 ml/min) by increasing the interval between doses from 12 to 24 hours.[16] Because of possible renal toxicity, serum concentrations should be determined regularly in patients whose creatinine clearance is less than 30 ml/min.[38]

Administration and Dosage The routine dosage in adults is trimethoprim 160 mg and sulfamethoxazole 800 mg, which is contained in two proprietary tablets taken twice daily. For children a paediatric suspension is available containing 40 mg trimethoprim and 200 mg sulfamethoxazole in each 5 ml. For children aged 6 weeks to 5 months, the dose is 2.5 ml; 6 months to 5 years, 5ml; and 6 to 12 years, 10 ml. Each dose is given twice daily. Preparations suitable for parenteral administration have recently been introduced for patients who cannot take oral therapy but these are not yet available in the United States.

Toxic Effects   The trimethoprim-sulfamethoxazole combination can cause all the undesirable side-effects of either alone, the most serious being hypersensitivity reactions which are probably due mainly to the sulphonamide component, and the haematological effects which may be due to either drug.

1. Skin rashes are the commonest form of hypersensitivity, occurring in 3.5 percent of patients in a recent survey.[74] Serious reactions such as Stevens-Johnson syndrome and exfoliative dermatitis have been described, but they are uncommon.[17] Drug fever, serum sickness, eosinophilic pneumonia, and vasculitis may occur rarely as allergic complications of sulphonamide therapy.
2. Gastrointestinal symptoms such as nausea, vomiting, and diarrhoea are among the most common side-effects (3.4 percent of patients) and are usually mild.
3. Haematological effects are uncommon but include serious complications such as acute thrombocytopenia[40] and agranulocytosis.[64] Depression of haemopoiesis occurs principally when abnormally high doses are used, following prolonged therapy or in patients who are prone to megaloblastic bone marrow changes such as pregnant women, the malnourished and elderly, or those receiving anticonvulsant therapy.[33]
4. Nephrotoxicity. Trimethoprim-sulfamethoxazole can sometimes affect renal function, most often when it is already compromised by other disease. The deterioration is usually but not always reversed when therapy is stopped and the preparation should be used cautiously in renal failure.[71]
5. The safety of trimethoprim-sulfamethoxazole in pregnancy is suspect because the preparation is teratogenic in animals. Both for this reason and because megaloblastic anaemia may be precipitated the combination should be avoided during pregnancy.[73]

Drug Interaction   Trimethoprim-sulfamethoxazole potentiates warfarin.[49] The mechanism of interaction is not known, but it is of practical importance and contraindicates the use of trimethoprim-sulfamethoxazole in warfarin-treated individuals unless they are under close laboratory supervision.

Table 5-5 / Major Clinical Indications for Trimethoprim-Sulfamethoxazole in Respiratory Infections

Priority	Indication
Drug of choice	*Pneumocystis carinii* pneumonia
Possible alternative	Bronchial infections or pneumonia in penicillin-allergic patients, or when initial treatment has failed

Clinical Use

Although they are not very common the potential seriousness of side-effects restricts the role of trimethoprim-sulfamethoxazole to the treatment of those respiratory infections for which less toxic drugs are excluded because of allergy or bacterial resistance (Table 5-5). Because of its dual action against the pneumococcus and *H. influenzae,* the compound is useful in treating acute exacerbations of bronchitis or pneumonia occurring in patients with chronic obstructive lung disease, and for these conditions it is the preferred alternative to ampicillin in penicillin-allergic individuals. It is also valuable as a "second-string" drug in cases where the response to ampicillin or a tetracycline has been inadequate.

Trimethoprim-sulfamethoxazole has been used effectively as an alternative to pentamidine in the treatment of *Pneumocystis carinii* pneumonia, and it may be the treatment of choice in view of the high incidence of side-effects from pentamidine.[58]

SODIUM FUSIDATE

This steroid antibiotic is obtained from a fungus, *Fusidium coccineum,* and has a high degree of activity against staphylococci, including penicillin-resistant and "methicillin-resistant" strains. Other Gram-positive cocci are comparatively insensitive. The drug inhibits bacterial protein synthesis by interfering with the translocation process necessary for orderly incorporation of amino acid units into the protein chain.

Sodium fusidate is readily absorbed from the gut and is well distributed throughout most tissues. It penetrates abscesses readily. It appears to be inactivated in the body, although some is excreted unchanged in the bile; little is excreted by the kidneys and no dosage adjustment is necessary when renal function is impaired.

Table 5-6 / Major Clinical Indications for Sodium Fusidate in Respiratory Infections

Priority	Indication
Possible alternative	Resistant staphylococcal pneumonia

The usual adult dosage is 0.5 g by mouth every 8 hours, and for children 20–40 mg/kg body weight per day in divided doses. An intravenous preparation of diethanolamine fusidate is available for use in severe infections, and it is administered by continuous infusion in isotonic saline via a largish vein to avoid the problems of venospasm and thrombosis. The drug is relatively free from side-effects, causing mild gastrointestinal symptoms and occasional slight rashes.

In respiratory infections it has a place in the treatment of resistant staphylococcal pneumonia (Table 5-6), usually in conjunction with another antibiotic such as cloxacillin, erythromycin, or rifampin in order to prevent the emergence of fucidin-resistant strains. Sodium fusidate is not at present available in the United States.

METRONIDAZOLE

Metronidazole has long been used for the treatment of protozoal infections such as trichomoniasis and amoebiasis, and has recently been introduced into the treatment of infections due to obligatory anaerobic bacteria. It acts as a powerful and rapid inhibitor of nucleic acid synthesis in susceptible organisms.[63]

Spectrum of Activity   The drug is highly active against *Fusobacterium, Bacteroides* species including *B. fragilis,* and against anaerobic Gram-positive cocci, and it is these organisms which are commonly implicated in aspiration pneumonia,[7] lung abscess,[8] and empyema.[9] Resistance is slow to develop.[60]

Clinical Pharmacology   Metronidazole is readily absorbed from the gastrointestinal tract after oral or rectal administration, and its bioavailability is not significantly reduced by concurrent ingestion of food. The drug is widely distributed to all tissues including the cerebrospinal fluid, abscess cavities, and empyema fluid, and it is only slightly bound to plasma proteins at therapeutic concentrations. It is metabolised by oxidation and glucuronide formation in the liver and largely excreted by the kidneys, about 70 percent being eliminated unchanged in the urine.[62] Some accumulation of inactive metabolites occurs in renal failure, but the results of one case report suggest that only small dosage modifications are necessary.[61]

Administration and Dosage   Metronidazole is usually administered orally or intravenously for bacterial or protozoal infections of the chest. The usual adult oral regimen is 400–800 mg 3 times daily for 5 to 10 days and in children the recommended dose is 7.5 mg/kg body weight 3 times daily (in the United States metronidazole tablets contain 250 mg). The intravenous preparation contains 500 mg of metronidazole in 100 ml, and the adult dose is 500 mg infused over 20 minutes 8-hourly. Rectal suppositories are available as an alternative to oral medication.

Toxicity   Gastrointestinal side-effects including an unpleasant taste, nausea, vomiting, and abdominal pain are likely to occur if the drug is given in high dosage for long periods. Peripheral sensory neuropathy has been described in a few cases, but this appears to resolve when treatment is stopped or reduced. A transient neutropenia has occasionally been observed during therapy. Malignant tumours have been reported after high dosage in mice, and the mutation rate of bacteria exposed to the drug is increased, but there has been no other evidence of carcinogenicity or mutagenicity; a retrospective epidemiological study by Beard of women treated with metronidazole for trichomonad infections failed to show a significant excess of cancer cases.[24] In a clinical study of its possible teratogenic effect, the overall incidence of congenital anomalies in the infants of treated patients was within normal limits but was higher than expected among those who received metronidazole during the first trimester.[96]

.   Drug interactions include a disulfiram-like reaction in some patients when metronidazole is taken with alcohol because of the accumulation of acetaldehyde in the blood, and the simultaneous administration of metronidazole and disulfiram can produce an acute psychosis.[108] A stereospecific interaction occurs between metronidazole and racemic or S($-$)-warfarin leading to prolongation of the prothrombin time.[92]

Clinical Uses   Metronidazole is now established as the best drug for all forms of amoebiasis,[101] and is highly effective in the treatment of pleural or pulmonary manifestations of the disease[31] (Table 5-7). Its place in the treatment of anaerobic bacterial infections of the lung is still controversial: some patients appear to respond satisfactorily to the drug,[116] but the experience of others has been disappointing.[110] At present the best initial treatment of anaerobic lung infections appears to be benzylpenicillin, with clindamycin as the drug of choice if *Bacteroides fragilis* is shown to be the predominant infecting microorganism.

Table 5-7 / Major Clinical Indications for Metronidazole in Respiratory Infections

Priority	Indications
Drug of choice	Pleuropulmonary amoebiasis
Possible alternative	Anaerobic chest infections due to *Bacteroides fragilis*

AMANTADINE

This synthetic antiviral agent has a small place in the armamentarium of the respiratory physician for the prophylaxis of Asian influenza. It has some action against rubella and parainfluenza viruses, but its only clinical application is against influenza A2 and other subtypes of influenza A.[89] The drug is thought to act by inhibiting the penetration of the virus particle into cells and by preventing virus uncoating,[68,93] but it is only effective as a prophylactic if given within a few hours of the start of symptoms,[128] although it may reduce their severity if started within 20 hours of onset.[47,118]

Amantadine is readily absorbed from the gastrointestinal tract, is widely distributed, and is excreted unchanged in the urine.[19] It has a relatively long duration of action (half-life 15 hours) and may accumulate if renal function is impaired. It causes central nervous system side-effects similar to the effects of amphetamine, such as nervousness, dizziness, light-headedness, poor concentration, slurring of speech, and insomnia; apart from its application in Parkinsonism, it should not be used in patients with epilepsy or other central nervous system symptoms. Nausea, vomiting, oedema, skin rashes, and livedo reticularis have also been described. Side-effects occur in 3 to 7 percent of people,[37] and there have been some isolated reports of possible serious adverse effects including teratogenicity,[90] heart failure,[125] and impairment of vision.[94] The drug should be avoided during pregnancy and used with great caution in patients with renal disease.[59]

The usual dose for adults and children over 10 years is 100 mg 2 times daily, and for younger children is 3 mg/kg body weight daily up to a maximum of 150 mg per day. Amantadine is administered by mouth and should be started as soon as possible after a single exposure to a known case of influenza A and should be continued for 10 days. It is only effective during the period of administration and should therefore be continued throughout the influenza epidemic for a month or more if repeated exposures are likely to occur.

There have been a number of studies to investigate the efficacy of amantadine in preventing or modifying the clinical course of experimentally induced or naturally acquired Asian influenza, and there is no doubt of its effectiveness both in prophylaxis and in the amelioration of symptoms.[65,113] There is also evidence that it reduces the disturbance of small airway function which results from influenzal infection.[78] Its place in clinical practice is less easy to define,[112] because the side-effects though generally slight are sufficiently frequent to discourage the use of amantadine in large-scale preventive programmes in which the protection afforded is successful in only 60 to 70 percent of subjects,[36,89] and the illness itself is usually mild. The drug has a possible role in the prevention of Type A influenza in elderly or high-risk patients in whom the disease is liable to be serious or even fatal,[82] although the greater incidence of side-effects among the elderly must be borne in mind, particularly if renal function is impaired. Its place in the treatment of severe Type A influenza is at present undefined.

ANTIFUNGAL CHEMOTHERAPY

Some pathogenic fungi occur most commonly as relatively harmless saprophytes at various sites in the human body. *Candida albicans,* for instance, is found in the mouth, the sputum, in the stools, on the perianal skin, and in the vagina without causing disease, although local irritation and inflammation may arise if the infection becomes florid as a result of broad-spectrum antibiotic therapy which suppresses the natural bacterial flora, or due to inhaled corticosteroid aerosols which facilitate fungal overgrowth in the oropharynx. *Aspergillus* species may also occur as saprophytes on various parts of the body, particularly in the external ear and the nasal sinuses, but these sometimes colonise the bronchial tree and produce the largely allergic manifestations of bronchopulmonary aspergillosis.[80] Other fungi such as *Histoplasma capsulatum* and *Coccidioides immitis* are readily inhaled as spores into the respiratory tract and in highly endemic areas a large proportion of the population will have been infected, as judged by skin test studies, although only about one-fourth of these will have experienced symptoms of a flu-like illness or mild pneumonitis.[43,127] These infections require only symptomatic treatment or, as in the case of local candidiasis, topical application of antifungal agents such as nystatin or amphotericin B, which avoids the serious toxicity of systemic antifungal therapy.

Disseminated infection by these and other fungal species is extremely rare in normal individuals but it occurs in people with compromised immunological defences due to serious disease, such as malignancy, severe nutritional

Table 5-8 / Systemic Fungal Infections[1,6,15,32,84,86,124]

Organism	Geographic Distribution	Treatment of Choice
Yeasts and yeast-like fungi		
Candida species	World-wide	5-FC* in mild infections if sensitive, otherwise combined amphotericin B and 5-FC
Cryptococcus neoformans	World-wide	Combined amphotericin B and 5-FC. Miconazole is a possible alternative.
Torulopsis glabrata	World-wide	Combined amphotericin B and 5-FC, or possibly 5-FC alone
Filamentous fungi		
Aspergillus species	World-wide	Amphotericin B
Mucoraceae e.g. Mucor species Rhizopus species	World-wide	Amphotericin B
Dimorphic fungi		
Histoplasma capsulatum	North America (Arkansas, Kentucky, Missouri, Tennessee), Central and South America, South East Asia	Amphotericin B; combination with rifampin may possibly be effective
Sporothrix schenckii	World-wide	Amphotericin B
Coccidioides immitis	S-Western United States (Arizona, California, Nevada, New Mexico, Texas, Utah)	Amphotericin B; miconazole is a possible alternative
Paracoccidioides braziliensis	Central and South America	Amphotericin B; miconazole is a possible alternative
Blastomyces dermatitidis	S-Eastern United States (Arkansas, Kentucky, Mississippi, North Carolina, Tennessee)	Amphotericin B; combination with rifampin may possibly be effective

*5-FC = Flucytosine (5-fluorocytosine)

deficiencies, and treatment with corticosteroids and cytotoxic or immunosup-pressant drugs. The incidence of systemic mycoses has therefore increased with the development of organ transplantation and sophisticated regimens of cytotoxic therapy for malignant disease.

The lungs are an important portal of entry for pathogenic fungi and consti-tute a major site for primary fungal lesions and for foci of infection dissemi-nated from elsewhere in the body. The pathogenic fungi which most common-ly cause systemic infection involving the respiratory tract are listed in Table 5-8 along with their geographical distribution. Only a small group of rather toxic drugs is available for the chemotherapy of systemic fungal infections. These are often fatal, and they require well-judged and intensive management to achieve a successful outcome of therapy.

Amphotericin B

This highly toxic antifungal agent originates from a soil actinomycete, *Strep-tomyces nodosus*. It is a polyene antibiotic consisting of a large conjugated double-bond ring linked to an amino-acid sugar, mycosamine. The drug is virtually insoluble in water but forms a complex with sodium desoxycholate which can produce a colloid dispersion in water suitable for intravenous ad-ministration.

Mechanism of Action   Amphotericin B binds to sterols which are present in fungal and mammalian cell membranes, causing an increase in the permeabil-ity of the cell which leads to the escape of small molecules such as nucleotides, amino acids and sugars, and the leakage of ions, notably potassium. This effect is fungicidal and presumably also accounts for the serious toxicity of amphotericin B to the host; indeed, the basis of its selective toxicity is not very clear but may be due to the drug's greater affinity for ergosterol, which is the principal sterol of fungal membranes, compared with cholesterol which fulfills a similar role in mammalian cells.[70]

The capacity of amphotericin B to increase the permeability of fungal cell membranes is responsible for its synergistic action with other antifungal agents by enabling them to penetrate the cells and exert their fungicidal effects. Syner-gy between amphotericin B and 5-fluorocytosine and between amphotericin B and rifampin has been demonstrated *in vitro*,[85] and the application of com-bined therapy in clinical trials appears promising,[123] permitting a reduction in the dosage of amphotericin B and the avoidance of serious side-effects. Ap-plication of this synergistic action with amphotericin B is being extended to other antibiotics such as the tetracyclines.[75]

Amphotericin B may be effective in the treatment of systemic mycoses due to all the organisms listed in Table 5-8, but there is some variability in the susceptibility of different species to the drug,[54] and *Aspergillus* species particularly are inclined to be resistant. Clinically important resistance to amphotericin B does not arise during therapy.

Clinical Pharmacology Because its absorption from the gastrointestinal tract is poor, amphotericin B is customarily administered by intravenous infusion although intrathecal administration is also indicated in the treatment of coccidioidal meningitis and some refractory cases of cryptococcal meningitis. During intravenous injection a peak serum level of 1.8–3.5 µg/ml is reached during the first hour of infusion and is maintained for 6 to 8 hours, followed by a more gradual fall in the serum concentration as the drug is distributed to more peripheral compartments. From there it is eliminated very slowly, with a half-life of about 15 days, renal excretion accounting for only 3 percent of elimination.[4] Renal insufficiency does not seem to affect serum levels or urinary excretion, and the fate of the major part of an infused dose of amphotericin B is unknown.

Administration[13] Amphotericin B is available as a complex with sodium desoxycholate; the complex forms a colloidal dispersion in glucose solution and is stable in most commonly available dextrose solutions. It is usually dissolved in 500–1,000 ml of 5 percent dextrose-in-water solution and administered over 4 to 6 hours, since more rapid infusion entails a possible risk of cardiotoxicity.[30] Treatment should begin with a 1 mg test dose administered over 20 to 30 minutes, and the pulse rate and the temperature should be recorded to monitor the occurrence of febrile reactions (rigors, anorexia, vomiting, and headaches) which can be reduced by adding 25–50 mg of hydrocortisone sodium succinate to the infusion fluid. Thrombophlebitis at the injection site can be minimised by adding heparin to the infusion. Dosage is increased by 5 mg increments on successive days up to about 0.6 mg/kg body weight over 1 or 2 weeks if renal function permits. Measurements of serum urea, electrolytes, creatinine clearance and blood count should be undertaken 2 times weekly since the final dosage and the total amount of amphotericin B which can be administered depend on the severity of the toxic effect produced. Once the regimen is stabilised it can be gradually changed to a double dose on alternate days in order to reduce the incidence of phlebitis.[18] Assays of amphotericin B serum concentrations have been advocated in order to determine individual dosage requirements based on the sensitivity of the patient's own fungal isolate,[41] but the techniques available for assessing amphotericin B susceptibility or blood levels are not reliable enough to provide a useful clinical guide to dosage.[13]

Toxicity Nephrotoxicity is the most important side-effect of therapy with amphotericin B and it occurs in nearly every patient treated, its severity being dose related.[28] Animal experiments show that the drug causes renal vasoconstriction with a decrease in glomerular filtration and progressive nitrogen retention,[29] while impairment of tubular function leads to excessive losses of potassium, bicarbonate, and water which sometimes produces a syndrome similar to renal tubular acidosis associated with nephrocalcinosis.[27,81] Potassium supplementation is often required because of the excessive renal loss. Mannitol has been used in an attempt to improve renal blood flow,[91,107] but its effectiveness has not been substantiated by controlled studies.[25] Renal damage is manifested by the appearance of casts and red and white blood cells in the urine, and therapy is guided by regular measurements of blood urea and creatinine clearance. A rise in these parameters is almost inevitable, but the level at which treatment should be prematurely halted is debatable; Bennett[13] suggests an upper limit of 50 mg/100 ml (8 mmol/l) for blood urea, and 3.5 mg/100 ml (0.3 mmol/l) for serum creatinine. Renal function usually returns when the drug is stopped, but permanent damage or irreversible renal failure may occur if large doses of the drug are used, and maintenance by renal dialysis may be required. Although caution is necessary in using amphotericin B, fear of nephrotoxicity should not prevent its use in life-threatening fungal infections when no alternative drug is available.[114]

Bone marrow depression by amphotericin B leads to a normocytic normochromic anaemia, unrelated to the degree of uraemia, which resolves on discontinuation of the drug.[122] Thrombocytopenia and leukopenia are said to be rare.[13] Cardiac arrest has been reported following overly-rapid infusion of the drug, and peripheral neuropathy has been described during intravenous therapy; neurological abnormalities are much more likely to occur during intrathecal therapy due to chemical arachnoiditis.

5-Fluorocytosine

5-Fluorocytosine is a fluorinated pyrimidine (Figure 5-2) which is available as a synthetic antifungal agent with a rather restricted range of activity but with a relatively low toxicity. It is active against yeast-like organisms including *Cryptococcus neoformans*, *Candida* species, and *Torulopsis glabrata*, but *Aspergillus* species are often resistant and it is ineffective against other systemic fungal pathogens. Moreover, many isolates of supposedly susceptible fungal species either turn out to be resistant *de novo* or they quickly develop resistance during a course of treatment, so that *in vitro* sensitivity testing on all strains is necessary before and during therapy. The major potential of 5-fluorocytosine lies in its additive or synergistic antifungal action with amphotericin B.

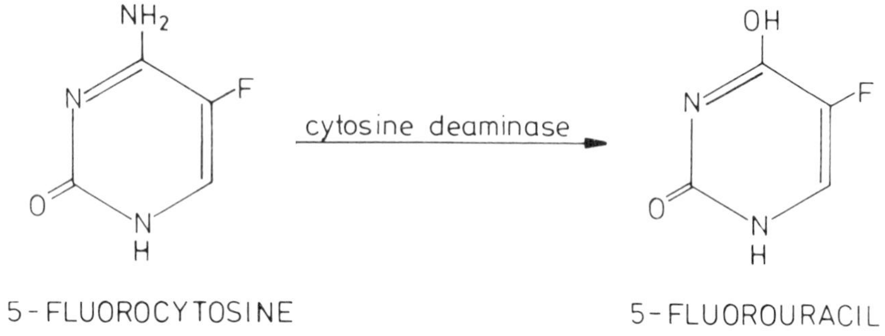

5-FLUOROCYTOSINE   5-FLUOROURACIL

Figure 5-2 *Conversion of 5-fluorocytosine to its active metabolite 5-fluorouracil.*

Mode of Action   5-Fluorocytosine is converted by cytosine deaminase in yeast cells to 5-fluorouracil (Figure 5-2) which is then further converted to 5-fluorouracil-ribose monophosphate and incorporated into RNA,[100] but the precise mechanism of the drug's fungicidal effect is uncertain.[14] 5-Fluorouracil is also highly toxic to mammalian cells, and the selective toxicity of 5-fluorocytosine may be attributable to a difference in the abilities of the host and the fungus to convert it to 5-fluorouracil, although some of the toxicity of the drug may be attributable to this metabolite.[39] 5-Fluorocytosine resistance due to fungal mutation can result by several mechanisms, including a reduction in the activity of the permease enzyme responsible for drug entry into the cell and loss of cytosine deaminase activity.[21,55]

Clinical Pharmacology   5-Fluorocytosine is well absorbed from the gastrointestinal tract and widely distributed in body fluids, including the CSF and bronchial secretions.[95] The serum half-life is 3 to 4 hours, but this is prolonged when renal function is impaired. There is no significant binding to serum proteins[20] and little metabolism in man, over 90 percent being excreted unchanged in the urine.[99]

Administration and Dosage   5-Fluorocytosine is available for oral administration in capsules containing 250 and 500 mg, the usual daily dose being 37.5–50 mg/kg body weight every 6 hours which in normal persons results in peak serum levels of 75–90 μg/ml. Modification of dosage is necessary when renal function is impaired using creatinine clearance as a guide, a commonly recommended regime being to double the dose interval from 6 to 12 hours if the creatinine clearance is between 20 and 40 ml/min, and to double it again if the creatinine clearance is less than 20 ml/min. The drug is removed by haemodialysis at the same rate as creatinine. In renal failure the optimal dose can only be determined by assaying the serum level,[67] aiming for a peak level not exceeding 100 μg/ml and trough levels maintained above 25 μg/ml. Prolonged blood levels above 100–125 μg/ml are frequently associated with leukopenia.[14]

Toxicity The commonest side-effects of 5-fluorocytosine are gastrointestinal symptoms, abnormalities of hepatic function, and bone marrow depression, each of which occur in 5 or 6 percent of cases. Nausea, abdominal bloating, and diarrhoea are the most frequent symptoms, but vomiting and severe diarrhoea occur occasionally, and mucosal necrosis or perforation of the bowel has been reported in a few cases.[49,106] Leukopenia and occasional thrombocytopenia, usually reversible, seem to occur most commonly in patients with impaired renal function, and this may be due to concurrent amphotericin B administration,[69] and is probably related to prolonged high blood levels of 5-fluorocytosine. Fatal aplastic anaemia has been described in a few cases,[87,104] although in some an underlying haemopoietic disorder may have played a part.

Transient elevation in hepatic enzyme levels may occur, but evidence suggests that hepatic necrosis seems to be extremely rare.[104] Most authorities advise weekly measurements of liver enzyme levels in patients on 5-fluorocytosine. Minor side-effects such as skin rashes and eosinophilia have been observed, and the drug is contraindicated in pregnancy because it is teratogenic in rats, although individual case reports of its use in pregnancy have been reassuring.[97,111]

Imidazoles

Three imidazole derivatives, clotrimazole, miconazole, and econazole are effective in the therapy of superficial fungal infections, and one of them, miconazole, appears to be of value in the treatment of systemic mycoses, having some activity against most of the major fungal pathogens.[115] The drug acts by damaging fungal cell membranes, but apparently in a different way from the polyene antibiotics.[13,1] Oral absorption is poor, but miconazole can be administered intravenously, being inactivated in the liver and excreted in the bile and urine.[98] Side-effects include anaemia, thrombocytosis, gastrointestinal symptoms, and thrombophlebitis at the injection site. Further controlled studies are necessary to evaluate the role of miconazole more fully. Ketoconazole, a newer derivative, is apparently effective when administered orally.[22]

Combined Therapy in Respiratory Mycoses

For many years amphotericin B has been the drug of choice in the treatment of severe life-threatening systemic fungal infections. It is so toxic that treatment is sometimes curtailed before optimum dosage has been achieved, and in these cases infection is liable to recur. Because it is relatively nontoxic 5-fluorocytosine may be the preferred choice in sensitive pulmonary infections due to *Aspergillus* species[5] and yeasts,[10,124] but the rapid development of resistance *in vitro* reduces its value in serious infections and has the additional disadvantage that if resistance develops, subsequent combination treatment using amphotericin B and 5-fluorocytosine loses its effectiveness.[14]

There is increasing clinical evidence that this combination of amphotericin B and 5-fluorocytosine is the initial regimen of choice in some serious systemic mycoses,[35] particularly in the treatment of the highly lethal cryptococcal meningitis.[15,123] There is some evidence from case reports which suggests that the combination is effective in pulmonary aspergillosis,[5,34] but comparative clinical studies are needed to establish its superiority over amphotericin B alone in the routine treatment of serious infections due to *Aspergillus* or *Candida* species. Therapy with these two antifungal agents has three advantages:

1. Their additive and possibly synergistic effect.[83]
2. The prevention of 5-fluorocytosine resistance developing during therapy.
3. The potential for using lower doses of amphotericin B and hence reducing the risk of nephrotoxicity.[123]

The effectiveness of combined therapy with amphotericin B and other chemotherapeutic agents such as rifampin, tetracyclines, and miconazole remains to be established by comparative clinical trials.

REFERENCES

1. AL-DOORY Y: The epidemiology of human mycotic diseases. Springfield, Ill: Charles C Thomas, 1975.
2. ALTEMEIER WA, AYOUB EM: Erythromycin prophylaxis for pertussis. Pediatrics 59: 623-625, 1977.
3. APPEL GB, NEU HC: The nephrotoxicity of antimicrobial agents. N Eng J Med 296: 663-670, 722-728, 784-787, 1977.
4. ATKINSON AJ, BENNETT JE: Amphotericin B pharmacokinetics in humans. Antimicrob Agents Chemother 13: 271-276, 1978.
5. ATKINSON GW, ISRAEL HL: 5-Fluorocytosine treatment of meningococcal and pulmonary aspergillosis. Am J Med 55: 496-504, 1973.
6. BAKER RD: Pulmonary mucormycosis. Am J Pathol 32: 287-313, 1956.
7. BARTLETT JG, GORBACH SL, FINEGOLD SM, The bacteriology of aspiration pneumonia. Am J Med 56: 202-207, 1974.
8. BARTLETT, JG, GORBACH SL, TALLY FP, FINEGOLD SM: Bacteriology and treatment of lung abscess. Am Rev Resp Dis 109: 510-518, 1974.

9. BARTLETT JG, GORBACH SL, THADEPALLI H, FINEGOLD SM: Bacteriology of empyema. Lancet 1: 338-340, 1974.

10. BARTLEY PC: Pulmonary candidiasis treated with 5-fluorocytosine. Aust NZ J Med 3: 189-192, 1973.

11. BASS JW, KLENK EL, KOTHEIMER JB, LINNEMANN CC, SMITH MHD: Antimicrobial treatment of pertussis. J Pediatr 75: 768-781, 1969.

12. BENNER EJ, MORTHLAND V: Methicillin-resistant *Staphylococcus aureus*. Antimicrobial susceptibility. N Engl J Med 277: 678-680, 1967.

13. BENNETT JE: Chemotherapy of systemic mycoses. N Engl J Med 290: 30-32, 320-323, 1974.

14. BENNETT JE: Flucytosine. Ann Intern Med 86: 319-322, 1977.

15. BENNETT JE, DISMUKES WE, DUMA RJ, MEDOFF G, SANDE MA, GALLIS H, LEONARD J, FIELDS BT, BRADSHAW M, HAYWOOD H, McGEE ZA, CATE TR, COBBS CG, WARNER JF, ALLING DW: A comparison of amphotericin B alone and combined with flucytosine in the treatment of cryptococcal meningitis. N Eng J Med 301: 126-131, 1979.

16. BENNETT WM, SINGER I, GOLPER T, FEIG P, COGGINS CJ: Guidelines for drug therapy in renal failure. Ann Intern Med 86: 754-783, 1977.

17. BERNSTEIN LS: Adverse reactions to trimethoprim-sulfamethoxazole, with particular reference to long-term therapy. Can Med Assoc J 112 (Suppl): 96S-98S, 1975.

18. BINDSCHADLER DD, BENNETT JE: A pharmacologic guide to the clinical use of amphotericin B. J Infect Dis 120: 427-436, 1969.

19. BLEIDNER WE, HARMON JB, HEWES WE, LYNES TE, HERMANN EC: Absorption, distribution and excretion of amantadine hydrochloride. J Pharmacol Exp Ther 150: 484-490, 1965.

20. BLOCK ER, BENNETT JE, LIVOTI LG, KLEIN WJ, MACGREGOR RR, HENDERSON L: Flucytosine and amphotericin B : haemodialysis effects on the plasma concentrations and clearance. Ann Intern Med 80: 613-617, 1974.

21. BLOCK ER, JENNINGS AE, BENNETT JE: 5-fluorocytosine resistance in *Cryptococcus neoformans*. Antimicrob Agents Chemother 3: 649-656, 1973.

22. BORELLI D, BRAN JL, FUENTES J, LEGENDRE R, LEIDERMAN E, LEVINE HB, RESTREPO-MA, STEVENS DA: Ketoconazole, an oral antifungal: laboratory and clinical assessment of imidazole drugs. Postgrad Med J 55: 657-661, 1979.

23. BRAUN P: Hepatotoxicity of erythromycin. J Infect Dis 119: 300-306, 1969.

24. BROGDEN RN, HEEL RC, SPEIGHT TM, AVERY GS: Metronidazole in anaerobic infections: a review of its activity, pharmacokinetics and therapeutic use. Drugs 16: 387-417, 1978.

25. BULLOCK WE, LUKE RG, NUTTALL CE, BHATHENA D: Can mannitol reduce amphotericin B nephrotoxicity? Double-blind study and description of a new vascular lesion in kidneys. Antimicrob Agents Chemother 10: 555-563, 1976.

26. BURCHALL JJ: Mechanism of action of trimethoprim-sulphamethoxazole: II. J Infect Dis 128 (Suppl) S437-S441, 1973.

27. BURGESS JL, BIRCHALL R: Nephrotoxicity of amphotericin B, with emphasis on changes in tubular function. Am J Med 53: 77-84, 1972.

28. BUTLER WT, BENNETT JE, ALLING DW, WERTLAKE PT, UTZ JP, HILL GJ: Nephrotox-

icity of amphotericin B. Early and late effects in 81 patients. Ann Intern Med 61: 175-187, 1964.

29. BUTLER WT, HILL GJ, SZWED CF, KNIGHT V: Amphotericin B renal toxicity in the dog. J Pharmacol Exp Ther 143: 47-56, 1964.

30. BUTLER WT, BENNETT JE, HILL GJ, SZWED CF, COTLOVE E: Electrocardiographic and electrolyte abnormalities caused by amphotericin B in dog and man. Proc Soc Exp Biol Med 116: 857-863, 1964.

31. CAMERON EW: The treatment of pleuropulmonary amebiasis with metronidazole. Chest 73: 647-650, 1978.

32. CARTWRIGHT RY: Antifungal therapy. Postgrad Med J 55: 583-700, 1979.

33. CHANARIN I, ENGLAND JM: Toxicity of trimethoprim-sulfamethoxazole in patients with megaloblastic haemopoiesis. Br Med J 1: 651-653, 1972.

34. CODISH SD, TOBIAS JS, HANNIGAN M: Combined amphotericin B - flucytosine therapy in *Aspergillus* pneumonia. JAMA 241: 2418-2419, 1979.

35. CODISH SD, TOBIAS JS, MONACO AP: Recent advances in the treatment of systemic mycotic infections. Surg Gynecol Obstet 148: 435-447, 1979.

36. COUCH RB, JACKSON GG: Antiviral agents in influenza - Summary of influenza workshop VIII. J Infect Dis 134: 516-527, 1976.

37. DAMESHEK W: Chloramphenicol aplastic anaemia in identical twins - A clue to pathogenesis. N Engl J Med 281: 42-43, 1969.

38. DENNEBERG T, EKBERG M, ERICSON C, HANSON A: Cotrimoxazole in the long-term treatment of pyelonephritis with normal and impaired renal function. Scand J Infect Dis (Suppl) 8: 61-66, 1976.

39. DIASIO RB, LAKINGS DE, BENNETT JE: Evidence for conversion of 5-fluorocytosine to 5-fluorouracil in humans: possible factor in 5-fluorocytosine clinical toxicity. Antimicrob Agents Chemother 14: 903-908, 1978.

40. DICKSON HG: Trimethoprim-sulphamethoxazole and thrombocytopenia. Med J Aust 2: 5-7, 1978.

41. DRUTZ DJ, SPICKARD A, ROGERS DE, KOENIG MG: Treatment of disseminated mycotic infections. A new approach to amphotericin B therapy. Am J Med 45: 405-418, 1968.

42. EYKYN S. PHILLIPS I, EVANS J: Vancomycin for staphyloccal shunt site infections in patients on regular haemodialysys. Br Med J 3: 80-82, 1970.

43. FIESE MJ: Coccidioidomycosis. Springifield Illinois: Charles C Thomas, 1958.

44. FINE PE: Mitochondrial inheritance and disease. Lancet 2: 659-662, 1978.

45. FINEGOLD SM: Therapy for infections due to anaerobic bacteria: An overview. J Infect Dis 135 (Suppl) S25-S29, 1977.

46. FINK TJ, GUMP DW: Chloramphenicol: An inpatient study of use and abuse. J Infect Dis 138: 690-694, 1978.

47. GALBRAITH AW, OXFORD JS, SCHILD GC, POTTER CW, WATSON GI: Therapeutic effect of 1-adamantanamine hydrochloride in naturally occurring influenza A_2/Hong Kong infection. A controlled double-blind study. Lancet 2: 113-115, 1971.

48. GEORGE WL, SUTTER VL, GOLDSTEIN EJC, LUDWIG SL, FINEGOLD SM: Aetiology of antimicrobial-agent-associated colitis. Lancet 1: 802-803, 1978.

49. HASSALL C, FEETHAM CL, LEACH RH, MEYNELL MJ: Potentiation of warfarin by co-trimoxazole. Lancet 2: 1155-1156, 1975.
50. HARDER EJ, HERMANS PE: Treatment of fungal infections with flucytosine. Arch Intern Med 135: 231-237, 1975.
51. HASSAM ZA, SHAW EJ, SHOOTER RA, CARO DB: Changes in antibiotic sensitivity in strains of Staphylococcus aureus, 1952-78. Br Med J 2: 536-537, 1978.
52. HAUSMANN K, SKRANDIES G: Aplastic anaemia following chloramphenicol therapy in Hamburg and surrounding districts. Postgrad Med J 50 (Suppl 5): 131-136, 1974.
53. HITCHINGS GH: Mechanism of action of trimethoprim-sulfamethoxazole: I. J Infect Dis 128 (Suppl): S433-S436, 1973.
54. HOEPRICH PD, HUSTON AC: Susceptibility of Coccidioides immitis, Candida albicans and Cryptococcus neoformans to amphotericin B, flucytosine and clotrimazole. J Infect Dis 132: 133, 1975.
55. HOEPRICH PD, INGRAHAM JL, KLEKER E, WINSHIP MJ: Development of resistance to 5-fluorocytosine in *Candida parapsilosis* during therapy. J Infect Dis 130: 112-118, 1974.
56. HOWARD AJ, HINCE CJ, WILLIAMS JD: Antibiotic resistance in Streptococcus pneumoniae and Haemophilus influenzae. Report of a study group on bacterial resistance. Br Med J 1: 1657-1660, 1978.
57. HUGHES DTD: Use of combinations of trimethoprim and sulphamethoxazole in the treatment of chest infections. J Infect Dis 128 (Suppl): S701-S705, 1973.
58. HUGHES WT: *Pneumocystis carinii* pneumonia. N Engl J Med 297: 1381-1383, 1977.
59. ING TS, DAUGIRDAS JT, SOUNG LS, KLAWANS HL, MAHURKAR SD, HAYASHI JA, GEIS WP, HANO JE: Toxic effects of amantadine in patients with renal failure. Can Med Assoc J 120: 695-698, 1978.
60. INGHAM HR, EATON S, VENABLES CW, ADAMS PC: *Bacteroides fragilis* resistant to metronidazole after long-term therapy. Lancet 1: 214, 1978.
61. INGHAM HR, RICH GE, SELKON JB, ROXBY CM, BETTY MJ, JOHNSON RWG, ULDALL PR: Treatment with metronidazole of three patients with serious infections due to *Bacteroides fragilis.* J Antimicrob Chemother 1: 235-242, 1975.
62. INGS RMJ, LAW GL, PARNELL EW: The metabolism of metronidazole (1-2'-hydroxy-ethyl-2-methyl-5-nitromidazole). Biochem Pharmacol 15: 515-519, 1966.
63. INGS RMJ, MCFADZEAN JA, ORMEROD WE: The mode of action of metronidazole in *Trichomonas vaginalis* and other micro-organisms. Biochem Pharmacol 23: 1421-1429, 1974.
64. INMAN WHW: Study of fatal bone marrow depression with special reference to phenylbutazone and oxyphenbutazone. Br Med J 1: 1500-1505, 1977.
65. JACKSON GG, STANLEY ED: Prevention and control of influenza by chemoprophylaxis and chemotherapy. Prospects from examination of recent experience. JAMA 235: 2739-2742, 1976.
66. KAPLAN SA, WEINFELD RE, ABRUZZO CW, MCFADEN K, JACK ML, WEISSMAN L: Pharmacokinetic profile of trimethoprim-sulfamethoxazole in man. J Infect Dis 128 (Suppl) S547-S555, 1973.

67. KASPAR RL, DRUTZ DJ: Rapid, simple bioassay for 5-fluorocytosine in the presence of amphotericin B. Antimicrob Agents Chemother 7: 462-465, 1975.
68. KATO N, EGGERS HJ: Inhibition of fowl plague virus by 1-adamantanamine hydrochloride. Virology 37: 632-641, 1969.
69. KAUFFMAN CA, FRAME PT: Bone marrow toxicity associated with 5-fluorocytosine therapy. Antimicrob Agents Chemother 11: 244-247, 1977.
70. KOTLER-BRAJTBURG J, PRICE HD, MEDOFF G, SCHLESSINGER D, KOBAYASHI S: Molecular basis for the selective toxicity of amphotericin B for yeast and filipin for animal cells. Antimicrob Agents Chemother 5: 377-382, 1974.
71. KUCERS A, BENNETT NM: Trimethoprim and Cotrimoxazole. in The Use of Antibiotics, 3rd Ed., p. 704-705. London: Heinemann, 1979.
72. LACEY RW: Lack of evidence for mutation to erythromycin resistance in clinical strains of Staphylococcus aureus. J Clin Pathol 30: 602-605, 1977.
73. LANCET: Co-trimoxazole and blood. Lancet 2: 950-951, 1973.
74. LAWSON DH, JICK H: Adverse reactions to co-trimoxazole in hospitalised medical patients. Am J Med Sci 275: 53-57, 1978.
75. LEW MA, BECKETT KM, LEVIN MJ: Antifungal activity of four tetracycline analogues against Candida albicans in vitro: potentiation by amphotericin B. J Infect Dis 136: 263-270, 1977.
76. LINDHOLM DD, MURRAY JS: Persistence of vancomycin in the blood during renal failure and its treatment by haemodialysis. N Engl J Med 274: 1047-1051, 1966.
77. LINES DR, VIMPANI GV, PEARSON CC: The use of 7-chlorolincomycin in the treatment of childhood respiratory disease. Med J Aust 1: 439-441, 1973.
78. LITTLE JW, HALL WJ, DOUGLAS RG: Small airways dysfunction in influenza A virus infection: therapeutic role and potential mode of action of amantadine. Ann NY Acad Sci 284: 106-117, 1977.
79. MARTELO OJ, MANYAN DR, SMITH US, YUNIS AA: Chloramphenicol and bone marrow mitochondria. J Lab Clin Med 74: 927-940, 1969.
80. McCARTHY DS, PEPYS J: Allergic broncho-pulmonary aspergillosis. Clinical Immunology: (1) Clinical features. Clin Allergy 1: 261-286, 1971.
81. McCURDY DK, FREDERIC M, ELKINGTON JR: Renal tubular acidosis due to amphotericin B. N Engl J Med 278: 124-131, 1968.
82. MEDICAL LETTER: Amantadine for high-risk influenza. Med Lett Drugs Ther 20: 25-26, 1978.
83. MEDOFF G, COMFORT M, KOBAYASHI GS: Synergistic action of amphotericin B and 5-fluorocytosine against yeast-like organisms. Proc Soc Exp Biol Med 138: 571-574, 1971.
84. MEDOFF G, KOBAYASHI GS: Pulmonary mucormycosis. N Engl J Med 286: 86-87, 1972.
85. MEDOFF G, KOBAYASHI GS: Amphotericin B. Old drug, new therapy. JAMA 232: 619-620, 1975.
86. MEDOFF G, KOBAYASHI GS: Strategies in the treatment of systemic fungal infections. N Engl J Med 302: 145-155, 1980.
87. MEYER R, AXELROD JL: Fatal aplastic anaemia resulting from flucytosine. JAMA 228: 1573, 1974.

88. Mintz U, Amir J, Pinkhas J, De Vries A: Transient perceptive deafness due to erythromycin lactobionate. JAMA 225: 1122-1123, 1973.

89. Monto AS, Gunn RA, Bandyk MG, King CL: Prevention of Russian influenza by amantadine. JAMA 241: 1003-1007, 1978.

90. Nora JJ, Nora AH, Way GL: Cardiovascular maldevelopment associated with maternal exposure to amantadine. Lancet 2: 607, 1975.

91. Olivero JJ, Lozano-Mendez J, Ghafary EM, Eknoyan G, Suki WN: Mitigation of amphotericin B nephrotoxicity by mannitol. Br Med J 1: 550-551, 1975.

92. O'Reilly RA: The stereoselective interaction of warfarin and metronidazole in man. N Engl J Med 295: 354-357, 1976.

93. Oxford JS: Specific inhibitors of influenza virus replication as potential chemo-prophylactic agents. J Antimicrob Chemother 1: 7-23, 1975.

94. Pearlman JT, Kadish AH, Ramseyer JC: Vision loss associated with amantadine hydrochloride use. JAMA 237: 1200, 1977.

95. Pennington JE, Block ER, Reynolds HY: 5-Fluorocytosine and amphotericin B in bronchial secretions. Antimicrob Agents Chemother 6: 324-326, 1974.

96. Peterson WF, Stauch JE, Ryder CD: Metronidazole in pregnancy. Am J Obstet Gynecol 94: 343-349, 1966.

97. Philpot CR, Lo D: Cryptococcal meningitis in pregnancy. Med J Aust 2: 1005-1007, 1972.

98. Plempel M: Pharmacokinetics of imidazole antimycotics. Postgrad Med J 55: 662-666, 1979.

99. Polak A, Eschenhof E, Fernex M, Scholer HJ: Metabolic studies with 5-fluorocytosine-6-^{14}C in mouse, rat, rabbit, dog and man. Chemotherapy 22: 137-153, 1976.

100. Polak A, Scholer HJ: Mode of action of 5-fluorocytosine and mechanisms of resistance. Chemotherapy 21: 113-130, 1975.

101. Powell SJ: Therapy of amebiasis. Bull NY Acad Med 47: 469-477, 1971.

102. Pratt WB: The inhibitors of cell wall synthesis. in Chemotherapy of Infection, Ch.2, p.22-84. New York: Oxford University Press, 1977.

103. Ray WA, Federspiel CF, Schaffner W: Prescribing of chloramphenicol in ambulatory practice. An epidemiological study among Tennessee Medicaid recipients. Ann Intern Med 84: 266-270, 1976.

104. Record CO, Skinner JM, Sleight P, Speller DCE: Candida endocarditis treated with 5-fluorocytosine. Br Med J 1: 262-264, 1971.

105. Riley HD: Vancomycin and novobiocin. Med Clin North Am 54: 1277-1289, 1970.

106. Robertson DM, Riley FC, Hermans PE: Endogenous Candida oculomycosis. Report of two patients treated with flucytosine. Arch Ophthalmol 91: 33-38, 1974.

107. Rosch JM, Pazin GJ, Fireman P: Reduction of amphotericin B nephrotoxicity with mannitol. JAMA 235: 1995-1996, 1976.

108. Rothstein E, Clancy DD: Toxicity of disulfiram combined with metronidazole. N Engl J Med 280: 1006-1007, 1969.

109. Rountree PM, Beard MA: Hospital strains of *Staphylococcus aureus*, with

particular reference to methicillin resistant strains. Med J Aust 2: 1163-1168, 1968.

110. SANDERS CV, HANNA BJ, LEWIS AC: Metronidazole in the treatment of anaerobic infections. Am Rev Resp Dis 120: 337-343, 1979.

111. SCHÖNEBECK J, SEGERBRAND E: Candida albicans septicaemia during first half of pregnancy successfully treated with 5-fluorocytosine. Br Med J 4: 337-338, 1973.

112. STUART-HARRIS C: Amantadine - What next? J Antimicrob Chemother 4: 295-297, 1978.

113. STUART-HARRIS CH, SCHILD GC: Influenza. The Viruses and the Disease. London : Arnold, 1976.

114. SYMMERS WC: Amphotericin pharmacophobia. Br Med J 4: 460-463, 1973.

115. SYMPOSIUM: New possibilities in the treatment of systemic mycoses. Reports on the experimental and clinical evaluation of miconazole. Proc R Soc Med 70 (Suppl 1): 1977.

116. TALLY FP, SUTTER VL, FINEGOLD SM: Treatment of anaerobic infections with me-tronidazole. Antimicrob Agents Chemother 7: 672-675, 1975.

117. TEDESCO F, MARKHAM R, GURWITH M, CHRISTIE D, BARTLETT JG: Oral vancomycin for antibiotic-associated pseudomembranous colitis. Lancet 2: 226-228, 1978.

118. TOGO Y, HORNICK RB, FELITTI VJ, KAUFMAN ML, DAWKINS AT, KILPE VE, CLAGHORN JL: Evaluation of therapeutic efficacy of amantadine in patients with naturally occurring A_2 influenza. JAMA 211: 1149-1156, 1970.

119. TOLMAN KG, SANNELLA JJ, FRESTON JW: Chemical structure of erythromycin and hepatotoxicity. Ann Intern Med 81: 58-60, 1974.

120. TSAI TF, FINN DR, PLIKAYTIS BD, McCAULEY W, MARTIN SM, FRASER DW: Legion-naires' disease: clinical features of the epidemic in Philadelphia. Ann Intern Med 90: 509-517, 1979.

121. TUAZON CU, LIN MYC, SHEAGREN JN: In vitro activity of rifampicin alone and in combination with nafcillin and vancomycin against pathogenic strains of *Staphylococcus aureus*. Antimicrob Agents Chemother 13: 759-761, 1978.

122. UTZ JP, BENNETT JE, BRANDRISS MW, BUTLER WT, HILL GJ: Amphotericin B toxicity. Ann Intern Med 61: 334-354, 1964.

123. UTZ JP, GARRIQUES IL, SANDE MA, WARNER JF, MANDELL GL, McGEHEE RF, DUMA RJ, SHADOMY S: Therapy of cryptococcosis with a combination of flucytosine and amphotericin B. J Infect Dis 132: 368-373, 1975.

124. VAIDYA GN, BERGER HW, GRANADA MG: Pulmonary infection due to Torulopsis glabrata: report of a case treated with flucytosine. Chest 69: 788-790, 1976.

125. VALE JA, MACLEAN KS: Amantadine-induced heart failure. Lancet 1: 548, 1977.

126. VAN MARION WF, VAN DER MEER JWM, KALFF MW, SCHICHT SM: Ototoxicity of erythromycin. Lancet 2: 214-215, 1978.

127. WARD JI, WEEKS M, ALLEN D, HUTCHESON RH, ANDERSON R, FRASER DW, KAUFMAN L, AJELLO L, SPICKARD A: Acute histoplasmosis: clinical, epidemiologic and serologic findings of an outbreak associated with exposure to a fallen tree. Am J Med 66: 587-595, 1979.

128. WEINSTEIN L, CHANG TW: The chemotherapy of viral infections. N Engl J Med 289: 725-730, 1973.

129. WESTENFELDER GO, PATERSON RY, REISBERG BE, CARLSON GM Vancomycin-streptomycin synergism in enterococcal endocarditis. JAMA 223: 37-40, 1973.
130. WORMSER GP, KEUSCH GT: Trimethoprim-sulfamethoxazole in the United States. Ann Intern Med 91: 420-429, 1979.
131. YAMAGUCHI H: Antagonistic action of lipid components of membranes from *Candida albicans* and various other lipids on two imidazole antimycotics, clotrimazole and miconazole. Antimicrob Agents Chemother 12: 16-25, 1977.
132. YUNIS AA, BLOOMBERG GR: Chloramphenicol toxicity: clinical features and pathogenesis. Progr Haematol 4: 138-159, 1964.
133. YUNIS AA, SMITH US, RESTREPO A: Reversible bone marrow suppression from chloramphenicol: a consequence of mitochondrial injury. Arch Intern Med 126: 272-275, 1970.

6

Antimicrobial Agents III: Pulmonary Tuberculosis

The treatment of pulmonary tuberculosis presents a fascinating challenge to the respiratory physician because modern chemotherapeutic agents offer the near certainty of cure, provided that a proven regimen of treatment is applied assiduously for a sufficient length of time. The difficulty lies in maintaining treatment with a combination of potentially toxic drugs for a long time, since the regimens which embody "standard" chemotherapy require sustained treatment for 9 to 18 months, although the efficacy of shorter regimens lasting 4 to 6 months is being actively investigated.[46,154]

Combination chemotherapy is essential in treating tuberculosis in order to prevent the emergence of resistance and to eradicate the infection in the shortest possible time, but the number of drugs used should be kept to the minimum which is compatible with these objectives in order to reduce the incidence of adverse reactions. Various treatment programmes have been compared in carefully controlled trials, and the regimens recommended later in this chapter are based on the results of such investigations. The essential factor in successful antituberculosis therapy is regular surveillance throughout the course of treatment by an experienced health care team, an aspect of management which increases in importance as the total dosage or duration of therapy are reduced in line with current recommendations for short-course chemotherapeutic regimens.

The drugs used in the treatment of pulmonary tuberculosis fall into two groups: the "first-line" drugs (isoniazid, rifampin, ethambutol, streptomycin, and pyrazinamide) which are the most effective and least toxic; and the "second-line" drugs (aminosalicylic acid [PAS], thiacetazone, ethionamide, cycloserine, capreomycin, viomycin-and kanamycin) which are mainly used in the retreatment of infections resistant to the first-line drugs or, in the case of thiacetazone, when cost is an important factor in the choice of regimen.

FIRST-LINE DRUGS

Isoniazid

Isoniazid is a highly effective bactericidal antituberculosis agent which is included in all current chemotherapeutic regimens against susceptible mycobacteria. The discovery of its antituberculosis action, based on the observation that nicotinamide was tuberculostatic, followed the experimental study of many pyridine derivatives including the congeners of isonicotinic acid; one of these, isonicotinic acid hydrazide (INAH, isoniazid) proved to be effective *in vitro* and *in vivo,* and it has become the mainstay of antituberculosis therapy.

Mechanism and Spectrum of Action   Isoniazid is effective against actively growing mycobacteria but less so against resting organisms. Its precise mode of action is unknown, but one possibility which has some experimental support is that isoniazid inhibits synthesis of mycolytic acids which are components of mycobacterial cell walls.[173] Such an action would explain the selective toxicity of isoniazid, since mycolytic acids are not present in animal cells or in other micro-organisms. The spectrum of activity of isoniazid is therefore confined to the mycobacteria, although some atypical mycobacteria are resistant. Even *M. tuberculosis* readily develops resistance to isoniazid if the drug is used alone for the treatment of tuberculosis. Except for preventive treatment in certain specific situations (see *Clinical Uses* below), isoniazid is therefore always used in conjunction with at least one other chemotherapeutic agent.

Clinical Pharmacology   Isoniazid is readily absorbed from the gastrointestinal tract and is nearly always administered by the oral route. A peak serum level of 10–15 μg/ml is achieved 1 to 2 hours after administering a large oral dose and the drug is widely distributed in all body tissues including pleural effusions and cerebrospinal fluid. It penetrates caseous tissue and macrophages, being effective against intracellular mycobacteria. The serum half-life varies according to the inactivator status of the patient which is genetically determined (see Chapter 1), being 0.5–1.0 hours in rapid inactivators and 2–4 hours in slow inactivators. Isoniazid is metabolised by acetylation in the liver to acetyl isoniazid[131] by the enzyme N-acetyltransferase, and it is excreted in the urine largely as its metabolites, acetylisoniazid and isonicotinic acid, although a small amount of the drug is excreted unchanged. Some dosage modification may be necessary in patients with severe renal failure (creatinine clearance less than 10 ml/min) if they are slow inactivators,[14] and in such cases the serum isoniazid level should be monitored.[20] It is not clear whether dosage adjustment is necessary in patients with impaired hepatic function, although there is some evidence that serum isoniazid levels are increased in chronic liver disease.[1]

The genetically determined variability in the rate of isoniazid acetylation has a significant effect on its clinical application. *In vitro* studies have shown that mycobacteria exposed to inhibitory concentrations of isoniazid for 10 hours or longer lose viability, but if inhibition is short-lived they slowly recover the capacity to synthesise mycolytic acid.[165] This observation may explain the loss of therapeutic effectiveness of isoniazid in patients who are rapid inactivators and who are treated by intermittent dosage regimens if the doses are spaced too far apart, that is, less often than twice weekly.[169] In contrast, the neurotoxic effects of isoniazid are more likely to occur in slow inactivators who have a greater tendency to accumulate the drug, particularly those treated by high dosage intermittent regimens, and some authorities advocate the administration of prophylactic pyridoxine to all patients receiving isoniazid therapy in order to prevent possible neuropathic side-effects.[176] It has been suggested that hepatotoxic metabolites are more likely to accumulate in rapid inactivators who would therefore be more liable to isoniazid induced hepatic necrosis,[122] but measurements have shown that the actual exposure of rapid inactivators to the relevant compound, acetylhydrazine, is no greater than that of slow inactivators,[56] and clinical studies confirm that there is no increased risk of hepatic toxicity among rapid inactivators of isoniazid whether treated with isoniazid alone or with a combination of isoniazid and rifampin.[41]

Administration and Dosage   Isoniazid is normally administered by mouth, either as tablets or as a syrup/elixir. A parenteral preparation is also available for intramuscular injection in patients who are vomiting or who are otherwise unable to take oral treatment. For daily therapy the usual dosage is 5 mg/kg body weight in adults to a maximum of 300 mg given as a single daily dose, while children tolerate higher doses and should be given 10–15 mg/kg per day. For those on a twice-weekly intermittent regimen, the dose is higher than the customary daily dose, usually 15 mg/kg body weight.[145] I personally favour the addition of 10 mg of pyridoxine daily to the regimen of all patients taking isoniazid, in order to avoid the possibility of neurotoxic side-effects. This precaution is particularly important in adults receiving large doses of 10 mg/kg or more of isoniazid per day or in those who may be predisposed to peripheral neuropathies by other conditions such as alcoholism or malnutrition. Combined preparations of isoniazid with rifampin, ethambutol, or aminosalicylic acid are widely used, having the advantages of reducing the number of tablets which the patient has to take and ensuring that therapy with a single agent is precluded.

Slow-release isoniazid preparations (matrix isoniazid) have been studied in an attempt to provide an effective once-weekly intermittent regimen, but these have proved unsatisfactory because the blood concentrations achieved in rapid isoniazid inactivators are inadequate except with doses which would be likely to cause toxicity in slow inactivators.[144]

Toxic Effects   The neurotoxic effects of isoniazid are related to the dosage of the drug and are more likely to occur in slow than in rapid inactivators. Peripheral neuropathy is attributed to deficiency of pyridoxine, which is excreted to excess in patients receiving isoniazid, and the neuropathy responds promptly to pyridoxine therapy. It is chacterised by tingling and numbness in the legs or feet, and occasionally in the hands.[74] Central nervous effects include dizziness which is usually related to high dosage, insomnia, restlessness and memory loss at ordinary dosage, and occasionally disabling loss of memory. The drug may precipitate fits in previously stable epileptics, and in excessive overdosage it may cause acute psychosis, convulsions, and coma. Muscle pains, arthropathy, and "frozen shoulder" are occasional symptoms of isoniazid toxicity.[130]

Hypersensitivity reactions are not common, but occasionally fever[94] or skin rashes may occur.[15] Isoniazid is one of the drugs which can induce the syndrome of systemic lupus erythematosus, and although this occurs very rarely, antinuclear antibodies can be found in a substantial proportion of patients treated with the drug.[3]

Probably the most important adverse effect of isoniazid is hepatotoxicity which usually occurs as a reversible asymptomatic elevation of serum transaminase but may occasionally be manifested as clinical jaundice preceded by gastrointestinal symptoms: rarely this leads to massive hepatic necrosis.[17] Hepatotoxicity may occur at any time during the course of isoniazid therapy in approximately 20 percent of individuals who receive the drug, and in about 5 percent it has to be withdrawn because continuing elevation of SGOT levels or clinical symptoms suggest that hepatocellular damage is developing.[29,147] In the great majority of patients the abnormalities subside without any alteration in the isoniazid regimen, and it is usual to persist with treatment unless the serum glutamic oxaloacetic transaminase (SGOT) value exceeds 5 times the upper limit of normal or if symptoms and signs of hepatitis develop.[30] Because progressive liver damage is more likely to occur in older patients[99] there is a school of thought which recommends that medication should be stopped in patients over 35 years of age who have any degree of biochemical abnormality but at present there is no evidence that harm comes from continued use of the drug when SGOT levels are mildly elevated. Biochemical monitoring has been advocated as a means of detecting liver toxicity at an early stage,[30] but the frequency with which non-significant biochemical abnormalities develop in isoniazid treated patients is too great for this to be a useful screening mechanism, and most clinicians rely on clinical evidence of jaundice as the best indication for premature withdrawal of the drug.

The development of isoniazid hepatotoxicity does not correlate with the plasma drug concentration and is probably unrelated to the inactivator status of the patient.[41] It is considered unlikely to be due to an allergic phenomenon,[123] and its exact mechanism is at present undefined. Isoniazid is commonly administered concurrently with other hepatotoxic antituberculosis agents, especially rifampin, and most evidence suggests that rifampin hepatotoxicity is enhanced by isoniazid,[108] particularly in slow inactivators who have higher isoniazid serum levels.[76,103]

Drug Interactions Concurrent administration of isoniazid inhibits the metabolism of diphenylhydantoin (phenytoin) leading to unexpectedly high serum diphenylhydantoin levels which cause toxic central nervous effects such as disorientation, drowsiness, lethargy, ataxia, nystagmus, psychotic behaviour, and coma.[121] It has been proposed that isoniazid interferes with the parahydroxylation of diphenylhydantoin, which is the rate-limiting step in diphenylhydantoin metabolism,[102] but the exact mechanism has not yet been defined. Slow isoniazid acetylators are more likely to be at risk,[21] but not invariably so, and determination of acetylator phenotype does not help in the management of patients who need to be treated with both drugs. In practice, dosage reduction of diphenylhydantoin from 300 to 100–200 mg daily is indicated if clinical signs of toxicity are encountered, and if facilities are available for measuring serum diphenylhydantoin concentration it is advisable to avoid levels greater than 20 µg/ml.

Clinical Uses Isoniazid is the most widely used of the antituberculosis agents because of its effectiveness, cheapness, and relative lack of toxicity. Used in combination with other chemotherapeutic agents it has an important place in the treatment of most mycobacterial infections, even those which are relatively resistant, such as *M. kansasii*.[80] Commonly used antituberculosis therapeutic regimens which include isoniazid are described in the last section of this chapter.

Isoniazid is used as a single agent in the preventive treatment of tuberculosis (sometimes called "disease prophylaxis"), in which chemotherapy is given to individuals who show evidence of infection although there is no sign of disease at the time.[60] The use of isoniazid alone for chemoprophylaxis has only very rarely led to the emergence of resistant strains of *M. tuberculosis*.[59] The indications for preventive therapy with isoniazid can be categorised as follows:

1. Household contacts of an active case of tuberculosis.
2. Radiological evidence of apparently inactive tuberculosis.
3. Positive tuberculin reactors: *either* recently converted from negative to positive within the past two years; *or* with increased susceptibility to the disease because of complicating factors such as long-term corticosteroid or immunosuppressive therapy, diabetes mellitus, or silicosis; or below the age of 35 years who have not received BCG vaccination.

The reason for giving preventive isoniazid therapy to positive reactors below the age of 35 is based on the argument that these individuals have a relatively high risk of developing active disease but little likelihood of suffering isoniazid hepatotoxicity, which occurs mainly in older age groups. The above criteria are based on the code of practice recommended by the American Thoracic Society and the U.S. Public Health Service Center for Disease Control joint statement,[6] and are illustrated diagramatically in Figure 6-1. Recent evidence suggests that they are followed fairly closely by metropolitan clinics in the United States.[111]

In Britain the practice of administering chemotherapy as a preventive measure is less rigidly defined but follows the same general pattern as described above,[96] although perhaps greater emphasis is placed on the preventive value of universal BCG vaccination of tuberculin-negative school children between the ages of 10 and 14 years.[24,157] Nevertheless it is common practice in Britain to give chemotherapy to children up to 6 years old with strong positive tuberculin reactions, especially if they have been identified as a result of contact examination, and often to older children who are found to be strongly tuberculin-positive as a result of school-entry or pre-BCG testing. The case for

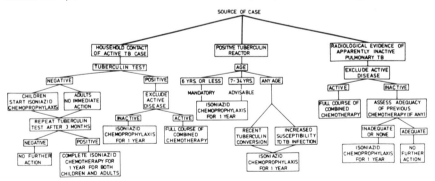

Figure 6-1 *Recommendations in the United States for the use of isoniazid in the preventive therapy of pulmonary tuberculosis.* Note. *Notwithstanding the indications depicted in the above diagram it is always necessary to consider possible contraindications before embarking on a 1-year course of chemoprophylaxis with isoniazid. These include: (1) previous reactions to isoniazid, (2) possible drug interactions with other medication, (3) excessive alcohol intake, (4) chronic liver disease, (5) pregnancy.*

giving preventive chemotherapy to all tuberculin-positive contacts and to people with apparently inactive radiographic lesions is also recognised,[23] but British physicians appear to be more reluctant than their American colleagues to offer year-long chemotherapy to people who are not ill, who have no complaints, and whose tuberculous infection presents only a very small risk.[26] The relatively high risk of tuberculosis among Asian immigrant communities in Britain provides a strong argument for giving chemotherapy to all with a moderate or strongly positive tuberculin reaction, but in such cases there is an increased likelihood that infection is due to an isoniazid-resistant organism, and an alternative regimen of chemoprophylaxis may be advisable for fear of failure with isoniazid alone.[58]

Single chemotherapy with isoniazid also has a place in the treatment of progressive BCG infection, which rarely complicates BCG vaccination. Such cases are usually characterised by regional lymphadenitis and localised abscesses.[156] Treatment with isoniazid in the usual dosage for 3 months is sufficient to control the infection.

Rifampin (Rifampicin)

Rifampin is a semi-synthetic derivative of the antibiotic rifamycin B, which was isolated from *Streptomyces mediterranei*. The drug has assumed increasing importance in antituberculosis chemotherapy because of its effectiveness in short-course treatment, one of the main drawbacks being its rather high cost which may amount to 90 percent of the total drug cost of some widely used therapeutic regimens.[70] Apart from its role in the therapy of tuberculosis rifampin is effective against a wide range of bacterial infections and offers considerable promise in treating some systemic mycoses. In the United States its use is currently limited to the treatment of pulmonary tuberculosis and to a minor role in treating nasopharyngeal carriers of *Neisseria meningitidis*, while in Britain and France rifampin is mainly used for tuberculosis chemotherapy. These limitations have the theoretical advantage of reducing the risk of encouraging rifampin-resistant strains of *Mycobacterium tuberculosis*, although one recent investigation of the prevalence of such strains in countries where rifampin is used unreservedly did not demonstrate a significant excess of resistant organisms.[2]

The drug is bactericidal and acts by inhibiting the activity of DNA-dependent RNA polymerase, which is the enzyme responsible for catalysing the polymerisation of certain ribonucleotides into RNA molecules, a step which transfers genetic data from DNA to RNA.[174] The selective toxicity of rifampin depends upon the relative insensitivity of mammalian RNA polymerases to the drug.[175]

Spectrum of Action   Rifampin is highly active against *Mycobacterium tuber-culosis* and *M. leprae,* but there is marked variation in its activity against other mycobacteria, some such as *M. kansasii* and *M. marinum* being usually susceptible while others such as the *avium-intercellulare* group are usually resistant. The drug is active against Gram-positive cocci including penicillin and methicillin-resistant *Staphylococcus aureus* and against *Neisseria* species which are highly sensitive, but in general it has a rather lower degree of activity against Gram-negative bacilli. Rifampin's potential for synergism, particularly with trimethoprim against Gram-negative pathogens[79] and with amphotericin B against fungi is the subject of current investigations.

Primary resistance to rifampin is low[113] but resistance develops rapidly during therapy among most micro-organisms which are initially sensitive, usually resulting from a single, large-step mutation which alters the conformation of DNA-dependent RNA polymerases and prevents rifampin binding.[97] In the therapy of tuberculosis it is therefore always used in combination with other drugs.

Clinical Pharmacology   The drug is readily absorbed from the gastrointestinal tract, but the presence of food diminishes absorption and rifampin is therefore usually administered on an empty stomach. After a normal oral dose of 600 mg, a peak blood level of about 7 µg/ml is reached after 1.5–3.0 hours, and effective therapeutic blood levels are maintained for 12–24 hours. The drug is widely distributed in all body tissues including CSF and pleural exudate,[19] and because it is lipid soluble it penetrates cells and kills intracellular micro-organisms. About 85 percent of the drug is protein bound.

Rifampin is partly deacetylated in the liver and is excreted in the bile in both the deacetylated form and as the unaltered drug. The latter is reabsorbed and recirculates through the liver, but the metabolite is very largely excreted in the faeces. Eventually about 60 percent of the drug is excreted in this way. Slight accumulation may occur in patients with hepatic dysfunction due to cirrhosis,[1] suggesting that care should be exercised in the use of rifampin in the presence of liver disease. Rifampin induces hepatic metabolising enzymes, including those responsible for its own metabolism, leading to a gradual reduction in the serum half-life during the first week of therapy, but this is insufficient to alter the therapeutic effectiveness of the drug and no dosage adjustment is necessary. Rifampin and its deacetylated metabolite are also excreted to a lesser extent in the urine,[101] but it does not accumulate in patients with impaired renal function and no reduction in dose is indicated.

Administration and Dosage   The drug is normally given by mouth in a single daily dose in the early morning 1 hour before breakfast. The usual

dose in adults is approximately 10 mg/kg body weight, often standardised
to 450 mg per day in those weighing less than 50 kg and 600 mg per day for
the remainder. In children the recommended dose is 10–20 mg/kg up to
a maximum of 600 mg daily. Rifampin is also used in intermittent twice-
weekly antituberculosis regimens using doses of 600 mg or 900 mg twice
weekly.[153]

Toxicity[72]   Although rifampin can cause a wide range of adverse effects, they
are relatively infrequent, and only rarely do they necessitate the drug's withdrawal. They include the following:

1. Gastrointestinal disturbances, such as nausea, abdominal distension,
    epigastric discomfort, and diarrhoea which seldom require a change of
    therapy.
2. Drug-induced hepatitis, which is sometimes difficult to attribute speci-
    fically to rifampin because the drug is commonly used in combination
    with other hepatotoxic agents, notably isoniazid. It usually takes the
    form of a transient elevation in liver enzymes during the early weeks of
    antituberculosis therapy which subsides spontaneously whether treat-
    ment is discontinued or not,[148] but the occasional development of a
    rising serum bilirubin level or clinical jaundice is the sign for immedi-
    ate withdrawal. Jaundice is more likely to occur in the elderly[110]
    and in alcoholics or those with pre-existing hepatic damage,[167] but the
    risk of hepatitis in patients with normal liver function appears to be
    slight.
3. Hypersensitivity reactions to rifampin are rare but various forms of
    rashes, urticaria, itching of the skin, and redness or watering of the
    eyes have been described, and these may necessitate withdrawal of
    rifampin from the treatment regimen.[32,126] Anaphylactic shock can also
    occur.[124]
4. Neurological symptoms of headache, drowsiness, dizziness, and atax-
    ia occur occasionally. A case has been reported of acute psychosis
    characterised by disorientation, confusion, agitation, delusions, and
    hallucinations which developed while the patient was receiving rifam-
    pin and rapidly resolved when the drug was withdrawn.[136]

Several other important adverse effects are largely but not entirely confined to patients treated with high-dosage intermittent regimens or who take
their treatment irregularly with long intervals between doses. These effects
include the following:

5. An influenza-like reaction ("flu syndrome"), characterised by fever,
    chills, muscle aching, nausea, and vomiting, may come on several

weeks or months after the commencement of therapy, usually precipitated 1 or 2 hours after the ingestion of a dose. It subsides spontaneously after a few hours but recurs with subsequent doses and is much more common in patients on once-weekly regimens who are taking higher doses, that is, 1,200 mg or more.[8,134] It is attributed to an immunological reaction, preventable by continuous treatment which is thought to result in the neutralisation of rifampin antibodies.[12] This can be avoided by reverting to daily administration.

6. Thrombocytopenia, which may be associated with bleeding, is another complication occurring most commonly with high-dose intermittent therapy,[18] and it appears to have an immunological basis. Because of the risk of bleeding, the drug is contraindicated if thrombocytopenia is observed.

7. Renal failure seems to occur when rifampin is taken intermittently or is resumed after an interval[62,143] and is usually due to acute tubular necrosis which may have an immunological basis, since high titres of antibodies to rifampin have been observed.[33] Withdrawal of the drug leads to recovery of renal function, but further use of rifampin is contraindicated.

Rifampin has several other biological effects which are of interest but which do not appear to affect the clinical use of the drug. It has been reported to have immunosuppressive effects on both humoral and cell-mediated immunity, but such changes that have been observed are readily reversed after treatment is discontinued. Therapy with rifampin is also associated with light-chain proteinuria in the majority of patients.[75] A harmless reddish discolouration of the urine and faeces, sometimes also affecting tears, saliva and sweat, may be produced by rifampin and its metabolites, and the patient should be warned of this possibility at the commencement of treatment, in order to allay unnecessary anxiety.

Drug Interactions   Because of its enzyme-inducing effect on the hepatic microsomal enzymes responsible for drug metabolism, rifampin increases the rate of elimination of several important drugs if administered concurrently with them. Included among these are the following:

1. Warfarin, leading to the need for an unusually high dose to maintain effective anticoagulation.[142]
2. Tolbutamide.[164]
3. Corticosteroids.[51]
4. Oestrogens, leading to menstrual irregularity and unwanted pregnancy in patients taking oral contraceptive agents.[155]

Concurrent administration of para-aminosalicylic acid impairs the absorption of rifampin, and careful spacing of these two drugs is therefore necessary when they are used together in the treatment of tuberculosis.

Clinical Uses The primary role of rifampin is in the treatment of mycobacterial infections in combination with one or more other chemotherapeutic agents. The regimens which are currently recommended for the treatment of pulmonary tuberculosis vary considerably in their content and duration from one country to the next, but there is growing recognition of the fact that the rifampin-isoniazid combination provides an essential element in most of the successful short-course regimens which have recently been on trial.[70] The place of rifampin in some widely used standard, intermittent, and short-course regimens is described in a later section of this chapter. Rifampin is also used in retreatment of patients who did not receive the drug during initial therapy[109,172] and in the therapy of extrapulmonary tuberculosis, for example, in tuberculous meningitis.[104] It has been included in treatment regimens for atypical mycobacteria, being often effective against *M. kansasii*.[53]

Although it is effective in the treatment of other infections which may cause pulmonary disease such as streptococcal or staphylococcal pneumonias, rifampin should generally be avoided for this purpose because other effective antibiotics are available and its use could delay the diagnosis of underlying tuberculosis or lead to the development of resistant mycobacteria. On the basis of *in vitro* evidence that *Legionella pneumophila* is highly susceptible to rifampin,[168] its use is justified in the treatment of legionnaire's disease that fails to respond to erythromycin or tetracycline. It has also proved effective in the treatment of the multiple-resistant pneumococcal pneumonia recently encountered in South African hospitals,[93] and against resistant staphylococcal endocarditis[128]: it is clearly right to use rifampin in the treatment of serious infection by susceptible organisms which are insensitive to the antibiotics conventionally used, but in such cases it is important to combine rifampin with another effective antibiotic in order to avoid the rapid emergence of resistance.

Rifampin is also recommended in the United States for the preventive treatment of nasopharyngeal carriers of meningococci. *Mycobacterium leprae* also responds to rifampin.

Ethambutol

The value of ethambutol in the initial treatment of tuberculosis is well established and the drug is used in most of the current standard regimens. It is a synthetic tuberculostatic agent which was discovered in 1961 and has the advantage of relative cheapness, low toxicity, and effectiveness by oral administration. Although its mode of action is uncertain, it is thought to inhibit RNA synthesis by mycobacteria.[63]

Spectrum of Activity The activity of ethambutol is limited to the mycobacteria. It is highly active against *M. tuberculosis,* and is usually active against *M. kansasii* and some strains of the *avium-intracellulare* group which are a rare cause of pulmonary infection. The prevalence of primary resistance of *M. tuberculosis* to ethambutol is very low in the United States[161] and in Britain,[113] but ethambutol-resistant strains develop readily if the drug is used on its own. It is therefore customarily used in combination with one or more other effective antituberculosis agents.

Clinical Pharmacology About 80 percent of an oral dose of ethambutol is absorbed, while the remainder is excreted unchanged in the faeces. After oral administration of a single dose of 25 mg/kg body weight a maximum serum concentration of 2–6 μg/ml is achieved after 2–4 hours falling to 0.4 μg/ml at 10 hours, the elimination half-life being just over 4 hours in patients with normal renal function.[43,105] Approximately 70 percent of the ingested dose is excreted unchanged by the kidneys and up to 15 percent is metabolised to inactive compounds which are also excreted in the urine.[129] Ethambutol is widely distributed in body tissues but it only achieves therapeutic levels in the cerebrospinal fluid in the presence of meningeal inflammation.[133] The drug is preferentially concentrated in red blood cells and is about 20–30 percent protein bound.[105]

Administration and Dosage Ethambutol is administered by mouth in a single daily dose of 15–25 mg/kg body weight in adults and children over 10 years of age. Below this age a dose of 35 mg/kg body weight has been recommended in order to achieve a peak serum concentration of more than 2 μg/ml,[91] but the risk of ocular toxicity and the difficulty of recognising it in small children should be borne in mind (see below).

Ethambutol is commonly used in the first two months of combined antituberculosis therapy in a dose of 25 mg/kg body weight and is then either stopped or in some regimens maintained at a lower dose of 15 mg/kg throughout the continuation phase of treatment to reduce the risk of ocular toxicity, which is dose related. To minimise this risk, my own practice is to use the 15 mg/kg dose schedule even during initial therapy, since it has proved to be clinically effective.[42]

Modification of ethambutol dosage is essential in patients with renal failure because elimination is largely dependent upon renal function. It can be achieved by giving the usual 25 mg/kg dose but prolonging the dosage interval to 36–48 hours in patients with a creatinine clearance of 10–50 ml/min, and to 48 hours or longer if the creatinine clearance is less than 10 ml/min.[14,92] As a guide to dosage in such patients it is important to measure serum ethambutol concentrations with the aim of obtaining a peak plasma level not greater than 5 μg/ml at 2 hours, declining to 0.5 μg/ml before the next dose. The clearance of

ethambutol is increased by peritoneal and haemodialysis, making dosage supplementation necessary. An alternative dosage schedule which has been recommended for the dialysis patient is 1.5 mg/kg body weight 3 times daily
increasing to 2.0 mg/kg for the predialysis dose.[34] This is said to achieve a
stable blood level of 2.0 μg/ml.

Toxic Effects   The most important adverse effect of ethambutol is *retrobulbar
neuritis,* causing either progressive loss of peripheral vision or impaired visual
acuity, particularly to green, which may progress to a central scotoma.[112] Optic
neuritis occurred in only 1 percent of patients treated with the customary
regimen (25 mg/kg daily for 2 months followed by a maintenance dose of 15
mg/kg),[11] but the continuation of the higher dose for 6 months led to a 5 percent
incidence of ocular complications.[9] The changes are usually but not always
reversed on withdrawal of the drug. A comprehensive ophthalmological examination should be carried out to provide a reference point before ethambutol
therapy is started, and patients should be questioned regularly about their
eyesight and warned to report any visual disturbance promptly.

The other complications of ethambutol treatment are rare. *Peripheral
neuropathy* can occur independently of isoniazid therapy,[170] and *nephrotoxicity* has been observed in 2 patients on combined antituberculosis therapy
whose renal function only recovered when ethambutol was withdrawn.[37]
Hyperuricaemia occurs in a substantial proportion of patients treated with the
drug due to a decrease in the renal clearance of uric acid,[135] and occasionally
acute gout may be precipitated.[150] *Allergic skin eruptions* have been
described.[127]

Clinical Uses   The combination of ethambutol with isoniazid is the most frequently used standard antituberculosis regimen in the United States,[10] and
ethambutol is an important component of the initial phase of therapy in the
standard 9-month regimen used in the United Kingdom at present.[117] It does not
contribute significantly to 6-month short-course chemotherapy,[68] and in this
role it is less effective than pyrazinamide in preventing relapse.[84] It appears to
be effective in twice-weekly intermittent chemotherapy when combined with
isoniazid after a 2- or 3-month initial phase of daily triple therapy,[5] and its
potential in this respect has been recently reviewed.[183]

Although isoniazid alone is usually all that is needed in chemoprophylaxis
of tuberculosis, some clinicians prefer to use a combination of isoniazid and
ethambutol,[96] and it is logical to do so if the patient originates from a community in which the prevalence of isoniazid resistance is high, such as among Asian
immigrants to Britain or oriental immigrants to the United States.[28] In the chemoprophylaxis of contacts of patients with isoniazid-resistant tuberculosis it
has been suggested that ethambutol may be used as an alternative preventive
agent.[58]

Ethambutol is effective in the retreatment of tuberculosis infections resistant to other chemotherapeutic agents and is used successfully in treating some atypical mycobacterial infections, such as those due to *M. kansasii.*[80]

Pyrazinamide

Although the bacteriostatic activity of pyrazinamide against tuberculosis was recognised as long ago as 1952,[181] until recently its use has largely been confined to the retreatment of infections resistant to the standard drugs, because of its low *in vitro* activity and significant record of hepatotoxicity. In the last few years there has been increasing clinical evidence to suggest that pyrazinamide can make an effective contribution to 6-month regimens,[45,84] possibly by using it only during the first 2 months of combined therapy.[154] The role of pyrazinamide is therefore undergoing reappraisal,[68] and it appears that the risk of hepatitis from the use of pyrazinamide in these short-course regimens is much lower than was suggested by earlier studies, in which larger doses were used for longer periods.

Pyrazinamide, which is a synthetic derivative of nicotinamide, has no antimycobacterial activity at neutral pH,[141] but it is effective against phagocytosed living tubercle bacilli, presumably due to the acid pH within macrophages.[31] It is active only against *Mycobacterium tuberculosis,* which rapidly develops resistance to pyrazinamide unless the drug is used in combination with other effective antituberculosis agents.

Clinical Pharmacology Pyrazinamide is readily absorbed from the gastrointestinal tract, and absorption is virtually complete. A peak serum concentration of up to 65 μg/ml is achieved within 2 hours of the oral administration of pyrazinamide in a single dose of 20 mg/kg body weight.[162] The serum half-life is approximately 6 hours.[54] The drug has been shown to penetrate the liver, kidneys, and lungs, and apparently it can reach therapeutic levels in the CSF of patients with tuberculous meningitis.[64] Pyrazinamide and its metabolites, pyrazinoic and 5-hydroxypyrazinoic acids, are filtered by the glomeruli, but nearly all of the unchanged drug is reabsorbed from the renal tubules while the metabolites are excreted in the urine. Pyrazinoic acid suppresses the tubular secretion of uric acid, which leads to hyperuricaemia and occasionally to clinical gout.[39] Pyrazinamide accumulates in jaundiced patients, (Krüger-Thiemer, 1961, quoted in reference 162), suggesting that it is metabolised in the liver.

Administration and Dosage Early trials of pyrazinamide showed that if the daily dose was maintained at 40–50 mg/kg body weight the incidence of hepatitis was unacceptably high, and it was this which led clinicians to discard it as a first-line drug.[73] This view has been revised by more recent assessments, which indicate that the likelihood of hepatic toxicity is very small when lower doses are used in 6-month regimens of combined chemotherapy.[69] The drug is available in tablets containing 0.5 g, which should be administered in an adult daily dosage of 20–35 mk/kg body weight, given in 2 or 3 divided doses, commonly 1 g twice daily or 0.5 g 3 times daily. It has also been used in intermittent regimens in a dose of 40–60 mg/kg taken twice or 3 times weekly or even 90 mg/kg body weight taken once weekly,[66] without serious incidence of side-effects.

Toxicity   The most important adverse effect of pyrazinamide is its tendency to cause hepatitis. As indicated above, the effect appears to be dose related,[171] and symptoms of hepatitis, liver enlargement, jaundice and, rarely, death due to hepatic necrosis have been described in patients treated for periods of 3 to 6 months with pyrazinamide in doses of 40–50 mg/kg body weight per day, that is, approximately 3 g per day.[115,171] More recent trials of its effectiveness and toxicity in various chemotherapeutic regimens in Hong Kong have demonstrated a very small incidence of jaundice in patients treated with lower doses of pyrazinamide, for example, 20–35 mg/kg body weight per day, although an increase in hepatic enzyme levels occurred in up to 9 percent of patients.[87] In the present state of knowledge it would seem sensible to avoid the use of pyrazinamide in people with impaired hepatic function, to withdraw the drug if serum enzyme (SGOT) levels become markedly elevated during the course of treatment, and to advise patients to report promptly all symptoms or signs suggestive of hepatic toxicity.

Arthralgia mainly affecting the shoulders, knees, and fingers occurs quite commonly during pyrazinamide administration,[87] and in patients on daily therapy it is associated with high serum uric acid concentrations.[90] However it differs from classical acute gout in the distribution of the arthritis, and it usually improves spontaneously after a few weeks; aspirin appears to be more effective than allopurinol in treating it symptomatically.

An interaction occurs between pyrazinamide and probenecid, which affects tubular excretion of uric acid and which may enhance urate retention when both drugs are administered concurrently.[182]

Clinical Uses   The use of pyrazinamide in the primary treatment of tuberculosis with modern short-course chemotherapeutic regimens is still being evaluated, but experience in many countries throughout the world both with daily and intermittent therapy has been highly encouraging,[68] and the incidence of troublesome or serious toxicity from pyrazinamide has been small with the dosage schedules now used. More evidence on the drug's toxicity is needed to show whether pyrazinamide has a place in routine antituberculosis regimens of the future.

At present pyrazinamide is occasionally used in the technically advanced countries for the retreatment of tuberculosis infections resistant to more effective and less toxic agents. In developing countries where drug-resistant tuberculosis is more common, satisfactory results have been obtained in retreatment regimens using pyrazinamide in various drug combinations with ethionamide and cycloserine,[89] and with PAS and streptomycin.[49]

Streptomycin

The clinical pharmacology of streptomycin and details of its administration and toxicity are described in the section dealing with the aminoglycosides in Chapter 4. The brief discussion which follows is confined to its use in the treatment of tuberculosis.

Until the introduction of rifampin and ethambutol into routine antituberculosis treatment within the last few years, streptomycin with isoniazid and PAS provided a standard chemotherapeutic regimen which was reliable and highly effective. The usual course was to give all three drugs during an initial phase lasting 2 to 4 months or at least until the sensitivities of the infecting organism had been ascertained, whereupon the streptomycin was generally stopped and the 2 oral drugs continued daily until a total duration of 18 months to 2 years of therapy had been completed. The advent of ethambutol provided a companion drug for isoniazid, which was better tolerated than PAS, while rifampin proved to be at least as effective as streptomycin—with the added advantages of oral administration. In developed countries where the high cost of rifampin-containing regimens is acceptable the effectiveness of treatment schedules containing isoniazid, ethambutol and rifampin in various combinations has led to the displacement of streptomycin from general use in the treatment of pulmonary tuberculosis to certain specific roles:

1. When oral drugs cannot be administered.
2. In retreatment of infections resistant to other drugs but sensivitive to streptomycin.
3. In treating large cavitary pulmonary lesions.[176]
4. In some short-course regimens.[68]
5. In some completely supervised twice-weekly regimens,[183] especially when the administration of the injection provides an excuse for supervision of concurrent oral therapy in out-patients who cannot be relied on to take medication.[145]

The need for intramuscular injections and the toxicity of streptomycin are sufficiently serious drawbacks to discourage its use for treating pulmonary tuberculosis when the other drugs are readily available, but amongst poorer populations and in developing countries where cost is a highly important consideration in the choice of therapy streptomycin still appears to play a useful and relatively inexpensive part in short-course and supervised intermittent regimens.[70]

Thiacetazone

Although more toxic and rather less effective than the others, thiacetazone currently has a place among the first-line antituberculosis drugs in developing countries because of its cheapness.[70] The drug is a thiosemicarbazone and is fairly active against *Mycobacterium tuberculosis*, although pretreatment sensitivities vary somewhat in different parts of the world; for example, strains from Britain and East Africa are considerably more sensitive than those from Hong Kong, Singapore, and Southern India,[36,55] while in some parts of West Africa thiacetazone-resistant strains are frequently isolated. As its toxicity also seems to vary considerably in different communities, it is generally recognised that the widespread use of thiacetazone in a new area should be preceded by a controlled clinical trial to establish the drug's efficacy. Resistance emerges during the course of treatment unless thiacetazone is used in conjunction with at least one other effective antituberculosis agent.

Thiacetazone is well absorbed from the gastrointestinal tract, peak serum concentrations of 1–2 µg/ml being obtained 4 to 6 hours after ingestion of a 150 mg dose. The estimated half-life in man is nearly 12 hours, about 20 percent of the dose being excreted unchanged in the urine.[55]

Administration and Dosage   The adult dose of thiacetazone is 150 mg given as a single daily dose, and it may be administered with isoniazid 300 mg as a single tablet. The suggested dosage in twice-weekly intermittent chemotherapy is 450 mg, combined with isoniazid 15 mg/kg body weight.[48]

Toxicity   In the doses recommended above the incidence of thiacetazone toxicity is low,[71] although there is some evidence to suggest that the frequency of adverse effects varies in different countries,[61] possibly due to differing standards of observation or interpretation.[119]

The commonest side-effects are anorexia, nausea, vomiting, and occasional diarrhoea.[118] Ototoxicity may lead to dizziness and rarely to ataxia,[71] while bone marrow depression can cause agranulocytosis and anaemia. Allergic skin rashes are not usually serious but may include Stevens-Johnson syndrome and exfoliative dermatitis, which necessitate withdrawal of the drug.[61] Hepatitis has been described in patients receiving thiacetazone but may have been attributable to a companion drug such as isoniazid.

Clinical Uses   The only indication for using thiacetazone in the primary treatment of pulmonary tuberculosis is in developing countries where cost is the predominant factor in determining the choice of tuberculosis treatment pro-gramme. It has been widely used in Africa and Asia, usually combined with isoniazid in a daily oral regimen lasting 18 months with streptomycin for the first 4 or 8 weeks. In East Africa this type of regimen was successful in over 90 percent of patients,[47] but was less effective in Singapore, where it proved to be too toxic.[152] Thiacetazone also has a possible role in twice-weekly intermittent treatment of pulmonary tuberculosis,[48] but it is ineffective in short-course regimens.[45]

SECOND-LINE DRUGS

The drugs which are briefly described in this section are all more toxic and are generally less effective than the first-line drugs, and their use is therefore largely confined to the retreatment of infections which are resistant to the usual anti-tuberculosis agents. As with the other drugs, resistance is likely to emerge during treatment unless at least one other effective drug is used concurrently.[141]

Sodium Aminosalicylate (PAS, para-aminosalicylic acid)

Until recently PAS was an essential component of the "classical" antituberculo-sis regimen, which also included streptomycin and isoniazid, but it has now been displaced from standard chemotherapy in the developed countries by ethambutol and rifampin, which produce fewer side-effects and fewer interrup-tions of treatment.[169]

PAS is a bacteriostatic drug which is effective only against *M. tuberculosis* and occasional strains of *M. kansasii*.[138] It inhibits mycobacterial growth by competing for para-aminobenzoic acid and preventing microbial synthesis of folate, an action similar to that of the sulphonamides against other bacteria.[137] It is well absorbed from the gastrointestinal tract and widely distributed in the body, including the pleural fluid and caseous tissue.[82] PAS has a half-life of 0.75 hours, being acetylated in the liver and excreted in the urine predomi-nantly as inactive acetylated compounds. The half-life is prolonged by im-paired renal function and the drug should be avoided in severe renal failure.[14] The usual daily dosage in adults is 12 g given in 2 divided doses, often com-bined with isoniazid.

The principal side-effects of PAS are due to gastrointestinal irritation which causes anorexia, nausea, vomiting, abdominal pain, and diarrhoea in 25–40 percent of cases. They are reduced if the drug is taken with food but are likely to discourage patients from adhering to the therapeutic regimen. Hypersensi-tivity reactions causing fever, rashes, lymphadenopathy, and eosinophilia have been described in up to 5 percent of patients,[151] and hepatitis progressing to hepatic necrosis may occur. Other side-effects include bone-marrow depression, hypokalaemia secondary to gastrointestinal disturbances,[116] and goitre.

Cycloserine

Cycloserine is an antibiotic with a bacteriostatic effect against mycobacteria and against some other organisms of which *Escherichia coli* is the most susceptible. The drug acts by inhibiting bacterial cell wall synthesis. It is readily absorbed from the gastrointestinal tract and widely distributed throughout body tissues, including the CSF. Cycloserine is excreted in the urine, about two-thirds being eliminated unchanged and the remainder eliminated as an unidentified metabolite.[159] It tends to accumulate in patients who have impaired renal function, and in such cases dosage adjustment is necessary. The usual dosage in adults is 250 mg twice daily, increased to 500 mg twice daily in seriously ill patients, but the higher dose may not be tolerated because of neurotoxicity.[22] Toxicity may be reduced by adjusting the dose to give plasma levels not exceeding 30 μg/ml.

The most important adverse effects of cycloserine are those affecting the central nervous system, including headache, insomnia, tremor, convulsions, and various psychotic disturbances. The incidence of major toxicity is high; for example, mental or neurological disturbance occurred in 16 percent of patients receiving cycloserine 500 mg daily as part of their retreatment regimen for resistant pulmonary tuberculosis in Hong Kong.[89] Peripheral neuropathy occurs rarely. The drug is contraindicated in epileptic patients and should be used cautiously in those with mental disturbances such as depression or anxiety. Toxic symptoms resolve when cycloserine is discontinued.

Ethionamide

This drug (alpha-ethyl thioisonicotinamide) is a derivative of isonicotinic acid, with activity against *Mycobacterium tuberculosis* but little activity against other mycobacteria. Ethionamide is well absorbed after oral administration and is widely distributed in the tissues, reaching significant concentrations in the CSF. It is probably largely metabolised in the liver,[78] less than 1 percent of the drug being excreted unchanged in the urine. Ethionamide is available in 125 mg and 250 mg tablets, the usual adult dosage being 250 mg twice daily, which may be increased to a maximum total daily dosage of 1.0 g depending on the patient's ability to tolerate the gastrointestinal side-effects. These may be minimised by taking the drug with meals or as a single bed-time dose.

The most common adverse effects of ethionamide are anorexia, nausea, and vomiting.[149,177] Depression and other psychological disturbances are quite common, and neurological symptoms such as headache, restlessness, visual and olfactory disturbances, tremors, convulsions, and peripheral neuropathy have been reported.[106,107] Allergic skin reactions, gynaecomastia, and alopecia have been described,[22] and hepatitis has been associated with ethionamide, particularly in diabetics.[132] It is teratogenic in animals and should be avoided during pregnancy.

Propionamide is the n-propyl derivative of ethionamide, with similar anti-tuberculosis activity and equivalent toxicity.[27] The drug has no advantages over ethionamide.

Capreomycin

This is a polypeptide antibiotic derived from *Streptomyces capreolus* with a bacteriostatic action against *Mycobacterium tuberculosis* and some *in vitro* activity against other mycobacteria.[163] It is effective against organisms resistant to the more commonly used antituberculosis drugs, but cross-resistance be-tween capreomycin and viomycin is the rule, and it frequently occurs between capreomycin and kanamycin.[114] Oral absorption is unsatisfactory and the drug is administered by intramuscular injection, achieving a peak serum level of about 30 μg/ml 2 hours after injection of the usual 1.0 g adult dose.[16] About half of the administered dose is excreted unchanged in the urine, while the remainder presumably is metabolised, although the mode and site of inactiva-tion is uncertain.

Capreomycin is given in a daily dosage of 15 mg/kg body weight, a commonly used adult dose being 1.0 g per day in a single intramuscular injection, usually for a period of 4 to 6 months.[7,9] Dosage reduction is advisable in patients with impaired renal function.

The adverse effects of capreomycin are rather similar to those of strep-tomycin and include *nephrotoxicity,* characterised by protein, casts, and cells in the urine, uraemia, and renal potassium loss causing hypokalaemia[9,83]; *oto-toxicity,* which may be manifested as vertigo, tinnitus, or deafness and is more liable to occur in the elderly; and *allergic reactions* such as eosinophilia, fever, and rashes.[120]

Viomycin

Viomycin is a bacteriostatic antibiotic obtained from *Streptomyces puniceus* with activity against *M. tuberculosis* which is one-fourth to one-half that of streptomycin.[138] It is effective against streptomycin-resistant organisms but ex-hibits cross-resistance with capreomycin and kanamycin.[114] It is administered by intramuscular injection in a daily dose of 1–2 g for a limited period of 2 to 3 weeks and thereafter in doses of 1–2 g 2 or 3 times per week.

Vestibular disturbances, deafness, nephrotoxicity, and allergic reactions have been described,[178] and use of viomycin should generally be avoided in conjunction with other ototoxic or nephrotoxic drugs, such as kanamycin and capreomycin, although it has been used successfully with streptomycin.[138] The therapeutic efficacy of viomycin appears to be low.[146]

TREATMENT OF PULMONARY TUBERCULOSIS

Until the advent of ethambutol and rifampin the "classical" regimen of chemotherapy for tuberculosis included streptomycin, isoniazid, and PAS for a period of 18 months, which was occasionally shortened to 12 months in patients with mild infection, and was prolonged to 2 years for those with severe cavitary disease.[35] Isoniazid and PAS were given throughout in a twice daily dosage scheme, while streptomycin was given daily by injection for the first 2 or 3 months of treatment. Initial treatment with three drugs provided a safeguard of two effective agents if the infecting organisms turned out to be resistant to one of the drugs, and it conformed with the concept of two phases in chemotherapy, an initial period of intensive drug therapy when the bacillary population is large, followed by a less intense phase of continuation therapy when the number of organisms has substantially decreased.[65] This regimen was highly successful when properly supervised, and it has been the standard against which modern regimens have been measured; it had the disadvantages of intramuscular injections of streptomycin, the lengthy dependence on patient compliance, and the significant toxicities of PAS and streptomycin. In developing countries a similar regimen was used, except that thiacetazone 150 mg was substituted for PAS as a companion drug to isoniazid because of its relative cheapness, but this drug has been little used in economically developed countries because of its greater toxicity and because of local variations in pretreatment sensitivity and toxicity in different parts of the world.

The benefits of ethambutol and rifampin are attributable to their greater efficacy and relative lack of adverse effects which have permitted the introduction of shorter and less toxic regimens. They have also led to the introduction of a wider variety of regimens of proven efficacy, and clinicians now have a choice of effective schemes of treatment which allow greater flexibility in circumventing adverse effects, improving supervision by means of intermittent administration, and shortening the duration of therapy. Nevertheless, the cardinal rules of therapy are unchanged, requiring careful attention to detail in the application of an approved regimen and skilled supervision throughout the duration of therapy to ensure that drugs are taken as prescribed.

Standard Chemotherapy

In the United States the most frequently used standard regimen is daily oral isoniazid and ethambutol for 18 months, with the addition of daily intramuscular streptomycin for the first 3 months in the case of extensive cavitary lesions or if the patient comes from an area where drug-resistant infection is prevalent.[10] The following modifications are accepted:

1. As an alternative for treating extensive disease, oral rifampin and isoniazid may be used throughout instead of the 3-drug regimen.[125]
2. If parenteral therapy is necessary during the early stage of treatment a combination of streptomycin and isoniazid may be used for the first 3 months.
3. PAS is preferable to ethambutol as a companion drug to isoniazid in young children because of the difficulty of recognising visual toxic symptoms in this age group.
4. Isoniazid with ethambutol is the preferred combination for the treatment of tuberculosis in pregnancy because of possible teratogenic effects of rifampin.[158]

A rather similar regimen is followed in Australia,[100] where initial daily 3-drug therapy with isoniazid and rifampin plus either streptomycin or ethambutol is given for 2 to 4 months, followed by continuation therapy with isoniazid and rifampin to complete 18 months of treatment. In Britain the standard treatment used at present for pulmonary tuberculosis is a 9-month short-course regimen (see below).

Intermittent Chemotherapy

The main indication for intermittent chemotherapy is in the treatment of individuals who cannot be relied on to take daily therapy unsupervised but who can be interviewed once or twice weekly and watched while they take their drugs. Generally speaking intermittent regimens are less toxic than daily ones,[183] and they can be combined with short-course chemotherapy (see below) to produce regimens which are highly effective in urban populations where every dose is supervised.[84]

Intermittent chemotherapy can be successful if given throughout the course of treatment,[140,169] even in short-course regimens of only 9 months[84,86]; but at present most authorities favour an initial phase of intensive daily therapy followed by a twice-weekly continuation regimen.[95,183] Some drugs, such as isoniazid, are unsuitable for once-weekly administration, and twice-weekly regimens are currently considered safer and more effective. The advantages of thrice-weekly schedules have yet to be defined.

An intermittent regimen which has been recommended in the United States[145] consists of daily conventional therapy for one to four months followed by twice-weekly isoniazid 15 mg/kg body weight by mouth plus streptomycin 25–30 mg/kg intramuscularly; or isoniazid 15 mg/kg plus ethambutol 50 mg/

kg, both orally, maintained for 18 months.[5] Recent reports show that prolongation of intermittent treatment beyond 1 year is unnecessary when fully supervised.[180] The twice-weekly combination of isoniazid 15 mg/kg plus rifampin 600 mg, with or without an initial phase of daily treatment, has produced good results with a low level of adverse effects,[153] although intermittent rifampin in higher dosage is more likely to cause systemic reactions.[57]

Short-course Chemotherapy

The advantages of short-course chemotherapy are summarised by Fox and Mitchison,[69] who draw attention to the reduction in cost and in chronic drug toxicity because the total quantity of drug used is less; the improvement in patient cooperation and in surveillance of therapy; and the diminished likelihood of relapse if patients default early from treatment. Evidence for the efficacy of short-course regimens for pulmonary tuberculosis comes from a series of experimental studies which set out to compare the frequency of bacteriological relapse following different chemotherapeutic regimens which were given for periods ranging from 4 to 12 months. These investigations have been reviewed by Fox[67,68] who concluded that in technically advanced countries a 9-month daily regimen consisting of rifampin and isoniazid, supplemented in the first 2 months by streptomycin or ethambutol,[25] should be adopted as the routine practice for the general run of patients. In Britain the current standard regimen is daily oral treatment for 9 months with a combination of rifampin 450–600 mg and isoniazid 300 mg, plus ethambutol 15–25 mg/kg body weight daily for the first 2 months.[117] The use of streptomycin instead of ethambutol for the initial phase of therapy is equally effective but leads to a greater incidence of side-effects.[25]

Shorter treatment regimens lasting 6 or even 4 months have shown considerable promise and are particularly relevant in developing countries where the problem of cost and the difficulties of lengthy supervision are overriding considerations. The use of four potent drugs (streptomycin, isoniazid, rifampin, and pyrazinamide) daily for 2 months, followed by a continuation phase of daily isoniazid and rifampin for 4 months appeared to be highly successful in a Singapore trial,[154] although the relapse rates after comparable regimens in which the continuation phase was reduced to 2 months was between 8 and 24 percent.[46] The most recent development in the effort to reduce the costs, inconvenience, and toxicity of antituberculosis chemotherapy has been the trial of 3-month and 2-month regimens of daily streptomycin, isoniazid, rifampin, and pyrazinamide for the treatment of patients for whom the diagnosis of pulmonary tuberculosis seems likely on clinical and radiological grounds but for whom microscopy of sputum reveals no acid-fast bacilli.[85] Observations after 1 year of follow-up suggest that those with negative cultures show a very low incidence of subsequent relapse if treatment is stopped after 2 or 3 months, but in those with positive cultures the incidence of relapse was at a level which would generally be regarded as unacceptable. The potential of these observations lies in the possibility of safely stopping treatment at 3 months if the initial cultures have proved negative, but a longer period of observation will be needed before reliable conclusions can be drawn.

The combination of intermittent treatment with short-course chemotherapy provides an alternative choice of regimen which minimises the total drug load and permits full supervision of every dose. A high level of effectiveness has been obtained by giving streptomycin, isoniazid, rifampin, and pyrazinamide daily for an initial phase of 1 to 2 months followed by a continuation phase consisting of twice-weekly streptomycin, isoniazid, and pyrazinamide to a total treatment duration of 6–8 months.[84,166] A similar type of regimen, largely unsupervised, has been tested in the United States, consisting of oral isoniazid (300 mg) and rifampin (600 mg) daily for 1 month, followed by isoniazid (900 mg) and rifampin (600 mg) twice weekly for a further 8 months.[44] There were 10 treatment failures, 5 due to death in the initial phase of treatment from overwhelming tuberculosis or from drug toxicity, and 5 with persistently positive sputum which was attributable in some to poor cooperation. More work is needed to demonstrate the superiority of this type of regimen over those already in widespread use in the developed countries.

Management

The management of pulmonary tuberculosis in the economically advanced countries is directed toward the eradication of infection in every person with active disease by administering a therapeutic regimen of proven efficacy for its full duration. The objective should be to achieve success with the least possible disturbance in the normal life of the patient or his family. The major management problems to be considered are (1) choice of regimen, (2) selection of patients for hospital treatment, (3) supervision of therapy, and (4) retreatment chemotherapy.

Choice of Regimen   In the routine management of pulmonary tuberculosis the initial regimen is customarily a standard schedule of treatment which has been shown by trial and experience to be effective in that population. Preliminary assessment is necessary to identify any factors which may give rise to modification of the standard regimen: those which should be routinely considered are listed in Table 6-1 but others may become apparent in the course of interviewing the patient. Once the decision is made the patient should be fully informed of the nature and duration of the therapeutic regime to which he is submitting himself, including the possibility and character of adverse effects, so that he

Table 6-1 / Common Factors That May Lead to Modification of the Standard Regimen for Antituberculosis Chemotherapy

Modifying Factor	Modification Recommended
Previous antituberculosis chemotherapy	Retreatment regimen; if possible, withhold treatment until sensitivities of the infecting micro-organisms have been ascertained.
Patient originates from an area where resistant organisms are common, (such as Asian or Hispanic communities, Oriental immigrants)	Always use three drugs in the initial phase of therapy, or until the sensitivities have been ascertained.
Unstable social background, due to psychiatric, domestic, or financial difficulties	Consider fully supervised intermittent chemotherapy regimen.
Pregnancy	Avoid rifampin during the first trimester.
Serious disturbance of vision, young children and the aged	Avoid ethambutol.
Impaired renal function	Modify dosage of streptomycin, ethambutol and PAS or avoid these drugs.
Impaired hapatic function	Avoid rifampin or monitor hepatic enzyme concentrations expectantly.

can adjust to the constraints which will be placed on him and learn the importance of strict adherence to the treatment schedule. These lessons will be
reinforced every time he reattends for follow-up interview.

Selection of Patients for Hospital Treatment   Hospital admission at the start of
therapy is not necessary for the routine management of pulmonary tuberculosis,[13,95] but certain categories of patients are best treated in hospital initially.
They include the following:

1. Very ill patients requiring supportive therapy and nursing care.
2. Uncooperative patients, such as those with unfavourable social or
   domestic circumstances, a history of poor cooperation, mental disturbance, alcoholism, or drug addiction. Hospital admission is usually
   necessary for the duration of the intensive initial phase of treatment
   which precedes a fully supervised out-patient intermittent continuation
   phase.
3. Patients with drug-resistant disease who require treatment with
   second-line drugs of high toxicity.
4. Infectious patients with highly susceptible domestic contacts such as
   tuberculin-negative children or family members with impaired immunological defence mechanisms. However there is strong evidence
   to show that the risk of infection to contacts is minimal once the index
   case has started treatment.[77]

The choice between hospital and out-patient therapy must depend on the
individual circumstances of the patient and the facilities which are available in
the locality for safe and efficient ambulatory care.

Surveillance of Therapy   It is important that the aims of treatment supervision
be clear:

1. To ensure adherence to the recommended regimen.
2. To detect evidence of adverse effects as early as possible, and take
   corrective steps if indicated.
3. To monitor recovery by regular clinical examination, smear, and culture examination of sputum, including sensitivity testing if compliance
   is suspect, and radiographic examination of the chest.
4. To terminate treatment as soon as the approved regimen has been
   completed.

Most clinicians with experience of treating pulmonary tuberculosis will have
developed their own schemes for achieving these objectives which suit local
circumstances.[10,117,160] It is important that the clinic facilities and personnel
should be able to respond rapidly to the problems posed by uncooperative

patients who fail to turn up for appointments by making telephone contact or by visiting the patient in his home. The maintenance of an unbroken therapeutic regimen becomes increasingly important as treatment schedules are shortened and the total number of doses is progressively reduced.

Once an approved regimen of treatment is completed, provided that the physician is satisfied that compliance has been good and there is adequate bacteriological, clinical, and radiological evidence of successful treatment, it is probably safe to discharge the patient from further follow-up.[50,88] Only patients who are known or thought to have had irregular chemotherapy or an inadequate duration of treatment should be followed for a limited period,[81] but routine chest radiography or sputum cultures rarely lead to the detection of reactivation disease, almost all cases presenting with symptoms.[4] The discharged patient must therefore be encouraged to return to the clinic promptly if he develops symptoms that might indicate a relapse.

Retreatment Chemotherapy   Recurrence of infection during or after a course of antituberculosis chemotherapy calls for a careful reassessment to determine the reasons for treatment failure (Table 6-2). Therapeutic errors such as single drug treatment, insufficient dosage, or inadequate duration of therapy are uncommon in the developed countries, but mistakes are occasionally made, particularly in those fields of medicine in which tuberculosis is nowadays rarely encountered[38]; in the developing countries such treatment errors have

Table 6-2 / Causes of Treatment Failure in Pulmonary Tuberculosis

Failure	*Cause*
Infection with resistant micro-organisms	Previous ineffectual treatment
	Primary resistance, most commonest in Developing countries, Recent immigrants from developing countries Asian and Hispanic communities in the United States
Choice of an inadequate regimen	Single drug therapy
	One or more drugs given in insufficient dosage
	Inadequate duration of therapy
Failure of adherence to the prescribed regimen	Inadequate explanation and/or supervision of therapy
	Intolerable side effects

been all too common and have led to a substantial pool of resistant organisms in some communities.[179] Primary resistance to one or more antituberculosis drugs occurs overall in less than 10 percent of infections in the highly developed countries of Europe and North America,[40,52] but within those populations the rate is considerably higher in certain communities, such as among Asian and Hispanic ethnic groups in the United States,[98] and among recent immigrants from countries with a high prevalence of the disease.[28] However a much more important reason for treatment failure is lack of cooperation with the recommended regimen, and the great majority of failures is found among individuals of low intelligence, vagrants, alcoholics, and drug addicts.

In planning the retreatment of patients who have had previous chemotherapy it is therefore necessary to take account of the ethnic and geographical origins of the individual, the social background, and the precise nature and duration of earlier treatment. The current sensitivities of sputum cultures should be obtained to enable the optimal drug regimen to be determined, and in general no treatment should be given until the results of reliable resistance tests are available. The following principles provide a guide to the successful chemotherapy of patients with resistant infection[36,139]:

1. Patients should be assessed prior to treatment for possible increased risks of hepatic or renal toxicity, and close monitoring for adverse effects should be maintained throughout, including measurements of plasma drug levels where necessary.
2. Treatment should begin with at least three drugs to which the organisms are known to be sensitive, using the most effective of the available drugs and taking into consideration their potential for toxicity in any given patient.
3. Drugs should be administered under strict supervision, initially in hospital. A parenteral drug is useful when patients progress to outpatient therapy since it provides an opportunity for supervising pill swallowing when the patient attends for injections.
4. Frequent tests of sputum microscopy, culture, and drug susceptibilities should be made during treatment.
5. Prolonged therapy for more than 18 months may be required and adjunctive surgery is occasionally indicated.

Since most patients with drug-resistant disease have acquired it because of failure to adhere to previously recommended therapy, the success of retreatment chemotherapy depends to a very large extent upon the establishment of a sympathetic relationship between doctor and patient.

REFERENCES

1. ACOCELLA G, BONOLLO L, GARIMOLDI M, MAINARDI M, TENCONI LT, NICOLIS FB: Kinetics of rifampicin and isoniazid administered alone and in combination to normal subjects and patients with liver disease. Gut 13: 47–53, 1972.

2. ACOCELLA G, HAMILTON-MILLER JMT, BRUMFITT W: Can rifampicin use be safely extended? Evidence for non-emergence of resistant strains of *Mycobacterium tuberculosis*. Lancet 1: 740–742, 1977.

3. ALCARCON-SEGOVIA D, FISHBEIN E, ALCALA H: Isoniazid acetylation rate and development of antinuclear antibodies upon isoniazid treatment. Arthritis Rheum 14: 748–752, 1971.

4. ALBERT RK, ISEMAN M, SBARBARO JA, STAGE A, PIERSON DJ: Monitoring patients with tuberculosis for failure during and after treatment. Am Rev Resp Dis 114: 1051–1060, 1976.

5. ALBERT RK, SBARBARO JA, HUDSON LD, ISEMAN M: High-dose ethambutol: its role in intermittent chemotherapy. A six year study. Am Rev Resp Dis 114: 699–704, 1976.

6. AMERICAN THORACIC SOCIETY: Preventive therapy of tuberculous infection. Am Rev Resp Dis 110: 371–374, 1974.

7. ANDREWS RH, JENKINS PA, MARKS J, PINES A, SELKON JB, SOMNER AR: Treatment of isoniazid-resistant pulmonary tuberculosis with ethambutol, rifampicin and capreomycin: a co-operative study in England and Wales. Tubercle 55: 105–113, 1974.

8. AQUINAS M, ALLAN WGL, HORSFALL PAL, JENKINS PK, WONG H-Y, GIRLING D, TALL R, FOX W: Adverse reactions to daily and intermittent rifampicin regimens for pulmonary tuberculosis in Hong Kong. Br Med J 1: 765–771, 1972.

9. AQUINAS M, CITRON KM: Rifampicin, ethabutol and capreomycin in pulmonary tuberculosis, previously treated with both first and second line drugs: The results of two years chemotherapy. Tubercle 53: 153–165, 1972.

10. BAILEY WC, RALEIGH JW, TURNER JAP: Treatment of mycobacterial disease. Am Rev Resp Dis 115: 185–187, 1977.

11. BARRON GJ, TEPPER L, IOVINE G: Ocular toxicity from ethambutol. Am J Ophthalmol 77: 256–260, 1974.

12. BASSI L, DI BERARDINO L, PERNA G, SILVESTRI LG: Antibodies against rifampin in patients with tuberculosis after discontinuation of daily treatment. Am Rev Resp Dis 114: 1189–1190, 1976.

13. BATES JH: Ambulatory treatment of tuberculosis—an idea whose time is come. Am Rev Resp Dis 109: 317–319, 1974.

14. BENNETT WM, SINGER I, GOLPER T, FEIG P, COGGINS CJ: Guidelines for drug therapy in renal failure. Ann Intern Med 86: 754–783, 1977.

15. BERTÉ SJ, DIMASE JD, CHRISTIANSON CS: Isoniazid, PAS and streptomycin intolerance in 1744 patients. An analysis of reactions to single drugs and drug groups plus data on multiple reactions, type and time of reactions, and desensitization. Am Rev Resp Dis 90: 598–606, 1964.

16. BLACK HR, GRIFFITH RS, PEABODY AM: Absorption, excretion and metabolism of

capreomycin in normal and diseased states. Ann NY Acad Sci 135: 974–982, 1966.

17. BLACK M, MITCHELL JR, ZIMMERMAN HJ, ISHAK KG, EPLER GR: Isoniazid-associated hepatitis in 114 patients. Gastroenterology 69: 289–302, 1975.

18. BLAJCHMAN MA, LOWRY RC, PETTIT JE, STRADLING P: Rifampicin-induced immune thrombocytopenia. Br Med J 3: 24–26, 1970.

19. BOMAN G, MALMBORG A-S: Rifampicin in plasma and pleural fluid after single oral doses. Eur J Clin Pharmacol 7: 51–58, 1974.

20. BOWERSOX DW, WINTERBAUER RH, STEWART GL, ORME B, BARRON E: Isoniazid dosage in patients with renal failure. N Engl J Med 289: 84–87, 1973.

21. BRENNAN RW, DEHEJIA H, KUTT H, VEREBELY K, MCDOWELL F: Diphenyl-hydantoin intoxication attendant to slow inactivation of isoniazid. Neurology 20: 687–693, 1970.

22. BRITISH MEDICAL JOURNAL: Drugs for tuberculosis. Br Med J 3: 664–667, 1968.

23. BRITISH MEDICAL JOURNAL: Chemoprophylaxis against tuberculosis. Br Med J 4: 63–64, 1974.

24. BRITISH THORACIC AND TUBERCULOSIS ASSOCIATION: Present effectiveness of BCG vaccination in England and Wales. Tubercle 56: 129–137, 1975.

25. BRITISH THORACIC AND TUBERCULOSIS ASSOCIATION: Short-course chemotherapy in pulmonary tuberculosis. Lancet 2: 1102–1104, 1976.

26. BRITISH THORACIC ASSOCIATION: A study of a standardised contact procedure in tuberculosis. Tubercle 59: 245–259, 1978.

27. BRITISH TUBERCULOSIS ASSOCIATION: A comparison of the toxicity of prothiona-mide and ethionamide. Tubercle 49: 125–135, 1968.

28. BYRD RB, FISK DE, ROETHE RA, GLOVER JN, WOOSTER LD, WILDER NJ: Tuberculosis in oriental immigrants. A study in military dependents. Chest 76: 136–139, 1979.

29. BYRD RB, HORN BR, GRIGGS GA, SOLOMON DA: Isoniazid chemoprophylaxis. Association with detection and incidence of liver toxicity. Arch Intern Med 137: 1130–1133, 1977.

30. BYRD RB, HORN BR, SOLOMON DA, GRIGGS GA: Toxic effects of isoniazid in tuberculosis chemoprophylaxis. Role of biochemical monitoring in 1000 patients. JAMA 241: 1239–1241, 1979.

31. CANETTI G: Host factors and chemotherapy. in Chemotherapy of Tuberculosis, Barry VC (ed) pp. 175–191. London: Butterworths, 1964.

32. CAYLEY FE, MAJUMDAR SK: Ocular toxicity due to rifampicin. Br Med J 1: 199–200, 1976.

33. CHAN WC, O'MAHONEY MG, YU DYC, YU RYH: Renal failure during intermittent rifampicin therapy. Tubercle 56: 191–198, 1975.

34. CHRISTOPHER TG, BLAIR A, FORREY A, CUTLER RE: Kinetics of ethambutol elimination in renal disease. Proceedings of the Clinical Dialysis and Transplant Forum 3: 96–100, 1973.

35. CITRON KM: The management of tuberculosis. Br J Hosp Med 5: 799–806, 1971.

36. CITRON KM: The chemotherapy of pulmonary tuberculosis. Br J Hosp Med 12: 731–735, 1974.

37. COLLIER J, JOEKES AM, PHILALITHIS PE, THOMPSON FD: Two cases of ethambutol nephrotoxicity. Br Med J 2: 1105–1106, 1976.
38. CROFTON J: Treatment of tuberculosis. Br Med J 1: 52, 1979.
39. CULLEN JH, EARLY LJA, FIORE JM: The occurrence of hyperuricaemia during pyrazinamide-isoniazid therapy. Am Rev Tuberculosis 74: 289–292, 1956.
40. DARBYSHIRE J, DAVIES P: Medical Research Council (1978–1979) survey of notifications of tuberculosis for England and Wales. Thorax 35: 231, 1980.
41. DICKINSON DS, BAILEY WC, HIRSCHOWITZ BI, EIDUS L: The effect of acetylation status on isoniazid (INH) hepatitis. Am Rev Resp Dis (Suppl) 115: 395, 1977.
42. DOSTER B, MURRAY FJ, NEWMAN P, WOOLPERT SW: Ethambutol in the initial treatment of pulmonary tuberculosis. Am Rev Resp Dis 107: 177–190, 1973.
43. DUME T, WAGNER C, WETZELS E: Pharmacokinetics of ethambutol in healthy subjects and in patients in terminal renal failure. Dtsch Med Wochenschr 96: 1430–1434, 1971.
44. DUTT AK, JONES L, STEAD WW: Short-course chemotherapy for tuberculosis with largely twice-weekly isoniazid-rifampin. Chest 75: 441–447, 1979.
45. EAST AFRICAN/BRITISH MEDICAL RESEARCH COUNCILS: Controlled clinical trial of short-course (6-months) regimens of chemotherapy for treatment of tuberculosis. Third report. Lancet 2: 237–240, 1974.
46. EAST AFRICAN/BRITISH MEDICAL RESEARCH COUNCIL: Controlled clinical trial of five short-course (4-months) chemotherapy regimens in pulmonary tuberculosis. First report of 4th study. Lancet 2: 334–338, 1978.
47. EAST AFRICAN/BRITISH MEDICAL RESEARCH COUNCIL FIFTH THIACETAZONE INVESTIGATION—THIRD REPORT: Isoniazid with thiacetazone (thioacetazone) in the treatment of pulmonary tuberculosis in East Africa. Third report of fifth investigation. Tubercle 54: 169–179, 1973.
48. EAST AFRICAN/BRITISH MEDICAL RESEARCH COUNCIL INTERMITTENT THIACETAZONE INVESTIGATION. A pilot stufy of two regimens of intermittent thiacetazone plus isoniazid in the treatment of pulmonary tuberculosis in East Africa. Tubercle 55:211–221, 1974.
49. EAST AFRICAN/BRITISH MEDICAL RESEARCH COUNCIL RETREATMENT INVESTIGATION—SECOND REPORT: Streptomycin plus PAS plus pyrazinamide in the retreatment of pulmonary tuberculosis in East Africa—second report. Tubercle 54: 283–290, 1973.
50. EDSALL J, COLLINS G: Routine follow-up of inactive tuberculosis, a practise to be abandoned. Am Rev Resp Dis 108: 851–853, 1973.
51. EDWARDS OM, COURTENAY-EVANS RJ, GALLEY JM, HUNTER J, TAIT AD: Changes in cortisol metabolism following rifampicin therapy. Lancet 2: 549–551, 1974.
52. EIDUS L, JESSAMINE AG, HERSHFIELD ES, HELBECQUE DM: A national study to determine the prevalence of drug resistance in newly discovered previously untreated tuberculosis patients as well as in retreatment cases. Can J Public Health 69: 146–153, 1978.
53. ELDER JL, EDWARDS FGB, ABRAHAMS EW: Tuberculosis due to Mycobacterium kansasii. Aust NZ J Med 7: 8–13, 1977.
54. ELLARD GA: Absorption, metabolism and excretion of pyrazinamide in man. Tubercle 50: 144–58, 1969.

55. ELLARD GA, DICKINSON JM, GAMMON PT, MITCHISON DA: Serum concentrations and antituberculosis activity of thioacetazone. Tubercle 55: 39–54, 1974.

56. ELLARD GA, MITCHISON DA, GIRLING DJ, NUNN AJ, FOX W: The hepatic toxicity of isoniazid among rapid and slow acetylators of the drug. Am Rev Resp Dis 118: 628–629, 1978.

57. EULE H, WERNER E, WINSEL K, IWAINSKY H: Intermittent chemotherapy of pulmonary tuberculosis using rifampicin and isoniazid for primary treatment: the influence of various factors on the frequency of side-effects. Tubercle 55: 81–89, 1974.

58. FAIRSHTER RD, RANDAZZO GP, GARLIN J, WILSON AF: Failure of isoniazid prophylaxis after exposure to isoniazid-resistant tuberculosis. Am Rev Resp Dis 112: 37–42, 1975.

59. FEREBEE SH: (1968). Long-term effects of isoniazid prophylaxis. Bull Int Union Tuberc 41: 161–166,

60. FEREBEE SH: Controlled chemoprophylaxis trials in tuberculosis. A general review. Adv Tuberc Res 17: 28–106, 1970.

61. FERGUSON GC, NUNN AJ, FOX W, MILLER AB, ROBINSON DK, TALL R: A second international cooperative investigation into thiacetazone containing regimens. Tubercle 52: 166–181, 1971.

62. FLYNN CT, RAINFORD DJ, HOPE E: Acute renal failure and rifampicin: Danger of unsuspected intermittent dosage. Br Med J 2: 482, 1974.

63. FORBES M, PEETS EA, KUCK NA: Effect of ethambutol on mycobacteria. Ann NY Acad Sci 135: 726–731, 1966.

64. FORGAN-SMITH R, ELLARD GA, NEWTON DAG, MITCHISON DA: Pyrazinamide and other drugs in tuberculous meningitis. Lancet 2: 374, 1973.

65. FOX W: Changing concepts in the chemotherapy of pulmonary tuberculosis. Am Rev Resp Dis 97: 767–790, 1968.

66. FOX W: General considerations in intermittent drug therapy of pulmonary tuberculosis. Postgrad Med J 47: 729–736, 1971.

67. FOX W: The modern management and therapy of pulmonary tuberculosis. Proc R Soc Med 70: 4–15, 1977.

68. FOX W: The current status of short-course chemotherapy. Tubercle 60: 177–190, 1979.

69. FOX W, MITCHISON DA: Short-course chemotherapy for pulmonary tuberculosis. Am Rev Resp Dis 111: 325–353, 1975.

70. FOX W, NUNN AJ: The cost of antituberculous drug regimens. Am Rev Resp Dis 120: 503–509, 1979.

71. FOX W, STARK AJ, TALL R, BHATIA JL, CLARKE JHC, DONIA TO, KRISHNASWAMI KV, OUSSEDIK N: A study of adverse reactions to high dosage intermittent thiacetazone. Tubercle 55: 29–40, 1974.

72. GIRLING DJ: Adverse reactions to rifampicin in antituberculosis regimens. J Antimicrob Chemother 3: 115–132, 1977.

73. GIRLING DJ: The hepatic toxicity of antituberculosis regimens containing isoniazid, rifampicin and pyrazinamide. Tubercle 59: 13–32, 1978.

74. GOLDMAN AL, BRAMAN SS: Isoniazid: a review with emphasis on adverse effects. Chest 62: 71–77, 1972.

75. Graber CD, Jebaily J, Galphin RL, Doering E: Light chain proteinuria and humoral immuno-incompetence in tuberculous patients treated with rifampin. Am Rev Resp Dis 107: 713–717, 1973.

76. Grönhagen-Riska C, Hellstrom P-E, Fröseth B: Predisposing factors in hepatitis induced by isoniazid-rifampin treatment of tuberculosis. Am Rev Resp Dis 118: 461–466, 1978.

77. Gunnels JJ, Bates JH, Swindoll H: Infectivity of sputum positive tuberculosis patients on chemotherapy. Am Rev Resp Dis 109: 323–330, 1974.

78. Hamilton EJ, Eidus L, Little E: A comparative study in vivo of isoniazid and alpha-ethylthioisonicotinamide. Am Rev Resp Dis 85: 407–412, 1962.

79. Hamilton-Miller JMT, Kerry DW, Brumfitt W: The use of antibiotic combinations in the treatment of Serratia marcescens infections. J Antimicrob Chemother 3: 193–194, 1977.

80. Harris GD, Johanson WG, Nicholson DP: Response to chemotherapy of pulmonary infection due to Mycobacterium kansasii. Am Rev Resp Dis 112: 31–36, 1975.

81. Hayden SP, Springett VH: An assessment of the place of follow-up in pulmonary tuberculosis. Br J Dis Chest 72: 217–221, 1978.

82. Heller A, Ebert RH, Kock-Weser D, Roth LJ: Studies with C^{14} labelled para-aminosalicylic acid and isoniazid. Am Rev Tuberc 75: 71–82, 1957.

83. Hesling CM: Treatment with capreomycin, with special reference to toxic effects. Tubercle 50 (Suppl): 39–41, 1969.

84. Hong Kong Chest Service/British Medical Research Council: Controlled trial of 6-month and 8-month regimens in the treatment of pulmonary tuberculosis. First report. Am Rev Resp Dis 118: 219–227, 1978.

85. Hong Kong Chest Service, Tuberculosis Research Centre, Madras, India and British Medical Research Council. Sputum-smear-negative pulmonary tuberculosis: Controlled trial of 3-month and 2-month regimens of chemotherapy. Lancet 1: 1361–3, 1979.

86. Hong Kong Tuberculosis Treatment Services/British Medical Research Council: Controlled trial of 6- and 9-month regimens of daily and intermittent streptomycin plus isoniazid plus pyrinazinamide for pulmonary tuberculosis in Hong Kong. Tubercle 56: 81–96, 1975.

87. Hong Kong Tuberculosis Treatment Services/British Medical Research Council: Adverse reactions to short-course regimens containing streptomycin, isoniazid, pyrazinamide and rifampicin in Hong Kong. Tubercle 57: 81–95, 1976.

88. Hopewell PD, Buckingham W, Elliott RC, Rosenblatt WF, Hsu KHK: Discharge of tuberculosis patients from medical surveillance. Am Rev Resp Dis 113: 709–710, 1976.

89. Horsfall PAL: Treatment of resistant pulmonary tuberculosis in Hong Kong with regimens of second-line drugs. Tubercle 53: 166–173, 1972.

90. Horsfall PA, Plummer J, Allan WGL, Girling DJ, Nunn AJ, Fox W: Double blind controlled comparison of aspirin, allopurinol and placebo in the management of arthralgia during pyrazinamide administration. Tubercle 60: 13–24, 1979.

91. HUSSELS H, KROENING U, MAGDORF K: Ethambutol and rifampicin serum levels in children: second report on the combined administration of ethambutol and rifampicin. Pneumonologie 149: 31–38, 1973.

92. JACKSON EA, McLEOD DC: Pharmacokinetics and dosing of antimicrobial agents in renal impairment, part 2. Am J Hosp Pharm 31: 137–148, 1974.

93. JACOBS MR, KOORNHOF JH, ROBINS-BROWNE RM, STEVENSON CM, VERMAAK ZA, FREIMAN I, MILLER GB, WITCOMB MA, ISAACSON M, WARD JI, AUSTRIAN R: Emergence of multiple resistant pneumococci. N Engl J Med 299: 735–740, 1978.

94. JACOBS NF, THOMPSON SE: Spiking fever from isoniazid simulating a septic process. JAMA 238: 1759–1760, 1977.

95. JOHNSTON RF, WILDRICK KH: The impact of chemotherapy on the care of patients with tuberculosis. Am Rev Resp Dis 109: 636–664, 1974.

96. JOINT TUBERCULOSIS COMMITTEE: Chemoprophylaxis against tuberculosis in Britain. Tubercle 54: 309–316, 1973.

97. KONNO K, OIZUMO K, OKA S: Mode of action of rifampicin on mycobacteria. Am Rev Resp Dis 107: 1006–1012, 1973.

98. KOPANOFF DE, KILBURN JO, GLASSROTH J, SNIDER DE, FARER LS, GOOD RD: A continuing survey of tuberculosis primary drug resistance in the United States: March 1975 to November 1977. Am Rev Resp Dis 118: 835–842, 1978.

99. KOPANOFF DE, SNIDER DE, CARAS GJ: Isoniazid-related hepatitis. A U.S. Public Health Service cooperative surveillance study. Am Rev Resp Dis 117: 991–1001, 1978.

100. KUCERS A, BENNETT NM: The use of antibiotics. 3rd Edn, p. 811. London: Heinemann, 1979.

101. KUNIN CM, BRANDT D, WOOD H: Bacteriologic studies of rifampin, a new semisynthetic antibiotic. J Infect Dis 119: 132–137, 1969.

102. KUTT H, WINTERS W, McDOWELL FH: Depression of parahydroxylation of diphenylhydantoin by antituberculosis chemotherapy. Neurology 16: 594–602, 1966.

103. LAL S, SINGHAL SN, BURLEY DM, CROSSLEY G: Effect of rifampicin and isoniazid on liver function. Br Med J 1: 148–150, 1972.

104. LANCET: Treatment of tuberculous meningitis. Lancet 1: 787–788, 1976.

105. LEE CS, GAMBERTOLGLIO JG, BRATER DG, BENET LZ: Kinetics of oral ethambutol in the normal subject. Clin Pharmacol Ther 22: 615–621, 1978.

106. LEES AW: Ethionamide, 750 mg daily, plus isoniazid, 450 mg daily, in previously untreated cases of pulmonary tuberculosis. Am Rev Resp Dis 92: 966–969, 1965.

107. LEES AW: Ethionamide, 500 mg daily, plus isoniazid, 500 mg or 300 mg daily in previously untreated patients with pulmonary tuberculosis. Am Rev Resp Dis 95: 109–111, 1967.

108. LEES AW, ALLAN GW, SMITH J, TYRELL WF, FALLON RJ: Toxicity from rifampicin plus isoniazid and rifampicin plus ethambutol therapy. Tubercle 52: 182–190, 1971.

109. LEES AW, ALLAN GW, SMITH J, TYRRELL WF, FALLON RJ: Retreatment of pulmonary tuberculosis with rifampin and ethambutol. Am Rev Resp Dis 105: 129–131, 1972.

110. LEES AW, ASGHER B, HASHEM MA, SINHA BN: Jaundice after rifampicin. Br J Dis Chest 64: 90–95, 1970.

111. LEFF A, HERSKOWITZ D, GILBERT J, BREWIN A: Tuberculosis chemoprophylaxis practice in metropolitan clinics. Am Rev Resp Dis 119: 161–170, 1979.

112. LEIBOLD JE: The ocular toxicity of ethambutol and its relation to dose. Ann NY Acad Sci 135: 904–909, 1966.

113. MACDONALD JB: *Mycobacterium tuberculosis* resistance to rifampicin and ethambutol: a clinical survey. Thorax 32: 1–4, 1977.

114. MCCLATCHY JK, KANES W, DAVIDSON PT, MOULDING TS: Cross-resistance in M. Tuberculosis to kanamycin, capreomycin and viomycin. Tubercle 58: 29–34, 1977.

115. MCDERMOTT W, ORMOND L, MUSCHENHEIM C, DEUTSCHLE K, MCKUNE RM, TOMPSETT R: Pyrazinamide-isoniazid in tuberculosis. Am Rev Tuberc 69: 319–333, 1954.

116. MCINTYRE PA: Hypokaliemia occurring during para-aminosalicylic acid therapy. Bull Johns Hopkins Hosp 92: 210–221, 1953.

117. MCNICOL M: Treatment of tuberculosis. J R Coll Phys Lond 13: 23–24, 1979.

118. MILLER AB, FOX W, TALL R: An international cooperative investigation into thiacetazone (thioacetazone) side-effects. Tubercle 47: 33–74, 1966.

119. MILLER AB, NUNN AJ, ROBINSON DK, FOX W, SOMASUNDARAM PR, TALL R: A second international cooperative investigation into thiacetazone side-effects. 2. Frequency and geographical distribution of side-effects. Bull WHO 47: 211–227, 1972.

120. MILLER JD, POPPLEWELL AG, LANDWEHR A, GREENE ME: Toxicology studies in patients on prolonged therapy with capreomycin. Ann NY Acad Sci 135: 1047–1056, 1966.

121. MILLER RR, PORTER J, GREENBLATT DJ: Clinical importance of the interaction of phenytoin and isoniazid. Chest 75: 356–358, 1979.

122. MITCHELL JR, THORGEIRSSON UP, BLACK M, TIMBRELL JA, SNODGRASS WR, POTTER WZ, JOLLOW DJ, KEISER HR: Increased incidence of isoniazid hepatitis in rapid acetylators: possible relation to hydrazine metabolites. Clin Pharmacol Ther 18: 70–79, 1975.

123. MITCHELL JR, ZIMMERMAN HJ, ISHAK KG, THORGIERSSON UP, TIMBRELL JA, SNODGRASS WR, NELSON SD: Isoniazid liver injury: clinical spectrum, pathology and probably pathogenesis. Ann Intern Med 84: 181–192, 1976.

124. NESSI R, DOMENICHINI E, FOWST G: 'Allergic' reactions during rifampicin treatment: a review of published cases. Scand J Resp Dis (Suppl 84): 15–19, 1973.

125. NEWMAN R, DOSTER BE, MURRAY FJ, WOOLPERT SF: Rifampin in initial treatment of pulmonary tuberculosis. Am Rev Resp Dis 109: 216–232, 1974.

126. NYIRENDA R, GILL GV: Stevens-Johnson syndrome due to rifampicin. Br Med J 2: 1189, 1977.

127. PASRICHA JS, KANWAR AJ: Skin eruption caused by ethambutol. Arch Dermatol 113: 1122–1123, 1977.

128. PEARD MC, FLECK DG, GARROD LP, WATERWORTH PM: Combined rifampicin and erythromycin for bacterial endocarditis. Br Med J 4: 410–411, 1970.

129. PEETS EA, SWEENEY WM, PLACE VA, BUYSKE DA: The absorption, excretion and metabolic fate of ethambutol in man. Am Rev Resp Dis 91: 51–58, 1965.

130. PERIMAN P, VENKATARAMANI TK: Acute arthritis induced by isoniazid. Ann Intern Med 83: 667–668, 1975.
131. PETERS JH, MILLER KS, BROWN P: Studies on the metabolic basis for the genetically determined capacities for isoniazid inactivation in man. J Pharmacol Exp Ther 150: 298–304, 1965.
132. PHILLIPS S, TASHMAN H: Ethionamide jaundice. Am Rev Resp Dis 87: 896–898, 1963.
133. PLACE VA, PYLE MM, DE LA HUERGA J: Ethambutol in tuberculous meningitis. Am Rev Resp Dis 99: 783–785, 1969.
134. POOLE G, STRADLING P, WORLLEDGE S: Potentially serious side-effects of high-dose twice-weekly rifampicin. Br Med J 3: 343–347, 1971.
135. POSTLETHWAITE AE, KELLEY WN: Studies on the mechanism of ethambutol-induced hyperuricaemia. Arthritis Rheum 15: 403–409, 1972.
136. PRATT TH: Rifampin-induced organic brain syndrome. JAMA 241: 2421–2422, 1979.
137. PRATT WB: The antimetabolites. in Chemotherapy of Infection, pp. 176–202, New York: Oxford University Press, 1977.
138. PYLE MM: Ethambutol and viomycin. Med Clin North AM 54: 1317–1327, 1970.
139. RADENBACH KL: Chemotherapy of chronic pulmonary tuberculosis with polyresistant bacteria with reference to ethambutol and capreomycin. Scand J Resp Dis 49 (Suppl 65): 195–206, 1968.
140. RAMAKRISHNAN CV, DEVADATTA S, EVANS C, FOX W, MENON NK, NAZARETH O, RADHAKRISHNA S, SAMBAMOORTHY S, STOTT H, TRIPATHY SP, VELH S: A four-year follow up of patients with quiescent pulmonary tuberculosis at the end of a year of chemotherapy with twice-weekly isoniazid plus streptomycin or daily isoniazid plus PAS. Tubercle 50: 115–124, 1969.
141. ROBSON JM, SULLIVAN FM: Antituberulosis drugs. Pharmacol Rev 15: 169–223, 1963.
142. ROMANKIEWICZ JA, EHRMAN M: Rifampicin and warfarin: a drug interaction. Ann Intern Med 82: 224–225, 1975.
143. ROTHWELL DL, RICHMOND DE: Hepatorenal failure with self-initiated intermittent rifampicin therapy. Br Med J 2: 481–482, 1974.
144. SARMA GR, KAILASAM S, MITCHISON DA, NAIR NGK, RADHAKRISHNA S, TRIPATHY SP: Studies of serial plasma isoniazid concentrations with different doses of a slow-release preparation of isoniazid. Tubercle 56: 314–323, 1975.
145. SBARBARO JA, BARLOW PB, CRAIG MW, JOHNSTON RF, REAGAN WP, REICHMAN LB: Intermittent chemotherapy for adults with tuberculosis. Am Rev Resp Dis 110: 374–376, 1974.
146. SCHAEFFELD HG, GARTHWAITE B, AMBERSON JB: Viomycin therapy in human tuberculosis. Am Rev Tuberc 69: 520–553, 1954.
147. SCHARER L, SMITH JP: Serum transaminase elevations and other hepatic abnormalities in patients receiving isoniazid. Ann Intern Med 71: 1113–1120, 1969.
148. SCHEUER PJ, SUMMERFIELD JA, LAL S, SHERLOCK S: Rifampicin hepatitis. A clinical and histological study. Lancet 1: 421–425, 1974.
149. SCHWARTZ WS: Comparison of ethionamide with isoniazid in original treatment cases of pulmonary tuberculosis. XIV. A report of the Veterans Administration—Armed Forces Cooperative Study. Am Rev Resp Dis 93: 685–692, 1966.

150. SELF TH, FOUNTAIN FF, TAYLOR WJ, SUTLIFF WD: Acute gouty arthritis associated with the use of ethambutol. Chest 71: 561–562, 1977.

151. SIMPSON DG, WALKER JH: Hypersensitivity to para-aminosalicylic acid. Am J Med 29: 297–306, 1960.

152. SINGAPORE TUBERCULOSIS SERVICES/BROMPTON HOSPITAL/BRITISH MEDICAL RESEARCH COUNCIL INVESTIGATION: A controlled clinical trial of the role of thiacetazone-containing regimens in the treatment of pulmonary tuberculosis in Singapore: second report. Tubercle 55: 251–260, 1974.

153. SINGAPORE TUBERCULOSIS SERVICES/BRITISH MEDICAL RESEARCH COUNCIL: Controlled trial of intermittent regimens of rifampicin plus isoniazid for pulmonary tuberculosis in Singapore. Lancet 2: 1105–1109, 1975.

154. SINGAPORE TUBERCULOSIS SERVICE/BRITISH MEDICAL RESEARCH COUNCIL: Clinical trial of six-month and four-month regimens of chemotherapy in the treatment of pulmonary tuberculosis. Am Rev Resp Dis 119: 579–585, 1979.

155. SKOLNICK JL, STOLER BS, KATZ DB, ANDERSON WH: Rifampicin, oral contraceptives and pregnancy. JAMA 236: 1382, 1976.

156. SPARKS FC: Hazards and complications of BCG immunotherapy. Med Clin North Am 60: 499–509, 1976.

157. SPRINGETT VH: Do we need BCG vaccination? Postgrad Med J 52: 584–586, 1976.

158. STEEN JSM, STAINTON-ELLIS DM: Rifampicin in pregnancy. Lancet 2: 604–605, 1977.

159. STOREY PB, McLEAN RL: A current appraisal of cycloserine. Antibiot Med Clin Ther 4: 223–232, 1957.

160. STOTT H: The treatment of pulmonary tuberculosis in the developing countries. Trans R Soc Trop Med and Hyg 72: 564–569, 1978.

161. STOTTMEIER KD, BAKER S: Primary drug-resistant tuberculosis in Massachusetts, 1975/76. N Engl J Med 296: 823, 1977.

162. STOTTMEIER KD, BEAM RE, KUBICA GP: The absorption and excretion of pyrazinamide. Am Rev Resp Dis 98: 70–74, 1968.

163. SUTTON WB, GORDON RS, WICK WE, STANFIELD LV: In vitro and in vivo laboratory studies on the antituberculous activity of capreomycin. Ann NY Acad Sci 135: 947–959, 1966.

164. SYVÄLAHTI EKG, PIHLAJAMAKI KK, IISALO EI: Half-life of tolbutamide in patients receiving tuberculostatic agents. Scand J Resp Dis (Suppl 88): 17, 1974.

165. TAKAYAMA K, ARMSTRONG EL, DAVID HL: Restoration of mycolate synthetase activity in Mycobacterium tuberculosis exposed to isoniazid. Am Rev Resp Dis 110: 43–48, 1974.

166. THIRD EAST AFRICAN/BRITISH MEDICAL RESEARCH COUNCILS STUDY: Controlled clinical trial of four short-course regimens of chemotherapy for two durations in the treatment of pulmonary tuberculosis. Am Rev Resp Dis 118: 39–48, 1978.

167. THOMPSON JE: The effect of rifampicin on liver morphology in tuberculous alcoholics. Aust NZ J Med 6: 111, 1976.

168. THORNSBERRY C, BAKER CN, KIRVEN LA: In vitro activity of antimicrobial agents on Legionnaires disease bacterium. Antimicrob Agents Chemother 13: 78–80, 1978.

169. TUBERCLE: PAS. Tubercle 54: 165–167, 1973.

169a.TUBERCULOSIS CHEMOTHERAPY CENTRE, MADRAS: A controlled comparison of a twice-weekly and three once-weekly regimens in the initial treatment of pulmonary tuberculosis. Bull WHO 43: 143–206, 1970.

170. TUGWELL P, JAMES SL: Peripheral neuropathy with ethambutol. Postgrad Med J 48: 667–670, 1972.

171. UNITED STATES PUBLIC HEALTH SERVICE: Hepatic toxicity of pyrazinamide used with isoniazid in tuberculous patients. Am Rev Resp Dis 80: 371–387, 1959.

172. VALL-SPINOSA A, LESTER W, MOULDING T, DAVIDSON PT, McCLATCHY JK: Rifampin in the treatment of drug-resistant *Mycobacterium tuberculosis* infections. N Engl J Med 283: 616–621, 1970.

173. WANG L, TAKAYAMA K: Relationship between the uptake of isoniazid and its action on in vivo mycolytic acid synthesis in *Mycobacterium tuberculosis*. Antimicrob Agents Chemother 2: 438–441, 1972.

174. WEHRLI W, NÜESCH J, KNÜSEL F, STAEHELIN M: Action of rifamycins on RNA polymerase. Biochim Biophys Acta, 157: 215–217, 1968.

175. WEHRLI W, STAEHELIN M: Actions of the rifamycins. Bacteriol Rev 35: 290–309, 1971.

176. WEINSTEIN L: Drugs used in the chemotherapy of tuberculosis and leprosy. In The Pharmacological Basis of Therapeutics, 5th Edn. Goodman LS, Gilman A (eds). pp. 1201–1223, New York: Macmillan, 1975.

177. WEINSTEIN HJ, HALLETT WY, SARAUW AS: The absorption and toxicity of ethionamide. Am Rev Resp Dis 86: 576–578, 1962.

178. WERNER CA, TOMPSETT R, MUSCHENHEIM C, McDERMOTT W: The toxicity of viomycin in humans. Am Rev Tuberc 63: 49–61, 1951.

179. WESSEL-AAS T: Practical aspects of work on tuberculosis in South Korea. Scand J Resp Dis 49 (Suppl 65): 73–79, 1968.

180. WHO COLLABORATING CENTRE FOR TUBERCULOSIS CHEMOTHERAPY, PRAGUE, A study of two twice-weekly and a once-weekly continuation regimen of tuberculosis chemotherapy, including a comparison of two durations of treatment. 2. Second report: The result at 36 months. Tubercle 58: 129–136, 1977.

181. YEAGER RL, MUNROE WGC, DESSAU FI: Pyrazinamide (aldinamide) in the treatment of pulmonary tuberculosis. Am Rev Tuberc 65: 523–546, 1952.

182. YU TF, PEREL J, BERGER L, ROBOZ J, ISRAILI ZH, DAYTON PG: The effect of the interaction of pyrazinamide and probenecid on urinary uric acid excretion in man. Am J Med 63: 723–728, 1977.

183. ZIERSKI M: Intermittent treatment regimens in pulmonary tuberculosis. Lung 156: 17–32, 1979.

7

Bronchodilator Drugs

There has been substantial progress in the therapy of asthma in the past two decades, not only because of the arrival of new agents such as the specific beta-2 adrenergic agonists and cromolyn sodium (disodium cromoglycate), but also because clinicians have learned to use long-established bronchodilator drugs such as theophylline in more effective ways. In addition there is increased awareness of variations in the patterns of asthma, such as asthmatic cough,[100] exercise-induced bronchoconstriction, and early morning wheeze,[145] which has led to a more discerning therapeutic approach. But in spite of these advances, asthma can still be a killing disease at any age, and even though recognition of the potentially fatal case may be difficult, some of the evidence suggests that doctors are still insufficiently aware of the scale and urgency of therapy which may be required in treating a dangerously severe attack.[32]

It is now well recognised that many patients with chronic asthma have persistent pulmonary dysfunction even after maximal therapy of the acute attacks, probably due to residual obstruction in the small airways.[25] With the advent of drugs which are capable of preventing attacks it has become possible for physicians to apply prophylactic therapy not only through environmental measures or by attempted hyposensitization but more effectively by long-term drug treatment with agents such as cromolyn sodium, beta-2 sympathomimetic aerosols, and topical corticosteroids. In this way the opportunity for preserving normal airway function and preventing chronic disabling lung disease has been greatly enhanced.

This change of emphasis in the therapy of asthma has led to a reappraisal in the United States of the way in which theophylline can be used as a prophylactic agent, while in Britain and elsewhere the use of inhaled preparations of cromolyn sodium, long-acting beta-2 sympathomimetic agents, anticholinergic agents, and corticosteroids has become the preferred method of preventive treatment in chronic asthma. In determining the best use of this bewildering array of powerful and potentially toxic drugs for the management of a chronic but unpredictable disease, it is of some help to the clinician if he can base his therapy on an understanding of the interplay of different pharmacological agents in the regulation of bronchial calibre.

REGULATION OF BRONCHIAL CALIBRE

The Autonomic Nerves

Bronchial smooth muscle is arranged in a continuous network which extends throughout the bronchial tree from the trachea to the alveolar ducts. It is controlled by the autonomic nervous system through the sympathetic nerves from the upper four or five thoracic segments of the spinal cord, and through the vagus nerve which carries parasympathetic fibres. The neurohumoral transmitter of the postganglionic sympathetic nerves is norepinephrine and that of the postganglionic parasympathetic nerves is acetylcholine. Sympathetic nerve stimulation causes relaxation of bronchial smooth muscle and sympathetic receptors also respond to circulating epinephrine or to exogenous catecholamines. On the other hand, vagus nerve stimulation leads to bronchoconstriction, and a similar effect can be obtained by inhaling parasympathomimetic agents such as acetylcholine and methacholine; as one would anticipate, atropine-induced cholinergic blockade decreases bronchoconstriction in asthmatic patients.

Ahlquist[1] classified sympathetic receptors (adrenoreceptors) into two distinct types: alpha receptors, stimulation of which produces excitatory responses including bronchoconstriction; and beta receptors, whose activation results mainly in inhibitory responses plus cardiac stimulation. Beta receptors were subsequently further subdivided[89] into beta-1 receptors (chiefly present in the heart) and beta-2 receptors (elsewhere, including the bronchi) (Table 7-1). On the basis of this classification bronchodilator drugs can be thought of, in terms of the autonomic pharmacology of bronchial smooth muscle, as follows:

1. Sympathomimetic (adrenergic) drugs
   (a) With mixed alpha and beta effects.
   (b) With beta effects, including beta-1 and beta-2.
   (c) With selective beta-2 effects.
2. Alpha-adrenergic blocking drugs.
3. Anticholinergic drugs (Table 7-2).

Table 7-1 / Some Effects of Adrenergic Receptor Stimulation in Man

Receptor Type	Effects of Stimulation
Alpha	Bronchoconstriction Vasocontriction of arterioles and veins Dilatation of the pupil Contraction of pilomotor muscles Hepatic glycogenolysis Contraction of sphincters of gastrointestinal tract and urinary bladder
Beta-1	Increase in heart rate and in cardiac muscle contractility Acceleration of A-V conduction Lipolysis—increase in free fatty acids
Beta-2	Bronchodilatation Vasodilatation Skeletal muscle tremor Muscle glycogenolysis Lactic acidaemia

Table 7-2 / "Autonomic" Classification of Bronchodilator Drugs

Autonomic Action	Drug	Nature of Action and Unwanted Effects
Sympathetic (adrenergic)	Epinephrine Ephedrine	Relaxation of bronchial smooth muscle (beta-2 effect). Unwanted alpha and beta-1 effects.
	Isoproterenol	Beta-2 bronchodilatation. Unwanted beta-1 effects.
	Selective beta-2 sympathomimetic agents (such as terbutaline and salbutamol)	Beta-2 bronchodilation. Unwanted beta-2 effects, for instance, muscle tremor, tachycardia.
Alpha-adrenoceptor blocking drugs	Indoramin Thymoxamine Phentolamine	Possibly cause relaxation of bronchial smooth muscle due to alpha-receptor blockade, but also have antihistamine and antiserotonin effects.
Anticholinergic drugs	Atropine Ipratropium bromide	Bronchodilatation due to para-sympathetic blockade

Although the above classification provides a useful framework for understanding the actions and unwanted effects of many of the most valuable bronchodilator drugs it does not account for the activity of theophylline and cromolyn sodium (disodium cromoglycate) in the treatment of asthma, or provide an explanation for the influence of humoral mediators such as histamine and the prostaglandins on bronchial smooth muscle. Further insight into the way bronchodilator agents act and interact can be obtained by considering the cellular processes which lead to smooth muscle relaxation or constriction, and their relationship to the chemical mediators which influence bronchomotor tone.

Cellular Function

Cyclic Nucleotides   Many of the drugs which influence bronchial calibre in asthmatic subjects can be seen to act through the mediation of the cyclic nucleotides and of calcium ions (Ca^{++}) which are considered to be important intracellular messengers not only in bronchial smooth muscle cells but also in tissue mast cells, in the secretory cells of the tracheobronchial mucosa, in vascular smooth muscle and endothelial cells, and in haematogenous cells capable of mediator secretion, such as the polymorphonuclear leucocytes and macrophages. It is now well established that beta-adrenergic compounds exert their effects by stimulating the activity of an enzyme located on the cell membrane, adenylcyclase, which transforms ATP into cyclic 3', 5'-adenosine monophosphate (cAMP). An increase in the concentration of cAMP influences the activity of a phosphokinase which, in turn, is responsible for further enzyme stimulation to give final expression of the adrenergic effect in that particular cell type; cAMP is degraded by a group of enzymes, the phosphodiesterases, which are inhibited by a number of drugs, including theophylline (Figure 7-1). In some types of cell augmentation of cAMP concentration leads to activation (for example, secretion by mammalian salivary gland) while in others it results in inhibition of activity as exemplified by the reduction of exocytotic secretion by mast cells or by the relaxation of bronchial smooth muscle.

Although Figure 7-1 depicts cAMP as occupying a central role in the enzymic interactions which influence cell activity other substances are known to be of great importance in intracellular control mechanisms. In many cell systems Ca^{++} plays the dominant role,[124] while in others there is some degree of interplay between the functions of Ca^{++} and cAMP.[16] For instance, in tissue mast cells the IgE-antigen reaction on the cell surface initiates a sequence of intracellular enzymic reactions which lead to the release of granules containing histamine and other chemical mediators.[79] The release of histamine and the slow-reacting substance of anaphylaxis (SRS-A) is inhibited by cAMP and by

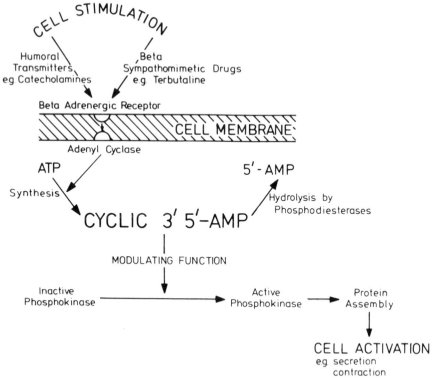

Figure 7-1 *Cell activation by beta-adrenergic stimulation, suggesting a central role for cyclic AMP.*

drugs which raise intracellular levels of cAMP,[18,88] but is stimulated by a flux of Ca^{++} into the cell,[54] possibly initiated by the IgE-antigen reaction at the cell surface[53] (Figure 7-2).

The existence of another system involving cyclic 3', 5'-guanidine monophosphate (cGMP) which is activated by cholinergic substances has been demonstrated more recently in a number of cell populations,[65] but the physiological role of this cyclic nucelotide is still unclear. It has been suggested that cAMP and cGMP have, in general, opposing roles in regulating the tone of smooth muscle[66] but several experimental observations indicate that this concept is an oversimplification; for example, it fails to account for the bronchodilator effect of phosphodiesterase inhibitions such as the methylxanthines which increase the intracellular level of *both* cAMP and cGMP. The complexity of the relationship between cAMP and cGMP is illustrated by observations in lung tissue *in vitro* that acetylcholine and bradykinin caused an increase in cGMP which provoked the release of prostaglandins, leading to a secondary increase

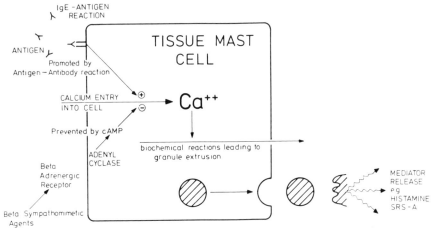

Figure 7-2 *The mast cell. Schematic diagram illustrating a hypothetical interaction between cAMP and Ca^{++} in the regulation of granule release (after Foreman and Garland, 1976).*

in cAMP.[139,140] A similar sequence of changes in cyclic nucleotide concentrations could be provoked by histamine in canine lung *in vivo*,[11] suggesting that these two messengers do not necessarily counteract one another but rather tend to buffer any abrupt deviation from equilibrium.

In terms of therapy it appears that agents which increase the intracellular concentration of cAMP such as beta-adrenergic compounds and methylxanthine phosphodiesterase inhibitors generally have a beneficial effect in asthma by relaxing bronchial smooth muscle, inhibiting the release of bronchoconstrictor mediators from mast cells and possibly influencing the production or clearance of bronchial secretion.[55,154] In contrast, agents which increase cGMP and/or reduce cAMP concentrations such as cholinergic drugs have an adverse effect but their antagonists, anticholinergics such as atropine or ipratropium bromide have some therapeutic applications as bronchodilators. The precise mode of action of cromolyn sodium is still unsettled, although the drug is known to have an effect through its ability to prevent the degranulation of mast cells and thus the release of mediators which initiate the asthmatic reaction[114] either indirectly by increasing the concentration of cAMP by phosphodiesterase inhibition,[126] or by preventing the ingress of Ca^{++} necessary for mediator release from the cell.[81]

Prostaglandins   An understanding of the role of naturally occurring chemical mediators in the regulation of bronchial calibre has been the origin of a long series of therapeutically useful bronchodilator drugs such as the sympathomimetic amines and the anticholinergic agents. Interest in the prostaglandins

(PGs) as a source for possible therapeutic agents has therefore been stimulated by experimental evidence that some are potent bronchoactive substances.

The prostaglandins are 20-carbon unsaturated fatty acids which can be synthesized by and released from virtually all mammalian cells. There are 8 prostaglandin families which vary according to the substituents on the 5-membered ring of prostanoic acid, the most relevant to this discussion being PGE_1 and PGE_2 which have been shown experimentally to relax airway smooth muscle and, as aerosols, to have a bronchodilator effect comparable to that of isoproterenol[39]; and $PGF_2\alpha$ which is a powerful bronchoconstrictor. Most prostaglandins are eliminated almost completely from circulating blood by one passage through the pulmonary vascular bed, but local release of PGEs and $PGF_2\alpha$ in lung tissue may occur as a result of a variety of stimuli, including anaphylaxis, hypoxia, embolisation, pulmonary oedema, and mechanical interference.[40,97] In addition to their effects on bronchial smooth muscle PGE_1 dilates arteries and veins whereas PGE_2 has no definite effect on arteries but constricts veins; while $PGF_2\alpha$ has a marked pressor effect on arteries and veins. It has been conjectured that release of prostaglandins and other mediators resulting from localised pathological processes in the lung might provide a mechanism for maintaining appropriate ventilation/perfusion ratios,[40] possibly based on differences in the relative rates of synthesis and catabolism of PGE_2 and $PGF_2\alpha$.[99]

The release of prostaglandins in the lung is provoked by mediators of allergic and inflammatory reactions such as histamine, bradykinin, and SRS-A, and conversely, prostaglandins of the E type inhibit the release of mediators from lung tissue, leucocytes, and mast cells. This interrelationship probably depends upon the cyclic nucleotide system since PGE_1 and, to a lesser extent, PGE_2 increase cAMP levels in experimental lung preparations presumably by stimulating adenylcyclase activity.[106,139] Aerosol preparations of PGE_1 and PGE_2 have been shown experimentally to produce short-lived bronchodilatation in healthy and asthmatic subjects,[75,136] although PGE_2 may occasionally induce bronchoconstriction.[98] This variability in response, and the highly irritant effect of these preparations on the upper respiratory tract, makes them unsuitable for therapeutic use, but the future development of prostaglandin analogues may provide useful agents for treating asthma.

SYMPATHOMIMETIC AGENTS

Sympathomimetic drugs have been used in the Western world for the treatment of asthma since the end of the nineteenth century, although the usefulness of a preparation obtained from a plant, of which ephedrine is the active principle, had been known to Chinese physicians for 4,000 years. Their major application is in the treatment of mild or moderately severe asthma, although epinephrine (adrenaline) has a special place in treating acute life-threatening bronchospasm of anaphylaxis, due to its extremely rapid action. The most recent development in the history of the sympathomimetic agents has been the introduction of analogues with longer durations of pharmacologic effect and greater selectivity for beta-2 activity, making the old stand-bys of epinephrine, ephedrine, and isoproterenol increasingly redundant in the routine treatment of asthma although still useful in selected clinical situations.

The parent compound of the sympathomimetic amines is β-phenyl-ethylamine which consists of a benzene ring and an aliphatic portion, ethyl-amine (Figure 7-3). Substitutions on the benzene ring, the α- and β-car-bon atoms and the terminal amino-group yield a wide range of compounds

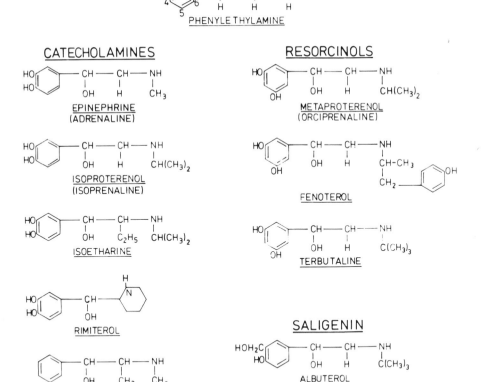

Figure 7-3 *Chemical structure of sympathomimetic bronchodilator agents.*

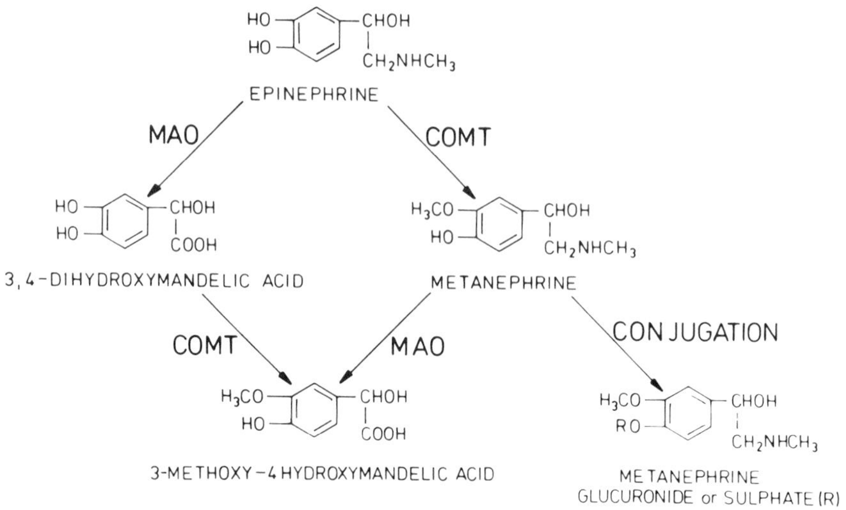

HO—⟨benzene⟩—CHOH
HO— |
                    CH_2NHCH_3

EPINEPHRINE

MAO   COMT

HO—⟨benzene⟩—CHOH H_3CO—⟨benzene⟩—CHOH
HO— | HO— |
                   COOH CH_2NHCH_3

3,4-DIHYDROXYMANDELIC ACID   METANEPHRINE

COMT   MAO   CONJUGATION

H_3CO—⟨benzene⟩—CHOH H_3CO—⟨benzene⟩—CHOH
HO— | RO— |
                   COOH CH_2NHCH_3

3-METHOXY-4 HYDROXYMANDELIC ACID   METANEPHRINE
                                          GLUCURONIDE or SULPHATE (R)

Figure 7-4   *Main pathways for the metabolism of epinephrine (adrenaline).*

with sympathomimetic activity. Norepinephrine, epinephrine, and isoproterenol have OH groups substituted in the 3 and 4 positions of the benzene ring, and because o-dihydroxybenzene is also known as *catechol,* sympathomimetic amines with these substitutions in the benzene ring are referred to as *catecholamines.* Catecholamines are largely metabolised by the enzyme catechol-o-methyltransferase (COMT) and also by monamine oxidase (MAO), being ultimately converted to the urinary excretion product 3-methoxy-4-hydroxy-mandelic acid (Figure 7-4).

Epinephrine (Adrenaline)

A benzoyl derivative of epinephrine was originally isolated from adrenal medullary tissue following the use of tablets of dessicated adrenal gland for the treatment of asthma. Its chemical structure (Figure 7-3) shows it to be a catecholamine, and it is ineffective when taken by mouth because it is largely inactivated by monoamine oxidase present in the gastrointestinal tract. In asthma the usual routes of administration are by aerosol or by subcutaneous injection, the intramuscular route being generally used only to administer a long-acting preparation of epinephrine in oil. Otherwise the drug has a short duration of action, being rapidly inactivated by the liver and excreted in the urine.

Epinephrine has beta-2 actions which confer its beneficial bronchodilator effect in asthma but it also has extensive adverse beta-1 and alpha effects which have led to its virtual displacement from the therapeutic scene in asthma in face of the introduction of specific beta-2 sympathomimetics. The most important of these side-effects are hypertension, tachycardia, and cardiac arrhythmias, including the risks of subarachnoid haemorrhage and ventricular fibrillation. Epinephrine is particularly liable to cause dangerous reactions in patients with hyperthyroidism, hypertension, and organic heart disease, but it may cause considerable discomfort in any case, producing symptoms of headache, palpitation, tremor, and anxiety.

For an acute asthmatic attack Epinephrine Injection U.S.P. (Adrenaline Injection B.P.) can be given slowly, subcutaneously in a dose of 0.1 ml of 1:1,000 solution per minute up to a total of 0.5 to 1.0 ml (equivalent to 0.5–1.0 mg), or administered by inhalation as a nebulised 1:100 solution. It is also included in numerous proprietary bronchodilator preparations which are administered by metered dose aerosol, either as epinephrine alone or as one constituent of a bronchodilator cocktail. The usual dose of epinephrine in these preparations is 0.16–0.20 mg per puff in the United States and 0.25–0.28 mg per puff in Britain and elsewhere.

The major modern-day indication for the use of epinephrine to treat bronchospasm is in the therapy of acute anaphylaxis, as may occur in hypersensitive individuals following bee and wasp stings, insect bites, ingestion of allergens, parenteral infusion of protein-containing products, injection of penicillins, and the like. Usually the drug is given subcutaneously as described above, and susceptible individuals may obtain valuable emergency protection by carrying a syringe preloaded with epinephrine which can be administered promptly if the need arises.

Ephedrine

Ephedrine is an alkaloid originally derived from the plant *ma huang* (from the species *Ephedra*) which was in use as a medicine in China in the second millennium B.C. Comparison of its chemical structure with that of epinephrine (Figure 7-3) shows that it lacks the catecholamine hydroxyl groups on the benzene ring, leading to relative loss of potency and resistance to the action of COMT; in addition the carbon methyl group results in resistance to MAO, so that the drug is effective when taken by mouth. It is metabolised to norephedrine by demethylation, but 60–75 percent is excreted unchanged in the urine. Some reabsorption occurs from the renal tubules depending on the degree of ionisation of the drug, which is mainly ionised at acid pH and therefore unabsorbed and excreted, but partially un-ionised at alkaline pH when there is significant reabsorption. Thus there are theoretical grounds for supposing that the handling of ephedrine and its half-life in the body may vary with the acid-base status of the patient, although measurements of half-life in patients taking ephedrine-containing tablets showed no relationship between ephedrine excretion rates and minor fluctuations in urinary pH.[153]

Ephedrine has some direct effect on adrenergic receptors but it also has an indirect action because it stimulates the release of endogenous catecholamines, an effect which may account for the development of tolerance in some patients,[74] due to depletion of available norepinephrine at nerve endings following 3 or 4 days treatment with rather high doses of ephedrine. Interruption of treatment for a few days may restore responsiveness. The drug has both alpha and beta effects with considerable nervous system stimulation, its actions being more prolonged though less potent than norepinephrine. The side-effects are similar to those of epinephrine, although hypertension and ventricular arrhythmias occur rarely. Ephedrine is likely to cause wakefulness in adults if taken at night and is best avoided in patients with benign prostatic hypertrophy, because it may precipitate urinary retention.

Ephedrine sulfate U.S.P. is the levoratory isomer, available in 25 and 50 mg tablets and capsules, and in a 4 mg/ml syrup. Ephedrine hydrochloride tablets B.P. are available in 15, 30, and 60 mg tablets, and Ephedrine Elixir B.P.C. contains ephedrine hydrochloride 15 mg in 5 ml. The usual dose for bronchospasm in adults is 15–60 mg every 3 or 4 hours, and for children up to 1 year 7.5 mg; 1–5 years 15 mg; and 6–12 years 30 mg.

The likelihood of side-effects and the development of tolerance have led to the displacement of ephedrine from regular use as a bronchodilator in favour of the specific beta-2 sympathomimetics and theophylline. A number of proprietary preparations containing ephedrine in combination with theophylline and a sedative such as a barbiturate or antihistamine have retained considerable popularity,[58] although there is little objective evidence of their superiority to theophylline alone.[151] The inclusion of barbiturates in such preparations is open to criticism because of their potential for inducing physical dependence, their liability for causing enzyme induction leading to clinically important drug interactions,[24] and their capacity for precipitating respiratory failure in patients with chronic obstructive lung disease. Indeed, it seems illogical to include *any* drug which can act as a sedative, hypnotic, or tranquilliser because of the risk of causing carbon dioxide narcosis in patients with respiratory failure.[31]

Isoproterenol (Isoprenaline)

Isoproterenol differs from epinephrine in having an isopropyl group substituted on the terminal amine group (Figure 7-3). This structural change alters the pharmacological properties to an almost exclusive beta-receptor activity which provides beta-2 bronchodilatation but also undesirable cardiovascular effects from its beta-1 action. The metabolism of isoproterenol depends upon the route of administration[34]: after oral ingestion the drug is absorbed from the gastrointestinal tract but is largely conjugated to an inactive sulphate derivative during its passage of the gut wall (Figure 7-5). The individual variability of this first-pass metabolism makes the effect of oral isoproterenol unpredictable and contraindicates its use by this route. After intravenous administration a greater proportion of the drug is metabolised by COMT to 3-o-methyl isoproterenol, and the initial half-life is short. It behaves as a non-selective beta-sympathomimetic agonist producing both cardiac stimulation and broncho-dilatation at the same dose level so that its value as a bronchodilator by the intravenous route is mainly limited by cardiovascular side-effects, although it has been used successfully in this way for the treatment of status asthmaticus.[158] The most effective method of administering isoproterenol therapeutically is by inhaled aerosol when it appears to provide adequate bronchodilatation in a dosage small enough to cause little likelihood of cardiac stimulation. By this route it begins to take effect in 3–5 minutes, reaching a peak within half an hour and lasting for about 2 hours.

The major adverse effects of isoproterenol arise from its beta-1 actions on the cardiovascular system, which cause palpitations, tachycardia, headache, and flushing of the skin. Anginal pain, ventricular arrhythmias, nausea, and tremor are a rare occurrence. Tolerance to the effect of isoproterenol has been described in animals and in humans,[33] and cross-tolerance between beta-receptor stimulants is a recognised phenomenon,[14,33,107] leading to the possibility that beta-receptor desensitisation due to tolerance from excessive use of beta-adrenergic stimulants in patients with asthma might upset a hypothetical

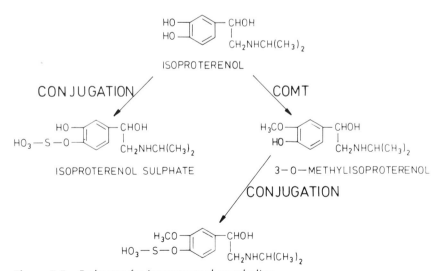

Figure 7-5 *Pathways for isoproterenol metabolism.*

balance between constrictor and dilator influences on bronchomotor tone and thus aggravate bronchoconstriction. Although the part played by these and other factors in the rise of asthma mortality in the 1960s is controversial, it is generally acknowledged that patients using isoproterenol and other beta-sympathomimetic aerosol preparations should be warned not to take repeated doses at short intervals.

The use of isoproterenol aerosols has declined since the introduction of the selective beta-2 sympathomimetic bronchodilators with longer duration of action and fewer cardiovascular side-effects, but a minority of patients with long-standing asthma have persisted with isoproterenol-containing preparations. There is a wide variation in the amount of isoproterenol base delivered per metered dose from different aerosol preparations, ranging from 40 μg per dose (for example, "Norisodrine Aerohaler 10%," available in the United States) to 500 μg per dose (for example, "PIB plus," available in the United Kingdom). A reasonable dose providing adequate bronchodilatation would be 2 inhalations of an aerosol giving 100 μg isoprenaline per metered dose.[118] The physician should be aware of the potency of the preparation he is prescribing and advise an upper limit to the number of inhalations, usually 1–3 inhalations 4 to 8 times a day. In the event of an asthmatic attack, the patient should be warned to obtain medical advice promptly if he ceases to obtain subjective benefit from the inhalation.

Now that wide experience has been gained in the use of selective beta-2 sympathomimetic aerosols such as albuterol (salbutamol) or terbutaline, there seems to be little place for the use of isoproterenol as a bronchodilator; the possible rare exception is the patient with well-controlled chronic reversible airway obstruction who has long been accustomed to an isoproterenol preparation.

Selective Beta-2 Sympathomimetic Bronchodilators

The search for the ideal bronchodilator agent has led to the synthesis and trial of numerous compounds based on the isoproterenol molecule with the objectives of prolonging bronchodilator activity and increasing beta-2 selectivity, thereby reducing the relative incidence of adverse effects arising from beta-1 stimulation. At present six drugs with a broadly similar range of pharmacological characteristics are widely prescribed—metaproterenol (orciprenaline), isoetharine, terbutaline, albuterol (salbutamol), fenoterol, and rimiterol (Figure 7-3).

Absence of one or both of the OH groups on the benzene ring prevents the action of catechol-o-methyltransferase (COMT), for example, in metaproterenol, terbutaline, albuterol, and fenoterol, while substitution on the alpha carbon atom blocks oxidation by monoamine oxidase (MAO), such as isoetharine. These alterations to the molecule greatly prolong the duration of action of these compounds and increase their oral effectiveness.

Some increase in selective beta-2 action can be produced by substitution in the alpha carbon atom of the catecholamine side chain—for example, isoetharine—but a greater degree of beta-2 selectivity is achieved by substitution on the amine head, for example, terbutaline, salbutamol, rimiterol, and fenoterol.[89] The tertiary butyl radical of terbutaline and salbutamol appears to be particularly potent in this respect. It is more difficult to estimate beta-2 selectivity in humans than in isolated organ preparations from experimental animals, because increase in heart rate, which is commonly taken as a crude indicator of beta-1 stimulation of the heart, may also be a secondary consequence of the fall in blood pressure which follows vasodilatation due to beta-2 effects on vascular smooth muscle.[47] Whether by residual beta-1 activity or by indirect beta-2 effects, therefore, all "selective" beta-2 sympathomimetic bronchodilators will have undesirable cardiovascular effects at sufficient dosage; their advantage over isoproterenol and other non-selective sympathomimetic bronchodilator agents lies primarily in the relative improvement in therapeutic index which beta-2 selectivity imparts. For example, experimental comparisons of "desirable" (that is, bronchodilatation) and "undesirable" (for example, fall in blood pressure and increased heart rate) effects between isoproterenol and the selective beta-2 sympathomimetic salbutamol after intravenous infusion in asthmatic patients show that for a given degree of bronchodilatation the increase in heart rate is approximately 5 times as great after isoproterenol than after salbutamol.[117] It is also important to bear in mind that in any population there is likely to be considerable variation in individual responsiveness to sympathomimetic stimulation so that some incidence of side-effects is likely even when recommended dosage regimens of selective agents are used. It is for this reason that the aerosol route of administration is so useful since it increases the therapeutic index by permitting a reduction in the total dose of drug administered while maintaining a useful bronchodilator effect.

Isoetharine   Isoetharine is a short-acting bronchodilator with a rapid onset of action and a duration of effect of 1 to 3 hours. An estimate of its potency as an aerosol suggested that isoetharine produced approximately half the bronchodilator effect of isoproterenol in similar dosage.[57] Animal experiments have shown that its cardiovascular effects are less than those of isoproterenol, but it causes some beta-1 stimulation. Side-effects include muscle tremor, headache, vertigo, and tachycardia. It is effective when taken by mouth and can be prescribed as a 10 mg slow-release tablet in Britain and elsewhere but not in the United States where it is only available as an aerosol. The metered dose preparation, known as Bronkometer or Bronchilator, contains 340 μg of isoetharine mesylate per puff, of which one to four are inhaled every 2 to 3 hours up to a recommended maximum of 12 puffs in a day. An aqueous solution called Bronkosol, containing 1 percent isoetharine hydrochloride, is also available in the United States for use with a hand nebuliser or for delivery by intermittent positive pressure breathing (IPPB).

Rimiterol   Like isoproterenol rimiterol is conjugated by sulphatase enzymes in the gut wall and is also a substrate for COMT so that it is inactive after oral administration and has a short half-life[49] when administered as an aerosol or intravenously. Rimiterol and isoproterenol are equipotent as bronchodilator aerosols in normal and asthmatic subjects,[132] and rimiterol is an effective bronchodilator by the intravenous route although less potent than isoproterenol.[95] The beta-2 adrenoreceptor selectivity of rimiterol is similar to that of salbutamol by the intravenous route of administration but greater than salbutamol when given in equipotent bronchodilating doses by IPPB in asthmatics.[36] Like other beta-2 selective bronchodilators it causes muscle tremor due to stimulation of skeletal muscle receptors.

At present the drug is available in Britain as a metered dose aerosol of rimiterol hydrobromide 200 μg per dose, but its most useful application may be as an intravenous bronchodilator in the treatment of severe asthma, because of its short half-life which permits rapid equilibration of its blood concentration and accurate monitoring.[96]

Metaproterenol (Orciprenaline)   This drug is similar structurally to isoproterenol except that the hydroxyl groups on the benzene ring are at positions 3 and 5 rather than at 3 and 4, making it resistant to the action of COMT or to sulphate conjugation and therefore active when given by mouth and long-lasting in its effects. As an intravenous preparation it has no advantage over isoproterenol, with which it is equipotent as a bronchodilator, but it is equally liable to produce cardiovascular side-effects. As an aerosol metaproterenol has a peak bronchodilator effect similar to isoprenaline, occurring somewhat later and lasting longer but without the tachycardia observed with isoproterenol.[29] It is comparable to salbutamol and terbutaline when given by mouth, producing a similar bronchodilator effect lasting about 4 hours, although metaproterenol caused a greater increase in heart rate.[110]

Metaproterenol sulphate is available as a 10 or 20 mg tablet taken 3 or 4 times daily, or as a syrup containing 10 mg in 5 ml. The metered dose aerosol contains 650 μg per puff (750 μg in Britain), and 1 to 3 inhalations are taken every 3 to 6 hours up to a maximum of 12 doses in 24 hours. It is also available outside the United States as a 5 percent solution for inhalation or as a solution for injection containing 0.5 mg per ml.

The pharmacological actions of metaproterenol differ little from those of isoproterenol, but it has the advantages of more prolonged action and oral effectiveness.

Terbutaline and Albuterol (Salbutamol)   These two drugs are so similar in their pharmacology and therapeutic applications that they are here discussed together, although albuterol is not currently available in the United States. Known as salbutamol, it is very widely used elsewhere, and in Britain it is probably prescribed as frequently as any single sympathomimetic bronchodilator. Both drugs have a similar molecular structure with a tertiary butyl substituent group at the amine head, but terbutaline is a resorcinol with hydroxyl groups at positions 3 and 5 on the benzene ring, while salbutamol has a saligenin substituent at the 3-hydroxyl position; these substitutions impart beta-2 selectivity and resistance to COMT and sulphate conjugation so that both have a predictable effect when given by mouth and have a long duration of action lasting 4 to 6 hours (Figure 7-3).

Comparison of intravenous salbutamol and isoproterenol in asthmatic patients showed that they were equipotent as bronchodilators,[147] but that salbutamol was approximately one-fifth as potent in causing a rise in heart rate.[117] Arner et al.[8] carried out a single dose study comparing intravenous injections of 0.25–0.5 mg of terbutaline with the same dose of metaproterenol, observing that a similar rise in heart rate and fall in peripheral resistance was produced by both drugs, but that the increase in systolic pressure, cardiac output, and stroke volume were all less with terbutaline, indicating less beta-1 activity. Arner[7] also showed that subcutaneous terbutaline was more potent than metaproterenol given by the same route of administration and had a longer effect, with slightly less cardiac stimulation. Salbutamol, which is now available on prescription in Britain for intravenous injection, appears to be an effective bronchodilator comparable to aminophylline in the early treatment of status asthmaticus when given by this route,[51,155] although it produces dose-related increases in heart rate, pulse pressure, and skeletal muscle tremor.[95] It has also been shown to produce a rise in free fatty acid levels and in plasma insulin, glucose, and lactate values[66,143] associated with a fall in plasma potassium, suggesting that there is a shift of potassium from the extracellular to the intracellular space.[90,108] The combination of sympathetic stimulation, hypoxia, and hypokalaemia might increase the danger of cardiac arrhythmias, and it has been suggested that if intravenous salbutamol is used in the management of severe asthma the plasma potassium level and the electrocardiogram should be carefully monitored.[90]

Both salbutamol and terbutaline are available for oral prescription, 5 mg of each showing a similar bronchodilator effect within 30 minutes, rising to a peak between 2 and 4 hours, and lasting for up to 6 hours. Both drugs cause an increase in heart rate and muscle tremor in some patients. A comparison of ephedrine 25 mg with terbutaline 5 mg showed that the latter produced greater bronchodilator effect in asthmatic patients but also caused a greater increase in heart rate and pulse pressure,[142] and a similar comparison between aminophylline 400 mg and terbutaline 5 mg revealed a comparable degree of bronchodilatation by both drugs coming on after 1 hour and lasting 7 hours with a similar incidence of tachycardia and other adverse effects.[157] A recent investigation suggested that cardiac arrhythmias are just as likely to develop in patients with chronic obstructive lung disease or asthma who are treated with oral terbutaline as with ephedrine or aminophylline.[9] Oral administration of salbutamol 4 mg to adult asthmatic and bronchitic patients has a similar effect to orciprenaline 20 mg and isoetharine 20 mg, resulting in significant bronchodilatation after 30 minutes with a peak effect at 2 to 3 hours and a duration of action of 4–6 hours. Tachycardia does not seem to be a problem in the day to day clinical use of salbutamol in the usual adult dosage of 2–4 mg 3 times daily, but muscle tremor is a troublesome side-effect which requires dosage reduction in a minority of patients.

Because it offers the advantage of minimising side-effects by reducing the dose, aerosol administration of salbutamol and terbutaline is the method of choice for using these drugs in the control or prevention of bronchoconstriction in chronic asthma or chronic obstructive pulmonary disease. Neither drug is available for administration by this route in the United States. The time scale for onset of action, peak effect, and duration of effect for both drugs is similar to that seen after oral administration, being slower in onset and longer in duration than isoproterenol but similar to metaproterenol. Used to prevent post-exercise asthma, salbutamol is more effective when given as a metered dose aerosol than by mouth.[4] Because of the possible dangers of fluorocarbon propellants and the difficulties which some patients find with the technique of pressurised aerosol inhalation, an aerosol powder form of salbutamol offers some advantage, administered by an inhalation-activated device (named a Rotahaler) which is considered easier to use, although the bronchodilator effect of salbutamol powder delivered in this way is slightly less, dose for dose, than for salbutamol given by pressurised aerosol.[71]

Administration of salbutamol by wet aerosol in a dose of 5–10 mg in 2 ml produces effective bronchodilatation with a liability to tachycardia at higher doses, and is equally effective whether given by Bird ventilator with or without IPPB or by Wright nebuliser. Smaller doses of 1.0 or 2.5 mg of salbutamol are also effective when delivered by IPPB,[127] and this method of administration is clearly of value if patients are unable to master the technique of pressurised aerosol inhalation. In patients with status asthmaticus, however, the response to salbutamol aerosol given by IPPB was shown to be unsatisfactory compared with intravenous administration,[156] emphasising that in severe asthma bronchodilators should be given parenterally.

Terbutaline sulphate is available in the United States as a tablet or for subcutaneous administration, the oral dose in adults being 2.5–5 mg 3 times daily; the subcutaneous preparation contains 1 mg/ml and is usually given in a dose of 0.25 mg repeated if necessary after 15–30 minutes; in children over 2 years the dose is 5–10 μg/kg body weight every 4–6 hours, to a maximum of 300 μg in 24 hours. Outside the United States terbutaline sulphate is also available for administration by parenteral injection, by aerosol using a metered dose inhaler or respirator solution, and as a syrup.

Salbutamol is a drug of choice outside the United States, being widely used as a metered dose aerosol containing 100 μg/puff in a dose of 2 puffs 4 times daily, or as a 2 or 4 mg tablet in a dosage of 2 to 4 mg 3 times daily. For children a syrup is available containing 2 mg in 5 ml. In addition a powder aerosol containing 200 or 400 μg/dose can be offered to patients who have difficulty in using the pressurised aerosol effectively. Salbutamol is also prepared in solutions for use with IPPB therapy and for parenteral injection or intravenous infusion.

Fenoterol This is a new adrenergic beta-receptor stimulant which is marketed outside the United States as a metered dose aerosol inhalant. Its structure (Figure 7-3) shows that it has a resorcinol nucleus which ensures prolonged activity, since it is not metabolised by COMT, and a hydroxyphenyl substituent on the isopropyl group which gives it beta-2 selectivity. It appears to be comparable to salbutamol[132] and to terbutaline[5] in producing bronchodilatation in asthmatic patients, possibly with a slightly longer duration of action.[103] In a few patients tremor and tachycardia were noticed after inhalation but were commoner after oral or intravenous administration. Further studies are necessary to determine the relative potency of fenoterol compared with other long-acting beta-2 sympathomimetic agents.

The recommended dose of fenoterol is 1–2 puffs of the metered dose aerosol 3 times daily. Each inhalation contains 200 μg of fenoterol hydrobromide.

Summary In clinical practice the main problem in the use of beta-2 sympathomimetic agents lies in the avoidance of overdosage because of their liability to cause cardiovascular side-effects and skeletal muscle tremor. This problem is aggravated if the patient is taking other sympathomimetic preparations concurrently, and it is not unknown for a combination of oral and aerosol preparations of the same drug to be prescribed without full appreciation of their additive toxic effects. Careful instructions to patients in the use of aerosols is mandatory, as is a warning to seek medical advice early if the treatment becomes ineffective in an acute attack of asthma. Despite these reservations the beta-2 sympathomimetic aerosols, particularly those with a longer duration of action such as terbutaline and salbutamol, currently provide an essential element in management of asthma[68] and are displacing isoproterenol, which is neither beta-2 specific nor long-acting and, it is suggested, no longer has a place in the rational management of asthma.[159]

ALPHA-ADRENOCEPTOR BLOCKING AGENTS

Alpha-adrenergic antagonists have been used experimentally to investigate the role of alpha-adrenergic activity in asthma, but as yet they have no place in therapy. Szentivanyi[141] suggested that in asthmatic patients there is an abnormal preponderance of alpha-receptors and a relative lack of beta-receptors in bronchial smooth muscle. Although it is difficult to demonstrate the presence of alpha-receptors in the tracheo-bronchial tree of humans, in asthmatics bronchoconstriction results from the administration of alpha-adrenergic stimulants such as phenylephrine[116,134] or methoxamine,[137] after beta-receptor blockade with propranolol. The mechanism of this effect is not fully understood, but it has been shown that alpha-adrenergic stimulation can cause an increase in the release of histamine and SRS-A in passively sensitised human lung.[82] It may be, therefore, that alpha-adrenergic stimulants cause bronchoconstriction either by the release of humoral mediators from mast cells or through the direct stimulation of alpha-receptors in bronchial smooth muscle.

Phentolamine, thymoxamine, and indoramin are alpha-adrenergic antagonists which have been used experimentally in asthma to reverse or prevent allergen- or exercise-induced bronchoconstriction[17] and to potentiate the bronchodilator effect of beta-adrenergic drugs.[115] None of these agents is specific for the alpha-receptor: phentolamine increases circulating catecholamine concentrations, and both thymoxamine and indoramin have antihistaminic properties. All alpha-receptor blocking agents tend to lower blood pressure and hence to cause a generalised homeostatic stimulation of the sympathetic nervous system; this maintains blood pressure and cardiac output but may also cause bronchodilatation. Thus it is at present uncertain exactly how these agents produce a bronchodilator effect, and their role in the treatment of asthma is undefined. Recent studies of asthmatic patients using prazosin, which is a specific alpha-receptor blocking drug, failed to show any bronchodilatation when compared with salbutamol,[10] suggesting that alpha-adrenergic mediated bronchoconstriction may not be important in asthma.

ANTICHOLINERGIC DRUGS

The rationale for using anticholinergic drugs in the treatment of bronchial asthma is based on the hypothesis of an irritant-bronchoconstrictor reflex,[61] whereby the allergen combines with antibodies in the surface of the bronchial epithelium, leading to the release of mediators which act on nervous receptors in the epithelium and elicit reflex bronchoconstriction by way of the vagus nerves.

Pharmacological studies using atropine as a parasympathetic blocking drug in patients with asthma and other chronic obstructive lung diseases have confirmed the importance of parasympathetic pathways,[133,161] but the clinical use of anticholinergic agents has been discouraged by the fear of side-effects, particularly mucus inspissation and increased airway obstruction, and by the ready availability of highly effective beta-sympathomimetic agents. There has been some reassessment of the clinical role of anticholinergic drugs recently in response to the introduction of a new agent, ipratropium bromide.[77]

Atropine This drug is a plant alkaloid (dl-hyoscyamine) (Figure 7-6), which is found in *Atropa belladonna* (deadly nightshade) and *Datura stramonium* (thorn-apple). It acts by competing with acetylcholine for cholinergic receptor sites, and if given systemically causes widespread effects by this mechanism, including blurring of vision due to paralysis of accommodation, alteration of heart rate, drying of salivary and respiratory tract secretions, and inhibition of bowel motility and of bladder contractions. Its therapeutic use in the treatment of bronchoconstriction is therefore limited to administration by inhalation, which reduces but does not eliminate unwanted effects. It is rapidly absorbed

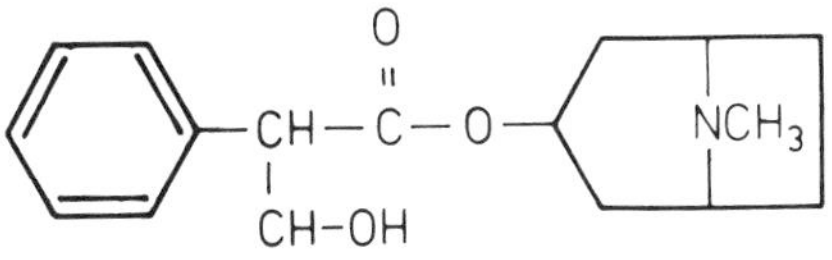

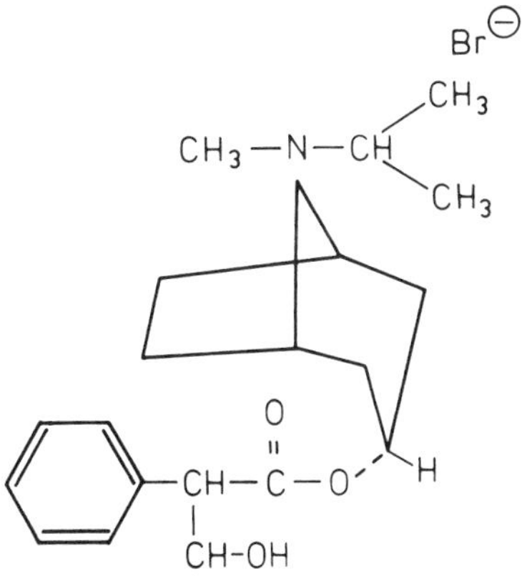

Figure 7-6 *Chemical structure of atropine and its quaternary ammonium derivative, ipratropium bromide.*

into the circulation from the gastrointestinal tract and from mucosal surfaces and is largely excreted in the urine within 12 hours, either unchanged or as an unidentified metabolite.[83]

The onset of action of atropine given by inhalation is 30–60 minutes and lasts for 2 or 3 hours.[27] The combination of atropine and isoprenaline in a pressurised aerosol was therefore useful before the advent of the long-acting beta-sympathomimetic drugs, and several combined preparations are marketed, consisting of atropine or its analogue, deptropine, with isoprenaline or adrenaline and sometimes other ingredients as well. These preparations offer no advantages over the selective beta-2 sympathomimetic bronchodilators and may cause dryness of the mouth, although few patients seem to be worried by this effect. A possible theoretical disadvantage is that drying of respiratory tract excretions may impair the clearance of bronchial mucus and aggravate small airway obstruction.

Ipratropium Bromide   This drug is a quaternary isopropyl-substituted derivative of atropine[43] (Figure 7-6) and is said to have some degree of bronchoselectivity which is increased when the drug is given by aerosol and is greater than that seen with atropine. The actions of ipratropium bromide are otherwise similar to those of atropine, and its therapeutic use is confined to aerosol administration. Absorption after oral administration is poor, a characteristic which tends to reduce the likelihood of side-effects arising from the major proportion of the aerosol dose, which is swallowed rather than inhaled. The drug is excreted in the urine and bile with an elimination half-life of 4 hours.[43]

Ipratropium bromide (Atrovent) is marketed in Europe as a metered dose aerosol containing 20 μg per puff, administered in an adult dose of 1 to 4 puffs 3 or 4 times daily. As with other anticholinergic preparations it should be used with caution in patients with prostatic hypertrophy, for fear of precipitating urinary retention.

The place of ipratropium bromide in the treatment of asthma and chronic obstructive lung disease is still uncertain, since at first sight the drug does not appear to have any advantage over the selective beta-2 sympathomimetic agents. The supposition that it decreases the rate of mucociliary clearance significantly has not so far been borne out by studies in isolated airway preparations[78] or in normal humans,[56] but further clinical evidence is needed to confirm these findings. The consensus of opinion from the early clinical trials comparing ipratropium bromide with beta-sympathomimetics seemed to indicate that the drug is more effective in the treatment of chronic bronchitis than of chronic asthma,[76] although it would be reasonable to make an objective trial of ipratropium bromide in chronic asthmatic patients who have become less responsive to sympathomimetic agents. Recent studies in chronic bronchitic patients suggest that ipratropium bromide aerosol (80 μg) has a comparable bronchodilator effect to salbutamol aerosol (200 μg) and that their effect is additive,[46] although a smaller dose of ipratropium bromide (40 μg) was not as effective as salbutamol (200 μg) in increasing the exercise tolerance of less seriously disabled patients.[91] More work is needed to confirm the additive effect of ipratropium bromide and selective beta-2 sympathomimetic drugs, and to define the type of patient likely to respond to the drug.

THEOPHYLLINE

Theophylline (1:3 dimethylxanthine) is a naturally occurring plant alkaloid which is closely related to caffeine. Its solubility is low and it is unsuitable for intravenous administration. Given by mouth, it tends to cause severe gastric irritation, and for this reason theophylline therapy has until recently largely depended upon the use of its salts, mainly theophylline ethylenediamine (aminophylline), choline theophyllinate (oxtriphylline), and theophylline sodium glycinate, all of which are converted to theophylline *in vivo*. Pharmaceutical innovations have now led to the introduction of anhydrous theophylline in microcrystalline form and of slow-release theophylline preparations, both of which are acceptable when taken by mouth. Prior to these developments a number of *N*-substituted derivatives of theophylline were used, such as etophylline, proxyphylline, acepifyline, and dyphylline, but these compounds do not dissociate to theophylline *in vitro* or *in vivo,* and little is known about their pharmacological properties in comparison with theophylline; for this reason their use is better avoided since they do not offer any advantage over theophylline.

Mode of Action Theophylline is a phosphodiesterase inhibitor and is supposed to exert a bronchodilator action by preventing intracellular inactivation of cAMP, thereby enhancing its relaxant effect in bronchial smooth muscle and its inhibitory effect on the release of bronchoconstrictor mediators from mast cells (see Figures 7-1 and 7-2). Thus its effect is similar to that of sympathomimetic drugs but is apparently achieved by a different intracellular mechanism. Theophylline has other pharmacological actions which include an increase in cardiac output, both by its inotropic effect on heart muscle and by stimulating heart rate; cerebral vasoconstriction and coronary artery vasodilatation; stimulation of the central nervous system, including the respiratory centre; and a direct diuretic action on the renal tubules.

Administration The treatment of asthma with theophylline has been radically changed by the introduction of simple, rapid methods for measuring plasma theophylline concentration which have permitted tight control of individual dosage requirements to be maintained over a long period.[73] In Britain and many other countries the need to make maximal effective use of theophylline has been diminished by the early availability of alternatives such as disodium cromoglycate, the long-acting specific beta-2 sympathomimetic drugs, and the corticosteroid aerosols. But in the United States there has been greater emphasis on the use of theophylline in developing therapeutic regimens for asthma. Many recent studies have confirmed the early observation that effective bronchodilatation is achieved with a serum or plasma theophylline concentration of 10 μg/ml,[144] and it appears that the bronchodilator effect increases with plasma concentrations over a range of 5–20 μg/ml,[104] although there is considerable individual variation in response at any given concentration.

Theophylline may be administered intravenously (as aminophylline), by mouth or per rectum. To obtain rapid relief of bronchoconstriction, a loading dose of aminophylline of 5.6 mg/kg body weight is administered intravenously over 20 minutes, followed by a maintenance infusion of 0.9 mg/kg each hour with the aim of achieving a plasma concentration of 10 μg/ml.[122] If there is no sign of toxicity but no improvement, these authors recommend a further loading dose of 3 mg/kg over 20 minutes and the maintenance infusion increased to 1.35 mg/kg in order to increase the plasma theophylline concentration to 15–20 μg/ml. In children and smokers the dosage requirement is slightly greater because the rate of elimination is increased but plasma clearance is reduced in patients with congestive heart failure, pneumonia, and severe airway obstruction, and dosages should be decreased according to the recommendations of Powell et al.[123] The loading dose should be halved if the patient has received theophylline therapy within the previous 24 hours. Measurement of plasma theophylline concentration is useful in these situations because individual variation in theophylline clearance is considerable.

There are numerous oral theophylline preparations available, either in the form of different salts which contain varying amounts of theophylline (for example, aminophylline contains 85 percent theophylline) or as anhydrous theophylline which is rapidly and completely absorbed after oral administration. Dosage requirements of any preparation should therefore be calculated in terms of its anhydrous theophylline content and should be based on dosage guidelines published by various authors,[111] which may be condensed as follows: 20 mg/kg per day in children of 1–8 years of age; 18 mg/kg per day in children of 9–16 years of age; and 15 mg/kg per day in adults of 17 years of age and over. These dosage recommendations need modification in the presence of factors which alter theophylline clearance. In the treatment of chronic asthma, oral theophylline should be used regularly every 6 hours in order to achieve a plasma theophylline concentration plateau in the required therapeutic range of 10–20 μg/ml within 1 to 2 days, using measurements of 1-second forced expired volume (FEV_1) or peak expiratory flow rate (PEFR) to assess the bronchodilator effect of the drug, and if possible plasma concentration estimations should be obtained as an additional guide to optimise dosage. Small dosage increments at the outset may help to avoid side-effects. Sustained-release theophylline preparations have recently been introduced, and they appear to have a number of advantages in that they decrease fluctuations in plasma theophylline concentration—a factor of clinical importance in children in whom theophylline elimination is rapid[152]; they can provide therapeutic drug concentrations on a 12-hour dose schedule,[102] and they are useful for overnight bronchodilatation in patients with nocturnal asthma.[2]

For prolonged effect, especially overnight, theophylline may be administered rectally as a suppository or as a solution, but absorption is variable and proctitis occurs occasionally. Many patients dislike rectal administration of drugs and in most circumstances the sustained-release oral preparations provide a reasonable alternative.

Clinical Pharmacology   Theophylline is readily absorbed from the gastrointestinal tract and is eliminated by biotransformation in the liver and by urinary excretion. Cigarette smoking increases theophylline elimination due to hepatic enzyme induction, and diminished theophylline metabolism attributable to decreased hepatocellular function occurs in hepatic cirrhosis and in pneumonia, congestive cardiac failure, and chronic pulmonary disease.[123] Even in the absence of hepatic or cardiac disease there is enormous individual variability in the metabolism of theophylline, with variations in half-life ranging from 3 to 12 hours in adults[80] and it is this unpredictability which makes theophylline a difficult drug to use effectively, except with the help of measurements of plasma theophylline concentration.

Toxicity   The toxicity of theophylline is largely related to dosage and plasma concentration. Serious toxic effects are uncommon at concentrations less than 20 μg/ml, although up to 15 percent of patients have unacceptable side-effects even when the plasma concentration does not exceed the usual therapeutic range. The most frequent adverse effects are anorexia, nausea, vomiting and abdominal discomfort, headache, anxiety and nervousness, but serious toxicity consisting of cardiac arrhythmias, cerebral seizures, and respiratory or cardiac arrest are nearly always related either to excessive dosage resulting in plasma theophylline concentrations of more than 40 μg/ml or to rapid intravenous administration leading to excessively high local concentrations of the drug in the heart or brain. Special care is necessary when using theophylline in patients with impaired hepatic function of whatever cause,[162] and intravenous bolus injection of aminophylline should be avoided or only given very slowly, at a rate no faster than 50 mg/min.

Theophylline is commonly prescribed in combination with beta-sympathomimetic agents such as ephedrine, isoproterenol, and terbutaline. Fixed dose combinations with ephedrine appear to increase toxicity in children without useful additive bronchodilator effect,[150] and the inclusion of a barbiturate in many of these proprietary preparations has additional disadvantages which are discussed earlier in this chapter. Because phosphodiesterase inhibitors and beta-sympathomimetic drugs are thought to achieve their bronchodilator effect by increasing intracellular cAMP through different mechanisms, there has been considerable interest in the possibility that combined treatment might have a synergistic effect. To date most clinical studies in asthmatic patients suggest that combined treatment with oral or intravenous theophylline and inhaled beta-2 sympathomimetic drugs have an additive rather than a synergistic effect.[26,94] The results of one such study also suggest that there may be a therapeutic advantage in using low doses of oral aminophylline and oral terbutaline in combination to achieve the same degree of bronchodilatation as could be obtained with high doses of either drug alone, in order to reduce the incidence of side-effects.[157]

The Place of Theophylline in Bronchodilator Therapy The usefulness of theophylline as a bronchodilator in the treatment of asthma has been greatly increased by the application of systematic methods for monitoring plasma theophylline concentrations, especially in the preventive management of childhood asthma.[149] It is a toxic drug with a low therapeutic index and requires expert handling, so that many clinicians prefer to use cromolyn sodium and aerosol preparations of long-acting beta-2 sympathomimetic agents or corticosteroids to prevent or control asthma in patients who are able to administer the inhaled preparations effectively.[159] Much has still to be learned about the value of slow-release theophylline preparations and the possible advantages of combining therapy with theophylline and beta-2 sympathomimetics, particularly in the management of the severe chronic asthmatic patient. Intravenous aminophylline retains an important role in the treatment of status asthmaticus, and modern methods of measuring plasma theophylline concentrations have increased the safety and effectiveness of administration by this route.

CROMOLYN SODIUM

Cromolyn sodium (disodium cromoglycate)[21] is a prophylactic antiasthmatic agent which has been widely used in Britain since 1968. It was introduced in 1973 to the United States, where its usefulness as a relatively non-toxic agent for the long-term prevention of many types of asthma has been increasingly recognised.

Structure-activity correlation studies based on khellin, a substance with smooth muscle relaxing properties derived from an eastern Mediterranean plant, *Ammi visnaga*, led to the synthesis of cromolyn sodium, which is a bis-chromone (Figure 7-7). The drug is a white hydrated powder which is moderately soluble in water but poorly soluble in lipid, so that less than 0.5 percent of the dose is absorbed after oral administration. In the treatment of asthma, cromolyn sodium is therefore administered in powder form by inhalation, less than 4 percent of the total dose being absorbed from the lung and the remainder being swallowed and excreted via the alimentary tract. The absorbed fraction is rapidly eliminated unchanged in the urine and bile in approximately equal amounts without significant accumulation in any tissue.[146]

Mode of Action The mode of action of cromolyn sodium is to inhibit the release of secretory granules containing chemical mediators such as histamine and SRS-A from mast cells following antigen challenge of tissues sensitised with specific IgE antibodies.[114] The action of the drug is not confined to the immediate (Type I) antigen-antibody reaction, for bronchial provocation tests with a number of inhaled allergens show that cromolyn sodium inhibits late reactions that are mediated by nonreaginic precipitating antibodies.[112,121] There is also considerable evidence that the drug can inhibit mast cell degranulation caused by non-antigenic stimuli, suggesting that cromolyn sodium prevents the release of pharmacological mediators in a non-specific way by temporarily stabilising the mast cell membrane. For example, it can also inhibit post-exercise asthma if given a short time before exercise, and some studies have suggested that the drug protects asthmatics against bronchoconstriction induced by alpha-receptor stimulation in the presence of beta-adrenergic receptor blockade,[37] and can inhibit the histamine hypersensitivity of bronchial smooth muscle in asthmatics.[3,87] The precise mechanism of action of cromolyn sodium at the cellular level is uncertain, but Foreman and Garland[53] have suggested that it prevents antigen-induced mediator release by interfering with Ca^{++} transport across the mast cell membrane (see Figure 7-2).

Administration Cromolyn sodium is available in capsules containing 20 mg of the powder, which is administered with a specially developed inhaler acti-

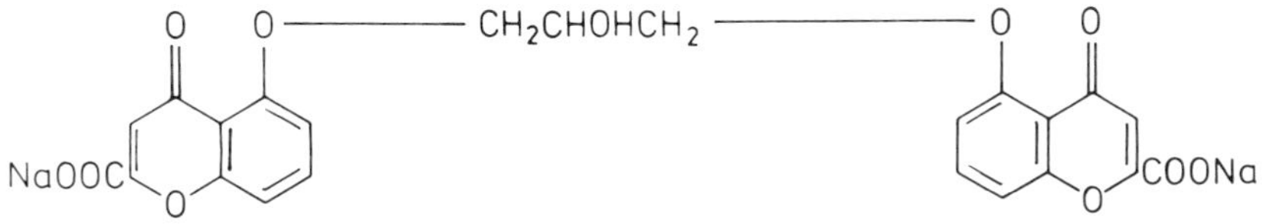

Figure 7-7 *Chemical structure of cromolyn sodium.*

vated by the inspired breath. The usual dose is one capsule 4 times daily, given in the first instance for a trial period of at least 4 weeks to allow an objective assessment to be made of its therapeutic efficacy.

Toxicity   Most of the adverse effects of cromolyn sodium are of minor importance, consisting of local effects such as irritation of the throat and trachea, dryness of the mouth and throat, or slight cough and wheeziness coming on immediately after inhalation of the dry powder. If necessary such symptoms can be minimised by prior inhalation of a bronchodilator aerosol. Nausea, muscle pains and weakness, or dermatitis occurred in 2 percent of 375 patients receiving treatment with cromolyn sodium,[130] but these symptoms subsided promptly when the drug was stopped. There have been a few accounts of immunologic reactions to cromolyn sodium which may be related to both cellular and humoral components of the immune response,[131] and these have included immediate hypersensitivity reactions, myopathy, myocarditis, pericarditis, and granulomatous rash with fever. Individual case reports of peripheral eosinophilia associated with pulmonary infiltrations,[93] pericarditis,[135] and granulomatous liver disease[125] have also been reported, but they seem to have subsided when the drug was discontinued although corticosteroids were also required to obtain complete resolution.

Clinical Use   Cromolyn sodium has two major applications in the management of asthma: the first is in the control of chronic perennial asthma and the second is in the prevention of asthma induced by exercise or specific allergens.
       Long-term studies in children[60] and in adults[23] have shown that cromolyn sodium controls asthmatic symptoms in 65–75 percent of patients with severe and persistant wheezing. Plainly, the drug fails to control symptoms in a minority of asthmatics, but in view of the relative absence of side-effects it should be standard practice to carry out a therapeutic trial with cromolyn sodium not only before corticosteroid therapy is instituted,[15] but also in corticosteroid-dependent patients to see whether the drug allows corticosteroids to be discontinued. It should be borne in mind that prophylactic treatment with cromolyn sodium has to be continuous, usually in the full dosage of 4 inhalations daily, and such treatment is unjustified on grounds of cost and inconvenience in patients who only suffer intermittent symptoms. The trial should be started when the asthma is in a reasonably stable phase and should be continued for at least 1 month at full dosage, the effectiveness of the drug being assessed objectively with the help of diary cards and daily peak expiratory flow measurements. The ability to reduce or discontinue corticosteroids may be another valuable indicator of its therapeutic usefulness. Once this has been established, prophylactic treatment with cromolyn sodium should be maintained at full dosage, although some patients find by experience that gradual

dose reduction to 2 or even 1 inhalation daily allows them to remain free of symptoms.[23] If there is no response to the drug it should be discontinued. Should cromolyn sodium be withdrawn from a patient who has gained benefit from the treatment, the dosage should be reduced progressively over several days—bearing in mind that asthmatic symptoms may recur. If the patient had previously been dependent on corticosteroid therapy, cromolyn sodium should not be discontinued without first reintroducing corticosteroids, because of the risk of precipitating an acute asthmatic attack.

Cromolyn sodium is often effective in preventing asthma brought on by exercise,[42] and it may be a useful alternative to beta-2 sympathomimetic aerosols in enabling children or adolescents to take part in games and sports.[59] It may also afford protection to atopic individuals exposed to known allergens, for instance, at times of high pollen and mould count.[52] The drug has an additional application in the prevention of allergic rhinitis,[22] for which it is used in a manner similar to its use in atopic asthma but administered by inhalation of the powder into each nostril with a special insufflator in a dose of 4 capsules daily.

There is no certain way of selecting those patients who will show an improvement in their asthma during treatment with cromolyn sodium except by carrying out a trial of therapy. In general, young patients with extrinsic asthma, especially those who show marked lability of symptoms, are more likely to show a favourable response, but this is not precluded by the absence of an atopic history.[109]

Other Cromolyn-like Compounds Several structurally related cromolyn-like compounds with better gastrointestinal absorption than cromolyn sodium have recently been undergoing investigation in the hope that oral administration would provide a higher degree of clinical effectiveness. The most promising of these, doxantrazole, has shown considerable anti-allergic activity in animals and in *in vitro* experiments with passively sensitised chopped human lung,[12] and it was shown to inhibit the acute bronchoconstrictor response to inhaled allergen in atopic asthmatic subjects.[72] This finding was not confirmed in another acute study,[119] or in a longer-term comparison of doxantrazole with cromolyn sodium and a placebo.[69]

PRACTICAL USE OF BRONCHODILATOR DRUGS

Use of Bronchodilator Aerosols

The administration of bronchodilator agents to the respiratory tract by inhalation of air-borne particles has the important advantage that the drug is applied close to the target tissue so that dissipation of its effect due to pharmacokinetic factors is minimised and the effective dose is small: for example, the effective bronchodilator dose of metaproterenol sulphate (orciprenaline) aerosol is 1.3 mg (2 puffs) compared with an oral dose of 20 mg. Some bronchodilator agents are poorly or erratically absorbed from the gastrointestinal tract but reliably and effectively absorbed as aerosols; isoproterenol (isoprenaline) is one of these, although it is now being superseded as a bronchodilator by the selective beta-2 sympathomimetic agents. A more relevant example is cromolyn sodium (disodium cromoglycate), which is non-absorbed when given by mouth but effective as a dry aerosol. Another advantage of aerosol therapy is that the rapid response rate makes it a highly practical way for asthmatics with intermittent wheeziness to treat themselves, and it also provides a simple means of administering life-saving epinephrine (adrenaline) treatment for subjects who are known to be highly sensitive to bee stings and other allergens.

Despite these advantages aerosol therapy has certain inherent drawbacks which need to be understood if this method of drug administration is to be used safely and effectively. Successful administration depends on the generation of drug-carrying particles of between 1 and 5 μm in diameter which penetrate to the small bronchi, most of those greater than 10 μm being deposited in the upper airways, mouth and pharynx, while those of 1 μm or less are likely to be exhaled again without deposition. Conventional pressurised aerosol dispensers produce a range of particle sizes, and experimental evidence shows that more than 90 percent of the supposedly inhaled dose is swallowed.[41] This non-inhaled "residue" may lead to adverse effects if the drug is subject to gastrointestinal absorption, especially if excessive and incautious use of the aerosol is prompted by an oncoming asthmatic attack.

Difficulties of Technique   The technique of aerosol administration has to be learned by the patient. A high inspiratory flow rate during inhalation of the aerosol reduces penetrance by causing impaction,[63] and an increased tidal volume increases penetrance if the flow rate remains constant.[120] Breath holding for a few seconds after inhalation may increase the deposition of particles which would otherwise remain airborne and be exhaled again. In patients with obstructive lung disease, there is a tendency for a greater proportion of the inhaled aerosol to be deposited earlier, presumably because the irregular flow in this condition increases impaction.[45] It is clear that a certain facility for coordination and breath control is needed if pressurised dispensers are to be used effectively, and some patients are unable to manage them, especially small children and the elderly. It is therefore important to ensure that lack of response to bronchodilator treatment is not simply due to faulty administration by seeing that all patients are adequately instructed and tested in the use of the aerosol dispenser.[113]

Failure of Delivery Due to Bronchospasm   Asthmatic patients who are maintained on aerosol preparations of beta-sympathomimetic and/or corticosteroid drugs but who are subject to intermittent exacerbations must be warned that if their regular therapy fails to prevent an oncoming attack it is mandatory to start alternative systemic therapy. This is because aerosol preparations can only reach their site of action via relatively clear airways, and the onset of airways obstruction may leave the patient without effective therapy. If they are dependent on corticosteroid aerosols, they should have ready access to oral corticosteroids when their conditions deteriorate, and if they use sympathomimetic inhalers they should be warned against taking excessive doses of the aerosol, since this will lead to gastrointestinal absorption and induce side-effects which may include cardiac arrhythmias.

Toxicity of the Propellant   Aerosol propellants are mainly halogenated hydrocarbons which are inhaled as gases together with the particles of drug. There is no evidence that the fluorocarbons used in aerosols are hepatotoxic or carcinogenic in humans, although a mixture of fluorocarbon with an enzyme inhibitor has been reported to cause hepatoma in mice.[48] Sensitisation of the heart to dysrhythmias induced by beta-adrenoceptor stimulation is a known hazard of anaesthesia with halothane, and it has been reported among pathologists engaged in the production of frozen sections using an aerosol of fluorocarbon-22.[138] When bronchodilator aerosols are used in conventional doses the level of fluorocarbon in the blood and heart are only about one-tenth of those associated with sensitisation to dysrhythmias but excessive use might result in dangerous levels, for example, 12–24 inhalations with successive breaths.[44] The possibility of this hazard is therefore further justification for cautioning patients against reckless use of bronchodilator aerosols.

Tissue Damage   A further theoretical objection to inhaled drugs is a possible long-term effect on the epithelium of the respiratory tract. There is at present no evidence that this is damaged by aerosols of cromolyn sodium, by metaproterenol, salbutamol, or by others of the beta-2 sympathomimetic drugs which have been in continuous use for many years. Oropharyngeal candidiasis is a well-recognised complication of aerosol corticosteroid therapy,[20] but appears not to produce epithelial changes or lead to fungal colonisation of the bronchial tree. Because pathological changes are seen in the skin during systemic or topical corticosteroid treatment, it has been argued that similar atrophic changes might occur in the ciliated epithelium of the bronchi after prolonged corticosteroid aerosol therapy, and although no evidence of damage attributable to such treatment has been observed over periods of up to 18 months,[6] there has yet been insufficient experience to exclude the possibility over a longer term.

Dangers of Overadministration   Unless they are properly warned, patients with asthma appear to be more willing to take extra doses of aerosols than of oral preparations, possibly because relief is obtained rapidly with inhaled preparations. Many of the objections to aerosol bronchodilator therapy arose from the epidemic of asthma deaths which occurred in some countries in the 1960s and was at one time thought to be associated with abuse of pressurised sympathomimetic aerosols, although the precise mechanism of the toxic effect is uncertain. Among the mechanisms canvassed were cardiac arrhythmias due simply to overdose, or to overdose coupled with hypoxia or to fluorocarbon sensitisation; due to a toxic metabolite of isoproterenol (3-0-methyl isoproterenol); or due to the development of tolerance to the effects of beta-receptor stimulation. The fact remains that isoproterenol now has little place in the rational management of asthma, and the selective beta-2 sympathomimetic agents, which are less cardiotoxic, have been used as aerosols more prudently and apparently without increased incidence of serious adverse effects for at least 15 years. There seems little doubt that several factors coincided to cause the increased asthma mortality of the 1960s, one of them being the tendency to rely on home relief with an aerosol which delayed patients from seeking early medical advice at the onset of a severe exacerbation.[85] The epidemic is a reminder to clinicians to instruct their patients on the dangers of excessive self-medication, to advise an upper limit on dosage of both sympathomimetic and corticosteroid aerosols, and to provide easy access to medical advice when serious asthma threatens.

Bronchodilator Delivery by IPPB   Intermittent positive pressure breathing (IPPB) was originally advocated as a means of providing ventilatory support in apnoeic subjects, although early observations suggested that it might assist patients with respiratory difficulty due to acute pulmonary oedema and asthma.[105] Protagonists of IPPB therapy now suggest that the method may be useful for promoting clearance of bronchial secretions, expanding collapsed pulmonary lobes or segments, and delivering bronchodilator aerosols.[128] It has been said that the use of IPPB to administer bronchodilators in acute asthma may lead to a deterioration in gas exchange[86] and may be associated with pneumothorax,[84] but in some centres it is used routinely, apparently with good effect.[35] In chronic obstructive pulmonary disease an improvement in pulmonary function has been observed when IPPB has been used with a nebulised bronchodilator,[129] but comparative studies have generally failed to show that it is superior to a hand nebuliser.[28,62] IPPB delivery of a bronchodilator may however be of benefit to patients who are unable to coordinate with a nebuliser or take a deep breath.[160]

Principles of Asthma Therapy

In the treatment of asthma the main objectives are to prevent attacks as far as possible, to reverse acute exacerbations, and to maintain normal airway function. As an initial step every effort should be made to avoid or reduce exposure to possible allergens and to protect the patient from known precipitating factors, but for the great majority of patients, effective avoidance is impossible to achieve and efforts to protect patients by immunotherapeutic procedures are seldom efficacious.[92] At the present time we have little understanding of the fundamental factors which initiate the bronchial hypersensitivity of asthmatic individuals, and the most effective therapeutic measures available are largely symptomatic, based on pharmacological agents which maintain bronchial dilatation throughout exacerbations of asthma until the disease goes into natural remission or the influence of a precipitating factor has receded. It is also recognised, however, that even when apparently symptom free some asthmatic patients can be shown to have significant impairment of lung function,[25,101] possibly due to repeated attacks which are never completely reversed. Thus an important objective of long-term prophylactic therapy with beta-2 selective sympathomimetic aerosols, oral theophylline, cromolyn sodium, and topical corticosteroids is to prevent attacks which might otherwise lead eventually to disabling lung damage.

To manage such a chronic fluctuating illness successfully it is important to obtain objective evidence of the therapeutic response, and to this end it is sometimes helpful to teach chronically ill patients how to keep a diary of symptoms and to make regular daily measurements of peak expiratory flow rate. Apart from their usefulness in demonstrating the effectiveness of treatment these records give the patient insight into the nature and behaviour of his disease and enable him to administer treatment in a rational and effective way with the minimum of medical surveillance. It is helpful if treatment can be seen as a cooperative endeavor in which the patient learns to adjust the regime to the variable behaviour of the disease, while the doctor provides occasional guidance and ensures rapid access to intensive care for patients with unstable asthma.

Because of the large number of effective bronchodilator agents available and the variable nature of the disease, it is impossible to lay down rigid rules about the choice of therapy at a particular stage of the disease. The following suggestions (Figure 7-8) are therefore based upon personal experience and upon recent authoritative publications which take account of the effectiveness of prophylactic pharmacological therapy, the superiority of selective beta-2 sympathomimetics over the more traditional sympathomimetic agents, and the improved therapeutic efficacy of aerosol over oral preparations.[30,50,67,68,148,159]

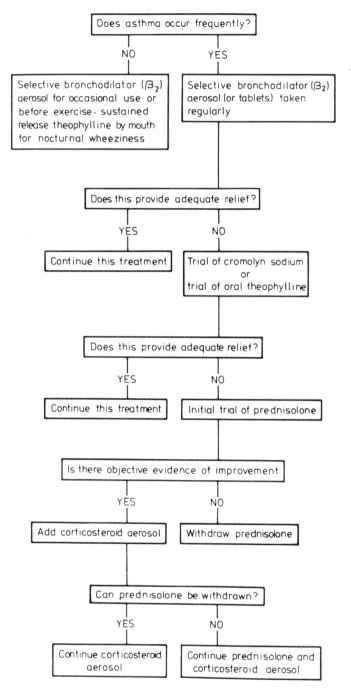

Figure 7-8 *Scheme for the rational choice of drugs in the treatment of asthma (after Gregg, 1977).*

Mild or Intermittent Bronchospasm   Patients with mild symptoms which only occur intermittently can usually be treated effectively with a selective beta-2 sympathomimetic metered dose aerosol which they employ as necessary, being cautioned appropriately against overdosage. I favour salbutamol or terbutaline because of their longer duration of action, but where these are not available metaproterenol or isoetharine may be substituted. Exercise-induced wheezing may be prevented by using a similar aerosol a few minutes prior to the beginning of exercise. The effect of most sympathomimetic preparations does not persist for long enough to prevent early-morning wheeze ("morning dipping"), but for such patients a sustained release theophylline preparation taken at bed-time is usually effective.

Persistent Bronchospasm   If bronchospasm is continuous the beta-sympathomimetic aerosol should be administered regularly in a dose of 2 puffs every 6 hours, or more frequently if a short-acting agent is used. Often the symptoms will be brought under control after a period of regular therapy and the patient can then revert to using the bronchodilator aerosols symptomatically. If they persist, however, two alternatives are available: either to add an oral theophylline preparation in round-the-clock therapy, undertaking regular measurements of plasma theophylline levels until the appropriate individual dosage regimen is established—a course favoured in the United States; or to institute a trial of cromolyn sodium therapy in regular dosage of 4 inhalations per day for at least a month, as is commonly preferred in Britain. Both procedures depend for success on a careful, objective assessment of the outcome, but both appear to be equally effective in expert hands.[70] The main disadvantage of theophylline is its low therapeutic index, while the problem with cromolyn is that 25–35 percent of patients fail to respond at all. It is an expensive drug and should not be continued if it proves ineffective.

Should the above measures fail to control bronchospasm it is then necessary to introduce corticosteroid drugs, and this is best done by giving oral prednisolone in a large initial dose of 30–60 mg per day to show convincingly that the treatment is effective on the basis of objective measurements of pulmonary function. Thereafter the oral dose should be reduced by decrements of 2.5–5 mg every 2 or 3 days to a minimum level which is sufficient to control symptoms. During the withdrawal of prednisolone, an aerosol corticosteroid preparation is introduced, for example, beclomethasone dipropionate in a dose of 2 puffs (100 μg) 4 times daily; this may enable the prednisolone to be withdrawn completely or at least help to minimise the dosage of systemic corticosteroids. Asthmatics who are maintained on combined prophylactic aerosol therapy with a topical corticosteroid and a sympathomimetic agent should be advised to inhale the bronchodilator preparation a few minutes before the corticosteroid, to ensure maximum penetration of the latter into a dilated bronchial tree. Oropharyngeal candidiasis occasionally complicates long-term corticosteroid aerosol therapy, but often it causes no symptoms or it responds quite quickly to local antifungal therapy with nystatin or amphotericin B lozenges; rarely does it requires discontinuation of the aerosol.

Asthmatic patients who are from time to time prone to disabling exacerbations of their bronchospasm often respond promptly to a short course of oral prednisolone, and if it is clear that wheeze is gradually becoming worse despite a reasonable increase in the use of their regular bronchodilator, such patients should be started on a short course of oral prednisolone, beginning with 30–40 mg to obtain control and then tapering the dosage gradually, with the aim of discontinuing the drug completely within 12 to 14 days. This routine is mandatory in those who are normally reliant on corticosteroid aerosol therapy, since the exacerbation of bronchospasm effectively prevents any aerosol from reaching the bronchi and the corticosteroid requirement of these patients can only be met by systemic administration. Most patients are able to recognise the danger signals of an impending attack and can be relied upon to administer such a course of treatment themselves if provided with a stand-by supply of prednisolone tablets, but it is important to ensure that those with severe or "brittle" asthma, whose disease is liable to sudden severe exacerbations, should have rapid access to expert care.[38]

One of the most difficult problems is the management of long-standing asthmatic patients who are never entirely free of symptoms and who gradually become more and more disabled over the years. Such patients usually obtain benefit from systemic corticosteroids, but a careful balance has to be struck between the relief of symptoms and the acceptance of side-effects which may in themselves aggravate exertional dyspnoea by causing obesity and fluid retention. Limitation of prednisolone dosage to 10 mg per day with a minimum of side-effects can often be achieved by maintaining continuous therapy with a long-acting beta-2 selective sympathomimetic aerosol, topical corticosteroids, and cromolyn sodium. Oral theophylline preparations or anticholinergic agents such as ipratropium bromide may also be tried in these difficult cases in order to determine the most effective regimen, using daily measurements of peak flow rate to provide objective evidence of the therapeutic response. Many such patients also suffer from chronic bronchitis and experience infective exacerbations from time to time which require antibiotic treatment as well as a temporary increase in systemic corticosteroid therapy.

Acute Severe Asthma   Patients should be warned that if they develop a severe acute attack of asthma which fails to respond to their usual bronchodilator therapy, they must alert their physician promptly. If the clinical state is fair and the patient has been able to continue working activities even if with great difficulty, it is reasonable to observe the effect of an increased dose of an inhaled sympathomimetic agent (preferably beta-2 selective), for example, 2 to 4 puffs of the metered dose which can be repeated every 2 hours. However, most patients will already have tried the effect of a modest increase in their normal medication before calling their doctor, and if this measure has been unsuccessful in obtaining control a slow intravenous injection of aminophylline should be given, bearing in mind the risk of toxicity which is greatest in hypoxic or elderly patients and in those with cardiovascular disease. Severe attacks of asthma may develop insidiously over a period of several days or with alarming suddenness, and in doubtful cases the safest course is urgent hospital admission for measurements of blood gases and ventilatory function and for monitoring the response to treatment. Because of the speed with which such patients may deteriorate, current thinking in Britain recommends that before sending the patient to hospital, the doctor should give an intravenous injection of 300 mg of hydrocortisone and a slow intravenous injection of 250 mg of aminophylline.[19] The clinical indications of a serious attack are disabling dyspnoea, which prevents movement from the chair or bed without difficulty, monosyllabic speech, severe disturbance of sleep, mental confusion or impaired consciousness, exhaustion, a tachycardia of 120 beats per minute or more, pulsus paradoxus, and central cyanosis. Severe functional abnormality is indicated by marked reduction in FEV_1 or peak flow rate and an increasing or raised arterial pCO_2 level which is an important indicator of failing alveolar-capillary gas exchange. These investigations should be carried out unfailingly at the outset of intensive treatment and repeated at intervals to monitor the effectiveness of therapy.

Once the patient is in hospital under regular supervision the usual regimen is to give aminophylline and hydrocortisone intravenously throughout the acute episode which may resolve in a few hours or persist for several days. Aminophylline is given in an initial loading dose over 20 minutes and maintained by continuous intravenous infusion (for dosage recommendations, see section on Aminophylline), the plasma theophylline concentration being measured to monitor individual dosage requirements. Hydrocortisone is given in an initial loading dose of 250–500 mg intravenously followed by 250 mg every 6 hours, and prednisolone tablets are started in a dose of 30 mg per day as soon as the patient is able to accept oral medication. Some authorities advise additional bronchodilator therapy with a beta-2 selective sympathomimetic aerosol which may be given either by metered dose inhaler or, if the patient is unable to cooperate sufficiently, with a simple Wright nebuliser or an IPPB device; but there is some evidence which suggests that inhaled bronchodilators are ineffective when given early in the treatment of acute severe asthma,[156] presumably because the drug fails to penetrate the obstructed bronchial tree.

Supportive therapy is essential. Fluid replacement is nearly always necessary because of respiratory fluid loss due to increased ventilation, and because severely dyspnoeic patients can take drinks only with difficulty. Occasionally a persistent metabolic acidosis calls for treatment with bicarbonate. Oxygen should be given, initially through a Venturi-type mask at a controlled concentration of 28 percent which may be increased to 40–50 percent provided that serial pCO_2 estimations show no evidence of carbon dioxide retention. Sedation should be strictly avoided. Complications such as cardiac failure, bronchopulmonary infection, or pneumothorax require appropriate treatment. The essential purpose of regular measurements of arterial blood gas tensions and respiratory flow rates is to ensure that the patient is maintaining effective ventilation throughout the acute episode. Should spontaneous ventilation become inadequate it is necessary to carry out endotracheal intubation and provide mechanical ventilatory support.

Bronchodilators in Chronic Bronchitis and Emphysema

Breathlessness is a major symptom of chronic obstructive lung disease associated with chronic bronchitis and emphysema, and it is frequently accompanied by wheeze, especially in acute infective exacerbations of the disease. The mechanism of bronchial narrowing in this disease differs, however, from that in chronic asthma, being variously due to mucous gland hypertrophy in the bronchial epithelium, excessive mucus production, and airway collapse resulting from emphysema. Although some degree of reversible bronchospasm commonly occurs in exacerbations of bronchitis, the contribution of this factor to ventilatory impairment is probably small compared with the effect of inflammatory changes in the bronchial mucosa and obstruction by excessive bronchial secretions. The value of bronchodilator agents is therefore limited in comparison with their effect in true bronchial asthma but nevertheless they play a significant part in the routine therapy of this disease.

The most widely used drugs are theophylline preparations and beta-2 selective sympathomimetics, the latter being commonly administered in aerosol form. Ipratropium bromide aerosol may turn out to be useful in some patients either alone or in combination with a sympathomimetic agent but more work is needed to prove its worth. Corticosteroids are not usually recommended in the treatment of chronic bronchitis but it is well recognised that among the population of middle-aged or elderly bronchitic patients with chronic productive cough and wheezy dyspnoea there is a minority who show a dramatic improvement when subjected to a trial of systemic corticosteroid therapy.[13] The practical steps which should be taken when carrying out a trial of this nature are described in Chapter 8.

REFERENCES

1. AHLQUIST RP: A study of adrenotropic receptors. Am J Physiol 153: 586–600, 1948.
2. AL-KHADER A, COLE RB, THOMPSON D: Two aminophylline preparations in nocturnal asthma. Br J Dis Chest 73: 169–172, 1979.
3. ALTOUNYAN REC: Changes in histamine and atropine responsiveness as a guide to diagnosis and evaluation of therapy in obstructive airways disease. in Disodium Cromoglycate in Allergic Airways Disease, Pepys J, Frankland AW (eds) pp. 47–53. London: Butterworths, 1970.
4. ANDERSON SD, SEALE JP, ROZEA P, BANDLER L, THEOBALD G, LINDSAY DA: Inhaled and oral salbutamol in exercise-induced asthma. Am Rev Resp Dis 114: 493–500, 1976.
5. ANDERSON G, WILKINS E, JARIWALLA AG: Fenoterol in asthma. Br J Dis Chest 73: 81–84, 1979.
6. ANDERSSON E, SMIDT CM, SIKJAER B, AINGE G, POYNTER D: Bronchial biopsies after beclamethasone dipropionate aerosol. Br J Dis Chest 71: 35–43, 1977.
7. ARNER B: A comparative clinical trial of different subcutaneous doses of terbutaline and orciprenaline in bronchial asthma. Acta Med Scand (Supple) 512: 45–48, 1970.
8. ARNER B, BERTLER A, KARLEFORS T, WESTLING H: Circulatory effects of orciprenaline, adrenaline and a new sympathomimetic β-receptor stimulating agent, terbutaline, in normal human subjects. Acta Med Scand (Suppl) 512: 25–32, 1970.
9. BANNER AS, SUNDERRAJAN EV, AGERWAL MK, ADDINGTON WW: Arrhythmogenic effects of orally administered bronchodilators. Arch Intern Med 139: 434–437, 1979.
10. BARNES PJ, IND P, DOLLERY CT: Inhaled prazosin in asthma. Thorax 35: 239, 1980.
11. BARNETT DB, CHESROWN SE, ZBINDEN AF, NISAM M, REED BR, BOURNE HR, MELMON KL, GOLD WM: Cyclic AMP and cyclic GMP in canine peripheral lung: regulation in vivo. Am Rev Resp Dis 118: 723–733, 1978.
12. BATCHELOR JF, FOLLENFANT MJ, GARLAND LG, GORVIN JH, GREEN AF, HODSON HG, HUGHES DTD, TATESON JE: Doxantrazole, an antiallergic agent orally effective in man. Lancet 1: 1169–1170, 1975.
13. BEEREL F, JICK H, TYLER JM: A controlled study of the effect of prednisone on air-flow obstruction in severe pulmonary emphysema. N Engl J Med 268: 226–230, 1963.
14. BENOY CJ, EL-FELLAH, MS, SCHNEIDER R, WADE OL: Tolerance to sympathomimetic bronchodilators in guinea-pig isolated lungs following chronic administration *in vivo*. Br J Pharmacol 55: 547–554, 1975.
15. BERNSTEIN IL, JOHNSON CL, TSE CSR: Therapy with cromolyn sodium. Ann Intern Med 89: 228–233, 1978.
16. BERRIDGE MJ: The role of cyclic nucleotides and calcium in the control of secretion. in Proceedings of the 6th International Congress of Pharmacology, Helsinki, Vol 1. Receptors and Cellular Pharmacology. Klinge E (ed) pp. 213–221, 1976.

17. Bianco S, Griffin JP, Kamburoff PL, Prime FJ: Prevention of exercise-induced asthma by indoramin. Br Med J 2: 18–20, 1974.
18. Bourne HR, Lichtenstein LM, Melmon KL: Pharmacologic control of allergic histamine release *in vitro*: evidence for an inhibitory role of 3', 5'-adenosine monophosphate in human leucocytes. J Immunol 108: 695–705, 1972.
19. British Medical Journal: Saving asthmatics. Br Med J 1: 1520–1521, 1979.
20. British Thoracic and Tuberculosis Association: A controlled trial of inhaled corticosteroids in patients receiving prednisone tablets for asthma. Br J Dis Chest 70: 95–103, 1976.
21. Brogden RN, Speight TM, Avery G: Sodium cromoglycate (cromolyn sodium): a review of its mode of action, pharmacology, therapeutic efficacy and use. Drugs 7: 164–282, 1974.
22. Brogden RN, Speight TM, Avery GS: Sodium cromoglycate (cromolyn sodium): II. Allergic rhinitis and other conditions. Drugs 7: 283–296, 1974.
23. Brompton Hospital/Medical Research Council Collaborative Trial Long-term study of disodium cromoglycate in treatment of severe extrinsic or intrinsic bronchial asthma in adults. Br Med J 2: 383–388, 1972.
24. Brooks SM, Werk EE, Ackerman J, Sullivan I, Thrasher K: Adverse effects of phenobarbital on corticosteroid metabolism in patients with bronchial asthma. N Engl J Med 286: 1125–1128, 1972.
25. Cade JF, Pain MCF: Pulmonary function during clinical remission of asthma. How reversible is asthma? Aust NZ J Med 3: 545–551, 1973.
26. Campbell IA, Middleton WG, McHardy GJR, Shotter MV, McKenzie R, Kay AB: Interaction between isoprenaline and aminophylline in asthma. Thorax 32: 424–428, 1977.
27. Cavanaugh MJ, Cooper DM: Inhaled atropine sulfate: dose response characteristics. Am Rev Resp Dis 114: 517–524, 1976.
28. Chang N, Levison H: The effect of a nebulised bronchodilator administered with or without intermittent positive pressure breathing on ventilatory function in children with cystic fibrosis and asthma. Am Rev Resp Dis 106: 867–872, 1972.
29. Choo-Kang YFJ, Simpson WT, Grant IWB: Controlled comparison of the bronchodilator effect of three β-adrenergic stimulant drugs administered by inhalation to patients with Asthma. Br Med J 2: 287–289, 1969.
30. Clark TJH: Adult asthma. in Asthma, Clark TJH, Godfrey S, (eds) Ch. 18, p. 367–394. London: Chapman and Hall, 1977.
31. Clark TJH, Collins JV, Tong D: Respiratory depression caused by nitrazepam in patients with respiratory failure. Lancet 2: 737–738, 1971.
32. Cochrane GM, Clark TJH: A survey of asthma mortality in patients between ages 35 and 64 in the Greater London Hospitals in 1971. Thorax 30: 300–305, 1975.
33. Conolly ME, Davies DS, Dollery CT, George CF: Resistance to β-adrenoceptor stimulants (a possible explanation for the rise in asthma deaths). Br J Pharmacol 43: 389–402, 1971.
34. Conolly ME, Davies DS, Dollery CT, Morgan CD, Paterson JW, Sandler M: Metabolism of isoprenaline in dog and man. Br J Pharmacol 46, 458–472, 1972.

35. COOKE NJ, CROMPTON GK, GRANT IWB: Observations on the management of acute bronchial asthma. Br J Dis Chest 73: 157–163, 1979.

36. COOKE NJ, KERR JA, WILLEY RF, HOARE MV, GRANT IWB, CROMPTON GK: Response to rimiterol and salbutamol aerosols administered by intermittent postive-pressure ventilation. Br Med J 1: 250–252, 1974.

37. COX JSG: Disodium cromoglycate. Mode of action and its possible relevance to the clinical use of the drug. Br J Dis Chest 65: 189–204, 1971.

38. CROMPTON GK, GRANT IWB, BLOOMFIELD P: Edinburgh emergency asthma admission service: report on 10 years' experience. Br Med J 2: 1199–1201, 1979.

39. CUTHBERT MF: Bronchodilator activity of aerosols of prostaglandins E1 and E2 in asthmatic subjects. Proc R Soc Med 64: 15–16, 1971.

40. CUTHBERT MF: Prostaglandins and respiratory smooth muscle, in The Prostaglandins, Cuthbert MF (ed). pp. 253–285, London: Heinemann, 1973.

41. DAVIES DS: Pharmacokinetics of inhaled substances. Postgrad Med J 51 (Suppl 7): 69–75, 1975.

42. DAVIES SE: Effect of disodium cromoglycate on exercise-induced asthma. Br Med J 3: 593–594, 1968.

43. DECKERS W: The chemistry of new derivatives of tropane alkaloids and the pharmacokinetics of a new quaternary compound. Postgrad Med J 51: (Suppl 7): 76–81, 1975.

44. DOLLERY CT, WILLIAMS FM, DRAFFAN GH, WISE G, SAHYOUN H, PATERSON JW, WALKER SR: Arterial blood levels of fluorocarbons in asthmatic patients following use of pressurised aerosols. Clin Pharmacol Ther 15: 59–66, 1974.

45. DOLOVICH MB, SANCHIS J, ROSSMAN C, NEWHOUSE MT: Aerosol penetrance: a sensitive index of peripheral airways obstruction. J Appl Physiol 40: 468–471, 1976.

46. DOUGLAS NJ, DAVIDSON I, SUDLOW MF, FLENLEY DC: Bronchodilatation and the site of airway resistance in severe chronic bronchitis. Thorax 34: 51–56, 1979.

47. DUNLOP D, SHANKS RG: Selective blockage of adrenoceptive beta receptors in the heart. Br J Pharmacol 32: 201–208, 1968.

48. EPSTEIN SS, JOSHI S, ANDREA J, CLAPP P, FALK H, MANTEL N: Synergistic toxicity and carcinogenicity of 'freons' and piperonyl butoxide. Nature 214: 526–528, 1967.

49. EVANS ME, PATERSON JW, SHENFIELD FM, THOMAS N, WALKER SR: The pharmacokinetics of rimiterol in asthmatic patients. Br J Pharmacol 49: 153P–154P, 1973.

50. FELDMAN NT, McFADDEN ER: Asthma therapy old and new. Med Clin North Am 61: 1239–1250, 1977.

51. FITCHETT DH, McNICOL MW, RIORDAN JF: Intravenous salbutamol in management of status asthmaticus. Br Med J 1: 53–55, 1975.

52. FORD RM: Disodium cromoglycate in the treatment of seasonal and perennial asthma. Med J Aust 2: 537–540, 1969.

53. FOREMAN JC, GARLAND LG: Cromoglycate and other antiallergic drugs: A possible mechanism of action. Br Med J 1: 820–821, 1976.

54. FOREMAN JC, MONGAR JL, GOMPERTS BD: Calcium ionophores and movement of calcium ions following the physiological stimulus to a secretory process. Nature 245: 249–251, 1973.

55. FOSTER WM, BERGOFSKY EH, BOHNING DE, LIPPMAN M, ALBERT RE: Effect of adrenergic agents and their mode of action on mucociliary clearance in man. J Appl Physiol 41: 146–152, 1976.

56. FRANCIS RA, THOMSON ML, PAVIA D, DOUGLAS RB: Ipratropium bromide: mucociliary clearance rate and airway resistance in normal subjects. Br J Dis Chest 71: 173–178, 1977.

57. FREEDMAN BJ, MEISNER P, HILL GB: A comparison of the actions of different bronchodilators in asthma. Thorax 23: 590–597, 1968.

58. GENERAL PRACTITIONER RESEARCH GROUP: A compound ephedrine preparation for asthma. Practitioner 190: 253–255, 1963.

59. GLASS RD: Experience with disodium cromoglycate in the treatment of asthmatic children. Med J Aust 1: 1382–1386, 1971.

60. GODFREY S, BALFOUR-LYNN L, KÖNIG P: The place of cromolyn sodium in the long-term management of childhood asthma based on a 3- to 5-year follow-up. J Paediatr 87: 465–473, 1975.

61. GOLD WM: The role of the parasympathetic nervous system in airways disease. Postgrad Med J 51 (Suppl 7): 53–62, 1975.

62. GOLDBERG I, CHERNIACK RM: The effect of nebulised bronchodilator delivered with and without IPPB on ventilatory function in chronic obstructive emphysema. Am Rev Resp Dis 91: 13–20, 1965.

63. GOLDBERG IS, LOURENÇO RV: Deposition of aerosols in pulmonary disease. Arch Intern Med 131: 88–91, 1973.

64. GOLDBERG ND, HADDOX MK, NICOL SE, GLASS DB, SANFORD CH, KUEHL FA, ESTENSEN R: Biologic regulation through opposing influences of cyclic GMP and cyclic AMP: the yin yang hypothesis. Adv Cyclic Nucleotide Res 5: 307–330, 1975.

65. GOLDBERG ND, O'DEA RF, HADDOX MK: Cyclic GMP. Adv Cyclic Nucleotide Res 3: 155–223, 1973.

66. GOLDBERG R, VAN AS M, JOFFE BI, KRUT L, BERSOHN I, SEFTEL HC: Metabolic responses to selective β-adrenergic stimulation in man. Postgrad Med J 51: 53–58, 1975.

67. GOLDSTEIN RS, SLUTSKY AS, REBUCK AS: Severe asthma: Prevention is better than cure. Drugs 16: 256–267, 1978.

68. GREGG I: The difficult asthmatic. Drugs 13: 35–45, 1978.

69. GRIBBIN HR, HARVEY JE, TATTERSFIELD AE: Trial of doxantrazole in asthma. Br Med J 1: 92, 1979.

70. HAMBELTON G, WEINBERGER M, TAYLOR J, CAVANAUGH M, GICHANSKY E, GODFREY S, TOOLEY M, BELL S, GREENBERG S: Comparison of cromoglycate (cromolyn) and theophylline in controlling symptoms of chronic asthma. Lancet 1: 381–385, 1977.

71. HARTLEY JPR, NOGRADY SG, SEATON A: Long-term comparison of salbutamol powder with salbutamol aerosol in asthmatic outpatients. Br J Dis Chest 73: 271–276, 1979.

72. HAYDU SP, BRADLEY JL, HUGHES DTD: Inhibitory effect of oral doxantrazole on asthma induced by allergen inhalation. Br Med J 3: 283–284, 1975.

73. HENDELES L, WEINBERGER M, JOHNSON G: Monitoring serum theophylline levels. Clin Pharmacokinet 3: 294–312, 1978.
74. HERXHEIMER H: Dosage of ephedrine in bronchial asthma and emphysema. Br Med J 1: 350–352, 1946.
75. HERXHEIMER H, ROESTCHER I: Effects of PGE_1 on lung function in asthma. Eur J Clin Pharmacol 3: 123–125, 1971.
76. HERZOG H: Comparison of anticholinergic agents other than bronchodilators and the effect of combining these drugs. Postgrad Med J 51 (Suppl 7): 146–148, 1975.
77. HOFFBRAND BI (ed): The place of parasympatholytic drugs in the management of chronic obstructive airways disease. Postgrad Med J 51 (Suppl 7):1975.
78. IRAVANI J, MELVILLE GN: Ciliary movement following various concentrations of different anticholinergic and adrenergic bronchodilator solutions in animals. Postgrad Med J 51 (Suppl 7): 108, 1975.
79. ISHIZAKA K, ISHIZAKA T: Mechanisms of reaginic hypersensitivity and immunotherapy. Lung 155: 3–22, 1978.
80. JENNE JW, WYZE E, ROOD FS, MACDONALD FM: Pharmacokinetics of theophylline. Clin Pharmacol Ther 13: 349–360, 1972.
81. JOHNSON HG, BACH MK: Prevention of calcium ionophore-induced release of histamine in rat mast cells by disodium cromoglycate. J Immunol 114: 514–516, 1975.
82. KALINER M, ORANGE RP, AUSTEN KF: Immunological release of histamine and SRS-A from the human lung. IV. Enhancement by cholinergic and alpha-adrenergic stimulation. J Exp Med 136: 556–567, 1972.
83. KALSER SC: The fate of atropine in man. Ann NY Acad Sci 179: 667–683, 1971.
84. KARETZKY MS: Asthma mortality associated with pneumothorax and intermittent positive pressure breathing. Lancet 1: 828–829, 1975.
85. KARETZKY MS: Asthma mortality: an analysis of one year's experience, review of the literature and assessment of current modes of therapy. Medicine 54: 471–484, 1975.
86. KARETZKY MS, BRANDSTETTER RD, MEYER RC, TEDALDI EM: Acute asthma. Part 1: a comparison of the immediate effects of six different modes of therapy. Am J Med Sci 267: 213–224, 1974.
87. KERR JW, GOVINDARAJ M, PATEL KR: Effect of alpha-receptor blocking drugs and disodium cromoglycate on histamine hypersensitivity in bronchial asthma. Br Med J 2: 139–141, 1970.
88. KOOPMAN WJ, ORANGE RP, AUSTEN KF: Immunochemical and biological properties of rat IgE. 3. Modulation of the IgE-mediated release of slow-reacting substance of anaphylaxis by agents influencing the level of 3', 5'-adenosine monophosphate. J Immunol 105: 1096–1102, 1970.
89. LANDS AM, ARNOLD A, MCAULIFF JP, LUDUENA FP, BROWN TG: Differentiation of receptor systems activated by sympathomimetic amines. Nature 214: 597–598, 1967.
90. LEITCH AG, CLANCY LJ, COSTELLO JF, FLENLEY DC: Effect of intravenous infusion of salbutamol on ventilatory response to carbon dioxide and hypoxia and on heart rate and plasma potassium in normal men. Br Med J 1: 365–367, 1976.

91. Leitch AG, Hopkin JM, Ellis DA, Merchant S, McHardy GJR: The effect of aerosol ipratropium bromide and salbutamol on exercise tolerance in chronic bronchitis. Thorax 33: 711–713, 1978.

92. Lichtenstein LM: An evaluation of the role of immunotherapy in asthma. Am Rev Resp Dis 117: 191–197, 1978.

93. Löbel H, Machtey I, Eldror MY: Pulmonary infiltrates with eosinophilia in an asthmatic patient treated with disodium cromoglycate. Lancet 2: 1032, 1972.

94. Marlin GE, Hartnett BJS, Berend N, Hacket NB: Assessment of combined oral theophylline and inhaled β-adrenoceptor agonist bronchodilator therapy. Br J Clin Pharmacol 5: 45–50, 1978.

95. Marlin GE, Turner P: Comparison of the β2-adrenoceptor selectivity of rimiterol, salbutamol and isoprenaline by the intravenous route in man. Br J Clin Pharmacol 2: 41–48, 1975.

96. Marlin GE, Turner P: Intravenous treatment with rimiterol and salbutamol in asthma. Br Med J 2: 715–719, 1975.

97. Mathé AA: Studies on actions of prostaglandins in the lung. Acta Physiol Scand (Suppl 441): 1976.

98. Mathé AA, Hedquist P, Holmgren A, Svanborg N: Bronchial hyperreactivity to prostaglandin $F_2\alpha$ and histamine in patients with asthma. Br Med J 1: 193–196, 1973.

99. Mathé AA, Hedquist P, Strandberg K, Leslie CA: Aspects of prostaglandin function in the lung. N Engl J Med 296: 850–855, 910–914, 1977.

100. McFadden ER: Exertional dyspnoea and cough as preludes to acute attacks of asthma. N Engl J Med 292: 555–559, 1975.

101. McFadden ER, Kiser R, DeGroot WJ: Acute bronchial asthma. Relations between clinical and physiologic manifestations. N Engl J Med 288: 221–225, 1973.

102. McKenzie S, Baillie E: Serum theophylline levels in asthmatic children after oral administration of a slow-release aminophylline preparation. J Int Med Res 7 (Suppl 1): 22–27, 1979.

103. Minette A: Ventilatory results and side-effects of salbutamol given by different routes in coal miners with reversible broncho-obstruction. Postgrad Med J 47 (Suppl): 55–61, 1971.

104. Mitenko PA, Ogilvie RI: Rational intravenous doses of theophylline. N Engl J Med 289: 600–603, 1973.

105. Motley HL, Werko L, Cournand A, Richards DW: Observations on the clinical use of intermittent positive pressure. J Aviat Med 18: 417–435, 1947.

106. Murad F, Kimura H: Cyclic nucleotide levels in incubations of guinea pig trachea. Biochim Biophys Acta 343: 275–286, 1974.

107. Nelson HS, Black JW, Branch LB, Pfuetze B, Spaulding H, Summers R, Wood D: Subsensitivity to epinephrine following the administration of epinephrine and ephedrine to normal individuals. J Allergy Clin Immunol 55: 299–309, 1975.

108. Nogrady SG, Hartley JPR, Seaton A: Metabolic effects of intravenous salbutamol in the course of acute severe asthma. Thorax 32: 559–562, 1977.

109. Northern General Hospital, Brompton Hospital and Medical Research Council Collaborative Trial: Sodium cromoglycate in chronic asthma. Br Med J 1: 361–364, 1976.

110. O'DONNELL TV, BUTLER GM, TOCKER MD: A comparison of orciprenaline and salbutamol administered orally in 12 adult asthmatic patients. Postgrad Med J 47 (Suppl): 115–118, 1971.

111. OGILVIE RI: Clinical pharmacokinetics of theophylline. Clin Pharmacokinet 3: 267–293, 1978.

112. ORIE NGM, BOOIJ-NOORD H, PELIKAN Z, SNOEK W, van LOOKEREN CAMAGNE, de VRIES K: Protective effect of disodium cromoglycate on nasal and bronchial reactions after allergen challenge: results in type I ("reaginic") and type III ("late") reactions. in Disodium Cromoglycate in Allergic Airways Disease, Pepys J, Frankland AW (eds). pp. 33–41. London: Butterworths, 1970.

113. OROHEK J, GAYRARD P, GRIMAUD CH, CHARPIN J: Patient error in use of bronchodilator metered aerosols. Br Med J 1: 76, 1976.

114. ORR TSC, POLLARD MC, GWILLIAM J, COX JSG: Mode of action of disodium cromoglycate, studies on immediate type hypersensitivity reactions using "double sensitization" with two antigenically distinct rat reagins. Clin Exp Immunol 7: 745–757, 1970.

115. PATEL KR: α-adrenoceptor blocking drugs in asthma. Br J Clin Pharmacol 3: 601–605, 1976.

116. PATEL KR, KERR JW: The airways response to phenylephrine after blockade of alpha and beta receptors in extrinsic bronchial asthma. Clin Allergy 3: 439–448, 1973.

117. PATERSON JW, COURTENAY EVANS RJ, PRIME FJ: Selectivity of bronchodilator action of salbutamol in asthmatic patients. Br J Dis Chest 65: 21–38, 1971.

118. PATERSON JW, SHENFIELD GM: Bronchodilators. B.T.T.A. Review, 4: 25–44, 61–74, 1974.

119. PAUWELS R, LAMONT H, VAN DER STRAETEN M: Further studies on the effect of oral doxantrazole on allergen-induced bronchospasm. Acta Allergol 31: 471–477, 1976.

120. PAVIA D, THOMSON ML, CLARKE SW, SHANNON HS: Effect of lung function and mode of inhalation on penetration of aerosol into the human lung. Thorax 32: 194–197, 1977.

121. PEPYS J, HARGREAVE FE, CHAN M, McCARTHY DS: Inhibitory effects of disodium cromoglycate on allergen-inhalation tests. Lancet 2: 134–137, 1968.

122. PIAFSKY KM, OGILVIE RI: Dosage of theophylline in bronchial asthma. N Engl J Med 292: 1218–1222, 1975.

123. POWELL JR, VOZEH S, HOPEWELL P, COSTELLO J, SHEINER LB, RIEGELMAN S: Theophylline disposition in acutely ill hospitalised patients. Am Rev Resp Dis 118: 229–238, 1978.

124. RASMUSSEN H, JENSEN P, LAKE W, GOODMAN DBP: Calcium ion as second messenger. Clin Endocrinol 5 (Suppl): 11s–27s, 1976.

125. ROSENBERG JL, EDLOW D, SNEIDER R: Liver disease and vasculitis in a patient taking cromolyn. Arch Intern Med 138: 989–991, 1978.

126. ROY AC, WARREN BT: Inhibition of cAMP phosphodiesterase by disodium cromoglycate. Biochem Pharmacol 23: 917–920, 1974.

127. RUFFIN RE, OBMINSKI G, NEWHOUSE MT: Aerosol salbutamol administration by IPPB: lowest effective dose. Thorax 33: 689–693, 1978.

128. Safar P: IPPB: indications and complications. In Advances in Respiratory Care and Physiology, Caldwell TB, Moya F (eds). pp. 96–108. Springfield, Illinois: Charles C Thomas, 1973.

129. Segal MS, Salomon A, Dulfano MJ, Hershfus JA: Intermittent positive pressure breathing. Its use in the inspiratory phase of respiration. N Engl J Med 250: 225–232, 1954.

130. Settipane GA, Klein DE, Boyd GK, Sturam JH, Freye HB, Weltman JK: Adverse reactions to cromolyn. JAMA 241: 811–813, 1979.

131. Sheffer AL, Rocklin RE, Goetzl EJ: Immunologic components of hypersensitivity reactions to cromolyn sodium. N Engl J Med 293: 1220–1224, 1975.

132. Shenfield GM, Patterson JW: Clinical assessment of bronchodilator drugs delivered by aerosol. Thorax 28: 124–128, 1973.

133. Simonsson BG, Jacobs FM, Nadel JA: Role of autonomic nervous system and the cough reflex in the increased responsiveness of airways in patients with obstructive airway disease. J Clin Invest 46: 1812–1818, 1967.

134. Simonsson BG, Svedmyr N, Skoogh BE, Andersson R, Bergh NP: In vivo and in vitro studies on alpha-receptors in human airways. Potentiation with bacterial endotoxin. Scand J Resp Dis 53: 227–236, 1972.

135. Slater EE: Cardiac tamponade and peripheral eosinophilia in a patient receiving cromolyn sodium. Chest 73: 878–879, 1978.

136. Smith AP, Cuthbert MF, Dunlop LS: Effects of inhaled prostaglandins E_1, E_2 and $F_2\alpha$ on the airway resistance of healthy and asthmatic man. Clin Sci Mol Med 48: 421–430, 1975.

137. Snashall PD, Boother FA, Sterling GM: The effect of α-adrenoreceptor stimulation on the airways of normal and asthmatic man. Clin Sci Mol Med 54: 283–289, 1978.

138. Speizer FE, Wegman DH, Ramirez A: Palpitation rates associated with fluorocarbon exposure in a hospital setting. N Engl J Med 292: 624–626, 1975.

139. Stoner J, Manganiello VC, Vaughan M: Effects of bradykinin and indomethacin on cyclic GMP and cyclic AMP in lung slices. Proc Nat Acad Sci USA 70: 3830–3833, 1973.

140. Stoner J, Manganiello VC, Vaughan M: Guanosine cyclic 3', 5'-monophosphate and guanylate cyclase activity in guinea pig lung: effects of acetylcholine and cholinesterase inhibitors. Mol Pharmacol 10: 155–161, 1974.

141. Szentivanyi A: The beta adrenergic theory of the atopic abnormality in bronchial asthma. J Allergy 42: 203–232, 1968.

142. Tashkin DP, Meth R, Simmonds DH, Lee YE: Double-blind comparison of acute bronchial and cardiovascular effects of oral terbutaline and ephedrine. Chest 68: 155–161, 1975.

143. Tickner TR, Cramp DG, Foo AY, Johnson AJ, Bateman SM, Pidgeon J, Spiro SG, Clarke SW, Wills MR: Metabolic response to intravenous salbutamol therapy in acute asthma. Thorax 32, 182–184, 1977.

144. Turner-Warwick M: Study of theophylline plasma levels after oral administration of new theophylline compounds. Br Med J 2: 67–69, 1957.

145. Turner-Warwick M: On observing patterns of airflow obstruction in chronic asthma. Br J Dis Chest 71: 73–86, 1977.

146. WALKER SR, EVANS ME, RICHARDS AJ, PATERSON JW: The fate of [14c] disodium cromoglycate in man. J Pharm Pharmacol 24: 525–531, 1972.
147. WARRELL DA, ROBERTSON DG, NEWTON HOWES J, CONNOLLY ME, PATERON JW, BEILIN LJ, DOLLERY CT: Comparison of cardiorespiratory effects of isoprenaline and salbutamol in patients with bronchial asthma. Br Med J 1: 65–70, 1970.
148. WEBB-JOHNSON DC, ANDREWS JL: Bronchodilator therapy. N Engl J Med 297: 476–482, 758–764, 1977.
149. WEINBERGER M: Theophylline for treatment of asthma. J Paediatr 92: 1–7, 1978.
150. WEINBERGER M, BRONSKY E: Evaluation of oral bronchodilator therapy in asthmatic children. J Paediatr 84: 421–427, 1975.
151. WEINBERGER M, BRONSKY E: Interaction of ephedrine and theophylline. Clin Pharmacol Ther 17: 585–592, 1975.
152. WEINBERGER M, HENDELES L, BIGHLEY L: The relation of product formulation to absorption of oral theophylline. N Engl J Med 299: 852–857, 1978.
153. WELLING PG, LEE KP, PATEL JA, WALKER JE, WAGNER JG; Urinary excretion of ephedrine in man without pH control following on administration of three commercial ephedrine sulphate preparations. J Pharm Sci 60: 1629–1634, 1971.
154. WHIMSTER WF, REID L: The influence of dibutyryl cyclic adenosine monophosphate and other substances on human bronchial gland discharge. Exp Mol Pathol 18: 234–240, 1973.
155. WILLIAMS SJ, PARRISH RW, SEATON A: Comparison of intravenous aminophylline and salbutamol in severe asthma. Br Med J 2: 685, 1975.
156. WILLIAMS S, SEATON A: Intravenous or inhaled salbutamol in severe acute asthma. Thorax 32: 555–558, 1977.
157. WOLFE JD, TASHKIN DP, CALVARESE B, SIMMONS M: Bronchodilator effects of terbutaline and aminophylline alone and in combination in asthmatic patients. N Engl J Med 298: 363–367, 1978.
158. WOOD D, DOWNES JJ, SCHEINKOPF H, LECKS HI: Intravenous isoproterenol in the management of respiratory failure in childhood status asthmaticus. J Allergy Clin Immunol 50: 75–81, 1972.
159. WOOLCOCK AJ: Inhaled drugs in the prevention of asthma. Am Rev Resp Dis 115: 191–194, 1977.
160. WU N, MILLER WF, CODE R, RICHBURG P: Intermittent positive pressure breathing in patients with chronic bronchopulmonary disease. Am Rev Tuberc Pulm Dis 71: 693–703, 1955.
161. YU DYC, GALANT SP, GOLD WM: Inhibition of antigen-induced bronchoconstriction by atropine in asthmatic patients. J Appl Physiol 32: 823–828, 1972.
162. ZWILLICH CW, SUTTON FD, NEFF TA, COHN WM, MATTHAY RA, WEINBERGER MM: Theophylline-induced seizures in adults. Correlation with serum concentrations. Ann Intern Med 82: 784–787, 1975.

8

Corticosteroids

In the field of respiratory medicine there are two sorts of pathological process that are susceptible to corticosteroid therapy. The first is reversible broncho-spasm, which is usually a manifestation of immediate (Type 1) hypersensitivity such as bronchial asthma or acute anaphylaxis but may also occur in chronic allergic bronchopulmonary aspergillosis,[69] and in late bronchial reactions attrib-uted to Type III allergic responses.[86] The second is widespread pulmonary fibrosis,[110] the final common pathway of a number of pathological processes in the lung which fall into four groups, namely, granulomatous disease, pulmonary exudative reactions, inorganic dust inhalation, and a miscellaneous group of unknown aetiology exemplified by cryptogenic fibrosing alveolitis.

In asthma and in at least some of the conditions which lead to widespread pulmonary fibrosis it is well recognised that the clinical manifestations of the disease are associated with abnormal immunological features[68]; for example, the Type III immune-complex reaction which characterises extrinsic allergic alveolitis, and the presence of granular deposits of IgG and C3 complement in the alveolar walls and capillaries of patients with cryptogenic fibrosing alveolitis of the cellular type.[34] It seems highly probable that the effectiveness of corticosteroids in controlling these conditions can be attributed to their in-hibitory influence on the immunologic and inflammatory response, although the variety and highly complex nature of these reactions make it difficult at present to determine the specific therapeutic action of corticosteroid drugs. In fact it is likely that they act in more than one way, since there is extensive evidence from *in vitro* experimentation that many different facets of immuno-logic and inflammatory reactions can be altered by corticosteroids.

ORIGIN AND STRUCTURE OF CORTISOL AND ITS ANALOGUES

The synthesis of corticosteroid hormones by the cells of the adrenal cortex is stimulated by adrenocorticotropic hormone (ACTH) which is secreted by the basophilic cells of the adenohypophysis in response to the release of cortico-tropin-regulatory hormone (CRH) from the hypothalamus. Stimuli that induce the release of ACTH are transmitted by nervous pathways which converge on the median eminence of the hypothalamus, and are initiated by a number of conditions which include cold, emotional stress, exercise, severe infections, and trauma. Circadian variation occurs in the rate of secretion of ACTH and corticosteroids, the output of cortisol being greatest in the early hours of the morning and declining during the day, with the lowest level occurring about midnight. Regulation of ACTH release also depends on a negative feedback control: corticosteroid administration inhibits ACTH release and in the long term induces both hyalinisation of the basophil cells of the adenohypophysis and atrophy of the adrenal cortex. An important clinical consequence of this process is that patients who have been treated with corticosteroids in high dosage for as little as 4 weeks are liable to suffer temporary suppression of the adrenal response to stress,[114] while those on longer-term therapy will experience prolonged inhibition of the hypothalamo-pituitary-adrenal axis (HPA) and extended loss of the stress response which may persist for as long as 12 months.[74]

The corticosteroids have been traditionally classified into glucocorticoids and mineralocorticoids, according to the dominant potency of the two categories. The mineralocorticoids, such as aldosterone, have their major action in influencing electrolyte balance and have little or no effect on carbohydrate metabolism or on the inflammatory response. The glucocorticoids, exemplified by cortisol, have a major function in physiological concentration of converting protein to carbohydrate, while at pharmacological dosage they have an anti-inflammatory action which provides their main therapeutic function and which seems to run parallel with their glucocorticoid effect. In the context of their clinical use as anti-inflammatory or anti-allergic agents, the glucocorticoids are commonly referred to indiscriminately as "corticosteroids."

The twenty-one-carbon atom structure of cortisol is shown in Figure 8-1. The characteristics of this structure which determine the glucocorticoid effect have been investigated by studies of structure-activity relationships, which show that the essential features are the ketone oxygen at C3, the unsaturated bond between C4 and C5, the hydroxyl group at C11, and the ketone oxygen at C20, presumably because this arrangement is necessary to fit the corticosteroid receptor. Substitutions at other sites on the cortisol molecule provide synthetic analogues which have an enhanced or diminished anti-inflammatory or mineralocorticoid activity compared with cortisol: for example, the introduction of an unsaturated bond between C1 and C2 produces prednisolone, which has a four-fold enhancement of anti-inflammatory activity, while further additions to the prednisolone molecule (Figure 8-1) produce dexamethasone, which has an even greater anti-inflammatory effect with diminution of sodium retentive activity. An additional consequence of these substitutions is to alter rates of metabolism and so influence the duration of corticosteroid activity in different compounds.

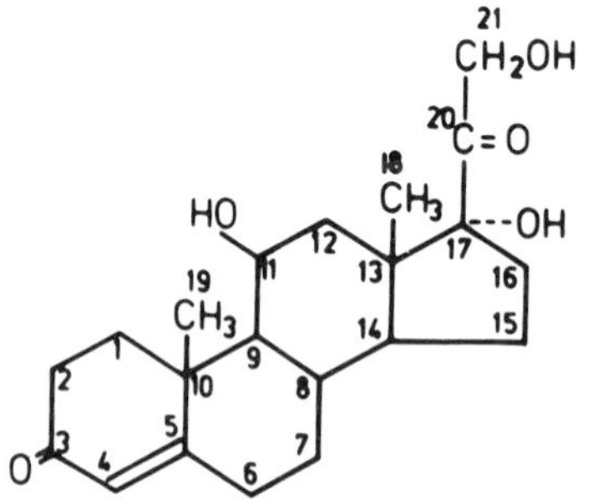

CORTISOL
(Hydrocortisone, 17-hydroxycorticosterone)

Mainly glucocorticoid effect
Minor mineralocorticoid effect
Biological half-life 8–12 hours

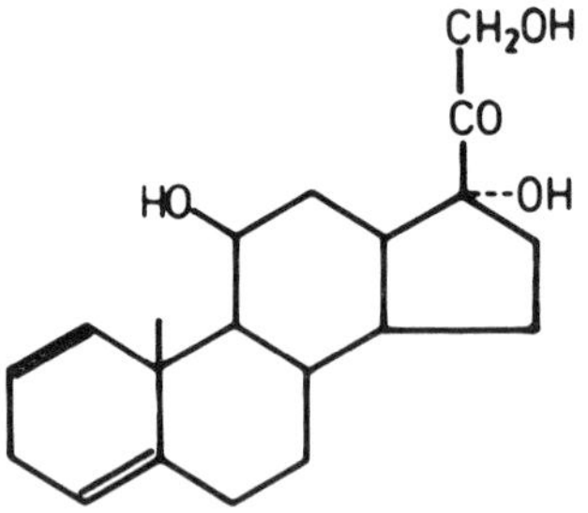

PREDNISOLONE

Mainly glucocorticoid effect
Slight mineralocorticoid effect
Biological half-life 18–36 hours

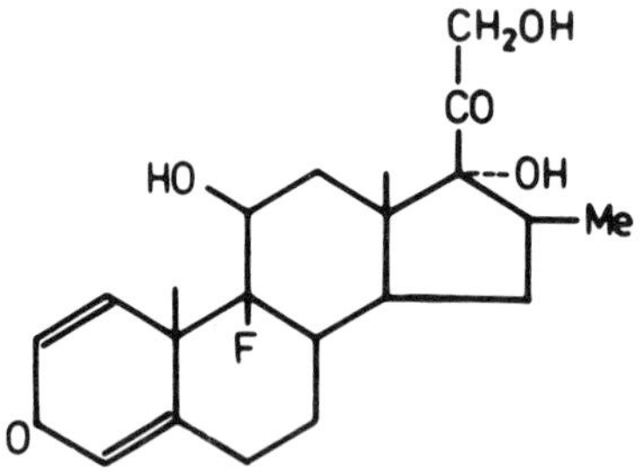

DEXAMETHASONE
(9 α–fluoro–16 α–methylprednisolone)

Major glucocorticoid effect
Minimal mineralocorticoid effect
Biological half-life 36–54 hours

Figure 8-1 *Chemical structure of cortisol and synthetic analogues.*

ACTIONS OF CORTICOSTEROIDS

The administration of glucocorticoids results in a wide range of effects which influence the metabolism of most tissues, and it has important therapeutic actions in immunologically-mediated and inflammatory disease processes. It seems likely that there is a physiological mechanism of glucocorticoid action which is common to all types of cell, by which the hormone penetrates the cell membrane and binds to a receptor protein, resulting in a corticosteroid-receptor complex which influences intra-cellular protein synthesis through the mediation of ribonucleic acid and leads to the glucocorticoid response appropriate to that particular cell. The therapeutic benefit of treatment with supraphysiologic doses of glucocorticoids has always to be considered in the light of the unwanted effects which are certain to occur if the drug is continued for long enough at sufficient dosage, and which are easily understood and recalled by considering the physiological actions of the glucocorticoid hormones.

Mechanism of Action

The mechanism of action of corticosteroid drugs in altering cellular function to produce an anti-allergic or anti-inflammatory effect is not certain, but three hypotheses have been advanced[108]:

1. Interaction with an intracellular corticosteroid receptor.
2. Stimulation of adenyl cyclase and cyclic 3'5' adenosine-monophosphate (cAMP).
3. Influence on cellular or lysosomal membrane stability.

The Corticosteroid Receptor Specific receptors for glucocorticoids are found in the cytoplasm of many glucocorticoid-responsive tissues,[78] and there is a substantial body of evidence which implicates the glucocorticoid-specific receptor interaction as the necessary preliminary to a glucocorticoid response in a variety of cell types as diverse as thymus, hepatic cells, fibroblasts, lymphoid cells, and macrophages. The essential features of this model of glucocorticoid action are depicted in Figure 8-2, which illustrates the critical concept that the physiological effects of steroid action are mediated through synthesis of specific messenger ribonucleic acids (mRNA) and proteins. The induced proteins (for example, enzymes) bring about the cellular reactions which are the expression of the glucocorticoid response in that particular cell type.

Corticosteroids and Cyclic AMP Whether the above model can be applied to all the known anti-inflammatory actions of the glucocorticoids is uncertain.

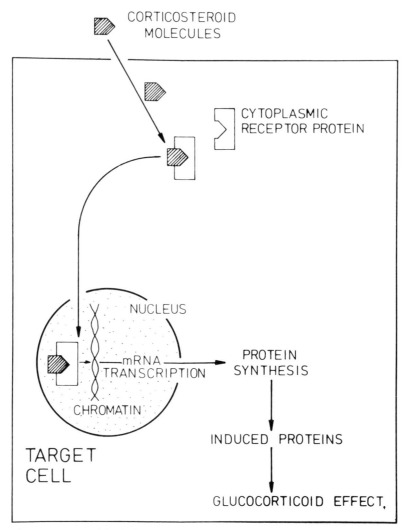

Figure 8-2 *Model of glucocorticoid mechanism of action.*

Many of the actions of cyclic AMP are facilitated or mimicked by glucocorticoids, and this could be explained if glucocorticoids acted by diminishing cyclic AMP phosphodiesterase activity as has been suggested,[70] thus increasing the intracellular level of cyclic AMP. Such an interaction would be highly relevant to the concept of cyclic AMP's important role in the pathogenesis of asthma (see Figure 7-2) and consistent with the possible therapeutic effect of corticosteroids in apparently restoring beta-receptor responsiveness in this disease.[37] Evidence that glucocorticoids might act in asthma by influencing cyclic AMP metabolism is based on *in vitro* studies of peripheral blood leucocyte preparations from symptomatic asthmatic patients, preparations which are known to show a decreased cyclic AMP response to beta-adrenergic agents compared with normal cells.[83] Treatment with glucocorticoids leads to recovery of the impaired cyclic AMP response, and this has been attributed to corticosteroid-induced adenyl cyclase stimulation[62] or to depression of cyclic AMP phosphodiesterase activity.[70,77]

In their extensive review, which took account of the possible mechanisms of action of glucocorticoids in many different tissues, Thompson and Lippman[108] admitted the similarity of the metabolic effects of cyclic AMP and glucocorticoids but drew attention to the differences in their mode of action. They concluded that cyclic AMP probably did not act as an intracellular mediator to effect the glucocorticoid response, but that glucocorticoids had an important permissive effect on the action of cyclic AMP.

Membrane Activity of Glucocorticoids   It has been suggested that corticosteroids may interact with the membranes of cell surfaces or of lysosomes, thereby modifying their surface configuration or stability. Such physical changes could account for the redistribution of mononuclear cells in the circulation which results from corticosteroid administration,[41] and for the suppression of lysosomal enzyme and mediator release which accounts for many of the physiological manifestations of immunological and inflammatory reactions.[123] However the corticosteroid concentrations at which·lysosomal stabilisation occurs[115] appear to be higher than would be reached under physiological conditions, and it is doubtful whether this mechanism is significant in the *in vivo* suppression of inflammatory reactions by corticosteroids at pharmacological dosage.[7,87]

Thus several mechanisms could explain the anti-inflammatory effect of glucocorticoids at a cellular level. Which is responsible for the beneficial effect of these drugs in immunological and fibrosing disease of the lungs is still uncertain, but they are probably not mutually exclusive.

Immunosuppressive and Anti-inflammatory Effects

Corticosteroids play an important part in the treatment of conditions such as asthma or extrinsic allergic alveolitis in which immunologic and inflammatory reactions initiate the disease process. Although they influence many aspects of these complex reactions, the evidence suggests that they act mainly in suppressing the inflammatory response whether this is due to antigen-antibody interaction or to some other form of tissue injury. It is worth bearing in mind that in general the inflammatory and immune responses have valuable protective functions in bringing about the healing of damaged tissue and in neutralising or removing toxic material, including micro-organisms, so that delay in wound healing and the facilitation of opportunist infections are among the important adverse effects of corticosteroid therapy.

The Immune Response   After the initial sensitisation of an immunologically reactive individual with an antigen, further exposure not only reinforces the immune response but also provokes hypersensitivity reactions. Four types of reaction are recognised,[28] three of which depend upon interaction of antigen with humoral antibody (humoral response) while the fourth involves antigen reacting with antibody-like molecules at the surface of cells (cell-mediated response). The key cell in both humoral and cell-mediated responses is the lymphocyte. Lymphocytes are divided into two classes, the B and T lymphocytes, both of which are derived from bone marrow stem cells. The B lymphocytes carry specific immunoglobulins on the surface membrane which interact with the appropriate antigen, resulting in the differentiation of the B lymphocyte into plasma cells which secrete specific humoral antibodies. The T lymphocytes are processed by the thymus gland in the course of maturation, the resultant cells being responsible for cell-mediated immunity after sensitisation by exposure to antigenic material. Both lymphocyte populations are stimulated by antigens through the mediation of macrophages which "capture" the antigen and process it, causing the antigenic information to be passed to the reactive cells which are part of the population of long-living circulating small lymphocytes. They are antigen-specific in the sense that one cell responds to one antigen only. When restimulated by antigen these cells divide and give rise to many sensitised lymphocytes which become the effector cells of the immune response.

The cell-mediated (Type IV) immune response, which includes delayed hypersensitivity, allograft rejection, and graft-versus-host disease, results from specifically sensitised T lymphocytes which react with antigen deposited at a local site, the classical example being the Mantoux reaction for tuberculin hypersensitivity. The reaction leads to the secretion of soluble mediators known as lymphokines which promote inflammation by attracting and localising macrophages and leucocytes at the reaction site.

The other three types of hypersensitivity response (Types I, II, and III) depend on the participation of the immunoglobulins which are humoral antibodies produced by plasma cells. The Type I reaction, which causes immediate hypersensitivity such as allergic rhinitis, asthma, and anaphylaxis is due to interaction between the antigen and tissue mast cells previously sensitised with antibody which is the immunoglobulin IgE. The hypersensitivity reaction leads to the release of a number of mediators, including histamine, SRS-A, kinins, serotonin, and some prostaglandins, all of which provoke the inflammatory response. The Type II reaction is initiated by circulating antibody which interacts either with an antigenic component of the cell membrane or with an antigen or hapten which has become intimately associated with the cell. The reaction usually involves the consumption of complement and leads to cell lysis: examples are Goodpasture's syndrome, the haemolytic anaemias of auto-immune disease such as systemic lupus erythematosus, and drug-induced thrombocytopenia due to sulphonamides or Sedormid. The Type III immune-complex reaction results from the interaction between circulating immunoglob-ulin antibody (usually IgG or IgM) and the antigen, either in the tissue spaces, causing precipitates around small blood vessels; or, when there is antigen excess, in the circulating blood, leading to the formation of soluble immune complexes which are deposited in basement membranes and the walls of blood vessels. Complement may be consumed in the course of the reaction. The resultant inflammation is responsible for such diseases as allergic broncho-pulmonary aspergillosis, extrinsic allergic alveolitis, and the nephritic lesions of systemic lupus erythematosus.

Corticosteroids depress the immune response in a number of ways. They produce transient depletion of monocytes[39] and lymphocytes[122] from the peripheral circulation, the latter effect being more marked among the T than the B lymphocytes and attributed to redistribution of the cells from the circula-tion to other body compartments.[40] It is reasonable to suppose that the exclu-sion of sensitised lymphocytes from the circulation reduces the effectiveness of the immune response, and although corticosteroids do not suppress already sensitised lymphocytes,[92] it is possible that they may still prevent futher recruit-ment of unstimulated lymphocytes and thus limit the immune process. In addition, they inhibit some aspects of lymphocyte and monocyte function which contribute to the immunological response, for instance, by interfering with the processing by macrophages of particulate antigens, such as transfused erythrocytes, or by suppressing the effects of lymphokines in recruiting ma-crophages and leucocytes to the inflammatory site, following cell-mediated immune reactions.[6,116] The reduction in complement levels which is produced by corticosteroid therapy[3] may inhibit some reactions mediated by humoral immune processes which are complement dependent. Corticosteroids may also influence the inflammatory process of immune-complex diseases by in-terfering with the transit of immune complexes across basement membranes.[46]

The Inflammatory Process   This rather vague term embraces the diverse man-ifestations of an extraordinarily complex mechanism which represents the fun-damental tissue reaction to injury. Some aspects of its complexity are revealed in recent reviews,[96,107] but in the current context we are interested in the process simply as it is influenced by corticosteroid therapy.

Inflammation is caused by all forms of tissue damage including trauma, heat or cold, ionising radiation, foreign bodies, ischaemia, invasion by micro-organisms, chemicals including endogenous substances such as histamine, and antigen-antibody reactions. In very general terms, the inflammatory reaction consists of vasodilatation, exudation of fluid due to increased permeability of vessels, emigration of leucocytes and macrophages from the blood into the perivascular space, and phagocytosis of tissue debris and micro-organisms by polymorphonuclear (PMN) leucocytes, monocytes, or tissue macrophages. Digestion of the engulfed particles is accomplished by proteolytic enzymes contained within cellular lysosomes, but at the same time some extracellular escape of lysosomal enzymes occurs which may aggravate tissue injury. Phagocytosing PMN leucocytes also release prostaglandins and thromboxanes, which are potent mediators of inflammation, leading to oedema and vasodilatation.[76] If the acute inflammatory response contains but fails to eradicate the irritant process completely, a chronic reaction develops which varies in histological character according to the nature of the underlying tissue injury (for example, the granulomatous reactions of sarcoidosis or berylliosis, or the fibrinoid necrosis occurring in immune-complex disease). In chronic inflammation the response is characterised by proliferation of cells, mainly lymphocytes, monocytes, and plasma cells but also eosinophils in hypersensitivity states. Epithelioid cells and multinucleate giant cells are typical of chronic granulomatous reactions, and they provide enhanced phagocytic activity; there is suggestive but not certain evidence that epithelioid cells derive from macrophages in cell-mediated hypersensitivity reactions.[109] Proliferation of capillaries and fibroblasts lead to the generation of new fibrous tissue which revitalises the injured area—although this process may fail to restore normal tissue function.

Corticosteroid administration produces a PMN leucocytosis which peaks 4–6 hours after giving the drug, due to increased release into the circulation from the bone marrow and diminished emigration from the blood to sites of inflammation. This inhibition of local PMN leucocyte accumulation is one of the most important effects of corticosteroids on the inflammatory response and is attributed to reduced leucocyte adherence to the vascular epithelium. Transient monocytopenia and eosinopenia also follow corticosteroid administration, while monocyte and macrophage accumulation is reduced by the inhibitory effect of corticosteroids on lymphokines which are released by cell-mediated immunological reactions, such as macrophage migration inhibitory factor (MIF), macrophage aggregating factor (MAF) and monocyte chemotactic factor (MCTF).[41] Escape of proteolytic enzymes from leucocyte lysosomes occurs in the course of phagocytosis and is a source of tissue damage which might be prevented by a membrane-stabilising effect of corticosteroids.[123] Although such an effect of glucocorticoids has been demonstrated experimentally, there is considerable doubt about its significance *in vivo* in pharmacological dosage.[108]

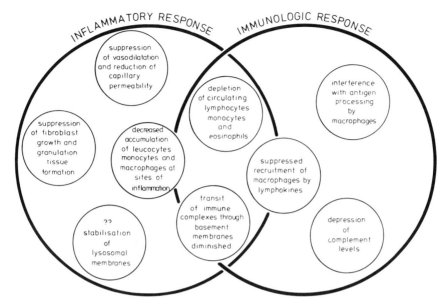

Figure 8-3 *The effects of corticosteroid therapy on the immunologic and inflammatory responses.*

Corticosteroid drugs also affect noncellular components of inflammatory reactions by suppressing vasodilatation and reducing capillary permeability. They inhibit fibroblast growth[90] and collagen synthesis,[80] and suppress granulation tissue formation[63]—effects which may contribute significantly to their therapeutic role in fibrosing conditions of the lung.

There is considerable overlap between the immunosuppressive and the anti-inflammatory effect of corticosteroid drugs, and this has been illustrated in Figure 8-3. Quite clearly, their action in controlling certain types of pulmonary disease cannot be ascribed to one particular effect but must involve many aspects of immunological and inflammatory reactions.

Glucocorticoid Effects on Metabolism

As indicated earlier in this chapter the anti-inflammatory effects of corticosteroid drugs appear to go hand-in-hand with their potential for exerting glucocorticoid effects on metabolic functions. Therefore their use in high dosage to control inflammatory and immunologic disease processes is inevitably accompanied by unwanted effects which result from their disturbing influence on normal metabolism. The following brief account of some of the metabolic effects of glucocorticoids provides background information for an understanding of the problems to be avoided or contended with in the successful management of corticosteroid therapy.

Carbohydrate and Protein Metabolism   The major effects of glucocorticoids are to mobilise tissue protein and enhance hepatic glyconeogenesis. Increased breakdown of tissue protein and inhibition of peripheral protein synthesis provide additional amino acid substrate for glyconeogenesis by hepatic enzymes, which are themselves induced by glucocorticoids. Increased glucagon secretion occurs, possibly as a consequence of the raised circulating amino acid level, and contributes to the enhanced synthesis of glucose. Peripheral utilisation of glucose is diminished by glucocorticoids due partly to a reduction in the activity of insulin receptors in insulin sensitive tissues.

   An exaggeration of these effects is seen with prolonged high-dose corticosteroid therapy which leads to muscle wasting and myopathy, thinning of the skin, increased vascular fragility, and hyperglycaemia with glycosuria. Frank diabetes mellitus may be precipitated in latent diabetics.

Lipid Metabolism   Glucocorticoids increase lipolysis which leads to the release of free fatty acids and glycerol. The free fatty acids inhibit uptake of glucose by peripheral tissues and provide an alternative source of energy, while glycerol may be used as a substrate for hepatic glyconeogenesis. The mobilisation of fats resulting from excessive levels of glucocorticoids in high dosage corticosteroid therapy or Cushing's syndrome leads to truncal obesity with depletion of peripheral fat stores due to differences in the sensitivity of adipose tissue in different parts of the the body to the action of glucocorticoids.

Bone Metabolism   The intestinal absorption of calcium is reduced and urinary calcium loss increased by glucocorticoids, leading to secondary hyperparathyroidism. In addition their catabolic action affects the protein matrix of bone, most markedly that of the vertebral bodies, diminishing calcium deposition and increasing the risk of vertebral collapse in patients on high dosage corticosteroids. Glucocorticoids inhibit osteoblast function and in children they reduce linear bone growth and delay epiphyseal closure so that normal growth is inhibited by excessive corticosteroid therapy.

Other Effects   Some additional actions of the corticosteroids may be significant in patients treated with these drugs. Some glucocorticoids have a slight mineralocorticoid function, for example cortisol and prednisolone, and induce sodium retention and potassium excretion although to a much lesser extent than the true mineralocorticoids, such as aldosterone; nevertheless, sodium retention with oedema often complicates their use, especially in patients with pre-existing cardiovascular disease. Hypertension rarely seems to occur as a result of prolonged glucocorticoid therapy, but it is common in Cushing's syndrome.

Most of the effects of corticosteroids on the formed elements of the blood have been described above. Besides causing a rapid PMN leucocytosis, corticosteroids increase the platelet count and red cell mass which in Cushing's syndrome is characteristically manifested by polycythaemia. Eosinophils and basophils are decreased in response to corticosteroids, probably as a result of redistribution out of the circulating blood in a similar manner to lymphocytes.[41]

Corticosteroids have important effects on the central nervous system but their metabolic basis is not clear. The effects on the CNS are considered below, among the other side-effects of therapy.

CLINICAL PHARMACOLOGY

Cortisol and its analogues are readily absorbed from the gastrointestinal tract and are therefore effective by mouth. They are also absorbed from sites of local application such as the skin, bronchial mucous membrane, and synovial spaces, and systemic side-effects can occur as a result of long-term applications over wide areas of the skin or from excessive aerosol dosage. Endogenous cortisol is largely protein-bound in plasma, approximately 80 percent to transcortin, a specific alpha globulin, which has a high affinity but low binding capacity for cortisol, and about 10 percent to albumin, which provides a low affinity, high capacity receptor. Less than 10 percent is unbound, but it is this portion of circulating cortisol which is available for biological activity in corticosteroid-sensitive tissues or for metabolism and excretion. Reduction in serum albumin level due to disease may lead to unexpectedly high levels of unbound corticosteroid and to an increased liability to side-effects in patients on high-dose therapy.[59,111] Corticosteroids are largely metabolised in the liver by glucuronide-conjugation and are excreted in the urine.

There are certain differences between the handling of cortisol and its synthetic analogues which presumably account for the variations in their biological potency and duration of action. Prednisolone and dexamethasone have lower affinities for transcortin than cortisol but have higher affinities for target tissue receptors, and both are metabolised more slowly than cortisol in the liver because of alterations to the glucocorticoid molecule. The net result of these differences is that the elimination half-lives of the cortisol analogues show considerable variation, for example, approximately 1.5 hours for cortisol, 3.5 hours for prednisolone, and 5.0 hours for dexamethasone.[5,72]

It is interesting that the biological activity of the glucocorticoids does not correspond very closely with plasma concentrations. Following a single intravenous injection of cortisol (4 mg/kg body weight) in acute asthma, there was a 6– to 8–hour delay before measurable improvement in bronchospasm was observed,[24] even though the plasma cortisol concentration declined steadily from its peak, which occurred within the first hour after administration. Furthermore, biological effects persist substantially beyond the duration of a raised plasma glucocorticoid concentration, as can be demonstrated by determining the biological half-life which is defined as the time taken for a measure of corticosteroid activity (for example, suppression of pituitary-adrenal function) to fall to half its initial level. There is a rough correlation between the biological half-life and the plasma half-life for different glucocorticoids, and between their relative anti-inflammatory potencies (Table 8-1).[73] A recent study suggests that the generally-accepted values given in Table 8-1 underestimate the relative potency of dexamethasone and overestimate the biological half-lives of dexamethasone and prednisolone.[72] The biological half-lives have been used as a guide to choice of drug in different treatment regimens, for example, to try and imitate the circadian variation of endogenous cortisol with twice daily cortisol tablets in replacement therapy, or to avoid continuous HPA suppression by alternate daily dosage with prednisolone in anti-inflammatory treatment.

The topical corticosteroids, beclomethasone dipropionate and betamethasone valerate have distinctive pharmacokinetic properties which account for their usefulness as aerosol preparations. Beclomethasone dipropionate has potent glucocorticoid activity if given intravenously but it also has high topical activity and is readily absorbed via the bronchial mucosa. The swallowed portion of the drug, which amounts to about 90 percent of the inhaled dose, is slowly absorbed from the gastrointestinal tract, although inactivation by first-pass metabolism in the liver has been suggested.[71] Systemic effects are avoided using inhaled doses of up to 1.0 mg per day,[22] but evidence of adrenal suppression has been elicited using doses of 1.6 to 2.0 mg per day.[20,45] Betamethasone has similar structure and properties to dexamethasone, and betamethasone valerate is an insoluble ester which, like beclomethasone propionate, has potent topical activity, although adrenal suppression results if large doses are

Table 8-1 / Glucocorticoid Drugs: Relative Potencies and Half-lives

Drug	Anti-inflammatory Potency	Equivalent Potency	Plasma Half-life (hours)	Biological Half-life (hours)
Cortisol	1	20	1.5	8–12
Prednisolone	4	5.0	3.5	12–36
Betamethasone	25	0.6	5.0	36–54
Dexamethasone	30	0.75	5.0	36–54

taken by mouth.[44] The virtue of both these corticosteroid aerosols lies in their very high topical activity, which provides a substantial bronchodilator effect at a dose which is well below the level of HPA suppression.[65]

PREPARATIONS

There is a wide choice of preparations available for glucocorticoid therapy in the treatment of allergic and inflammatory diseases, and it is advisable for the prescriber to make use of a selected group with which he can become thoroughly acquainted.

ACTH   At the present time ACTH is mainly used as a diagnostic agent in the investigation of adrenal insufficiency. Its effectiveness in the treatment of acute asthma is dependent upon the responsiveness of the adrenal cortex, which may be impaired by prior glucocorticoid therapy, while in the long-term control of chronic asthma the necessity for expensive daily intramuscular injections has obvious disadvantages. Dosage regulation is less easy than with oral preparations and ACTH is more liable to cause salt and water retention than synthetic glucocorticoids. A commonly used ACTH preparation is Repository Corticotropin Injection U.S.P. (Corticotropin Gelatin Injection B.P.) given in a dose of 40 units once daily intramuscularly, but in Britain it has largely been superseded by the synthetic analogue Tetracosactrin Zinc Injection B.P., which is a synthetic peptide containing 24 of the 39 amino acids present in natural corticotropin. Allergic reactions are less frequent and the duration of action may be up to 48 hours. This preparation can be given intramuscularly or intravenously in a dose of 0.5 to 1 mg every second or third day initially. A similar preparation, Cosyntropin for injection (Cortrosyn) is available in the United States for diagnostic purposes.

Intravenous Corticosteroids   Intravenous hydrocortisone is part of the standard treatment regimen in acute severe asthma and other life-threatening allergic reactions. Hydrocortisone sodium succinate injection U.S.P. and B.P. is usually given as a single bolus injection intravenously, as soon as the seriousness of the patient's state is recognised, in a dose of 250 mg, followed by 250 mg every 4 to 6 hours by intravenous infusion or regular bolus injections. In order to maintain the plasma cortisol concentration in the range 100–150 μg/100 ml Collins and his colleagues[24] recommend in severe asthma an initial loading dose of 4 mg of hydrocortisone per kg body weight by bolus injection followed by 3 mg per kg body weight 6-hourly by continuous intravenous infusion; this allows the plasma cortisol concentration to be sustained with a smaller total daily dose than with intermittent injections and may reduce the hazards of electrolyte disturbance and fluid retention. There appear to be no advantages in giving higher doses of corticosteroids in severe asthma.[11]

Oral Therapy The preferred oral corticosteroid is prednisolone. This is the biologically-active compound to which prednisone is metabolised by the liver, and there are therefore theoretical grounds for using it when impaired liver function is a possibility. Otherwise there is no basis for choosing between prednisolone and prednisone. Prednisolone and prednisone tablets are available in strengths ranging from 1 to 50 mg per tablet, but the most generally useful are the 1, 2.5, and 5 mg tablets, and these include enteric-coated preparations which are sometimes found to be more acceptable by patients who experience dyspeptic symptoms with the plain tablets. Dosage regimens for oral corticosteroid therapy are discussed later in this chapter.

Aerosols The aerosol corticosteroid preparations which are currently available in Britain are betamethasone valerate (Bextasol) and beclomethasone dipropionate (Becotide). The latter is somewhat more potent and seems to be the preferred preparation, being available in the United States since 1976 as the proprietary drug Vanceril. Both drugs are delivered by metered dose aerosol from pressurised containers holding about 200 doses or "puffs"; each puff of beclomethasone dipropionate contains 50 μg, and of betamethasone valerate 100 μg. The usual treatment regimen for both drugs is 2 puffs 4 times daily. Higher dosages may be tried if necessary, but these increase the likelihood of opportunist infection of the oropharynx due to *Candida albicans*.

PROBLEMS OF CORTICOSTEROID THERAPY

The complications of corticosteroid therapy have already been referred to frequently in earlier sections of this chapter, and clearly they constitute a major difficulty in the use of these drugs. (For a comprehensive review, see reference 32.) Patients on long-term therapy are constantly at risk of developing side-effects which can be minimised only by careful surveillance and relentless determination on the part of both physician and patient to maintain effective treatment at the lowest possible dosage.

Adrenal Suppression

Systemic treatment with glucocorticoids in a dosage of 20 mg of cortisol or 5 mg of prednisolone per day, or more, for longer than a few days leads to suppression of the hypothalamo-pituitary-adrenocortical axis which may be prolonged for up to 12 months after high-dosage, long-term therapy.[74,94] Over-rapid withdrawal leads to a recurrence of symptoms and leaves the patient exposed to the extreme hazard of adrenal insufficiency in the face of stress such as an acute severe attack of asthma.[19,27] A variety of lesser manifestations have also been described, including tiredness, weakness, nausea, anorexia, arthralgia, muscle pains, skin desquamation, hypotension, and hypoglycaemia. Withdrawal of long-term corticosteroid treatment should therefore be carried out slowly and under careful supervision.

Metabolic Side-effects

Metabolic side-effects are largely attributable to enhanced glucocorticoid action on responsive tissues. These include the following:

1. Redistribution of body fat leading to truncal obesity, buffalo hump, and moon face.
2. Tissue protein catabolism leading to muscle wasting, myopathy, thinning of the skin, and increased fragility of vessel walls.
3. Hyperglycaemia and glycosuria, with the emergence of latent diabetes which may rarely manifest diabetic ketosis[2]; hyperlipidaemia is commonly associated.[4]
4. Osteoporosis, sometimes leading to vertebral collapse. It is widely thought to result from corticosteroid administration, but this contention is difficult to prove. In a critical review Dujovne and Azarnoff[35] suggest that glucocorticoids may be an exacerbating factor in those who are predisposed to osteoporosis, for example, in postmenopausal women and chronic arthritic or immobilised patients.
5. Disturbance of growth due to a reduction in the rate of skeletal growth and maturation in children,[112] whose physical development is frequently impaired in any case by underlying diseases such as chronic asthma or renal disease.
6. Dependent oedema, usually mild, due to the slight mineralocorticoid effect of some glucocorticoids, which causes sodium retention and potassium loss.

Anti-inflammatory Side-effects

The suppressive effect of prolonged corticosteroid therapy on normal immunologic and inflammatory processes exposes the patient unduly to the hazards of infection. This has been well substantiated in animals, and although it is more difficult to demonstrate unequivocally in humans (because many of the dis-

eases for which corticosteroids are administered themselves predispose to infection) there appears to be a correlation between dosage level and enhanced
susceptibility to infection.[31] It is generally supposed that latent tuberculosis may
become reactivated during corticosteroid therapy, but many such patients are
already affected by other diseases which alter immune responsiveness[30,98]; and
in asthmatics, treatment with corticosteroids does *not* seem to increase the
incidence of tuberculosis.[60,101] There is an increased liability for patients on
chronic corticosteroid treatment to develop infection with opportunist micro-
organisms such as Gram-negative bacteria and fungi which are relatively infrequent pathogens in uncompromised individuals. The increased incidence of
candidiasis of the oropharynx in patients taking aerosol corticosteroids regularly is a case in point, illustrating the opportunistic nature of the infection and the
relationship of incidence to dosage level.[12,65]

Miscellaneous Side-effects

Gastrointestinal Effects   A small proportion of patients taking corticosteroids
may experience nausea or vomiting, and the results of a drug surveillance
programme suggest that corticosteroids do occasionally induce gastrointestinal
bleeding in hospital patients without known predisposing illness.[54] Careful
controlled trials have not demonstrated that they cause an increased incidence
of peptic ulceration.[26] Corticosteroid-induced pancreatitis occurs rarely, but
fatal cases have been described.[81] The incidence of perforation of the colon in
patients with diverticulitis is also increased,[104] and clinical recognition of these
complications may be masked by the anti-inflammatory effects of corticosteroids.

Psychiatric Disturbances   Corticosteroids can produce almost any form of
psychiatric disorder. Euphoria and slight mood changes are quite common, but
almost any psychological disturbance ranging from insomnia, nervousness,
and anxiety to manic depressive or schizophrenic psychoses and attempted
suicide have been described[47]; the disturbances are thought to be determined
by the individual's pre-treatment personality. Such adverse reactions appear to
be dose related.[10]

Ocular Complications   Glaucoma and posterior subcapsular cataracts occur
in patients receiving both ocular and systemic corticosteroid therapy although
they usually regress when treatment is discontinued. The risk of glaucoma is
greatest in genetically predisposed or highly myopic individuals, and in susceptible patients irreversible glaucoma and blindness have been described.[43]

Drug Interactions

Enzyme Inducing Agents   Because the main route of corticosteroid inactivation is glucuronide conjugation in the liver, agents which augment the activity
of hepatic uridine diphosphate glucuronyl transferase are likely to increase the
rate of clearance of corticosteroids from the plasma and reduce their clinical
effectiveness. These include phenobarbital (phenobarbitone),[13] diphenylhydantoin (phenytoin),[88] and rifampin (rifampicin).[36] This effect of anticonvulsants
is greatest upon corticosteroids with longer plasma half-lives, such as dexamethasone, but the degree of hepatic enzyme induction is variable and
unpredictable in any individual. When concurrent administration of a drug
with enzyme-inducing properties and a corticosteroid is unavoidable, it is
recommended that the corticosteroid dose is doubled.[55] Careful surveillance of
the clinical response is important.

Concomitant administration of ephedrine increases the rate of clearance
of dexamethasone and presumably other corticosteroids,[14] an effect which has
been attributed both to hepatic enzyme induction and to increased hepatic
blood flow. Alternative bronchodilators should therefore be used for asthmatics on corticosteroid therapy, particular care being taken to avoid combined
preparations containing both ephedrine and phenobarbital.

Salicylates   Corticosteroid administration increases the rate of metabolism of
salicylates so that higher doses have to be given[50]; reduction in corticosteroid
dosage may then lead to salicylate intoxication unless the dosage of salicylates
is reduced appropriately.[57]

Both corticosteroids and aspirin occasionally induce gastrointestinal
bleeding severe enough to require blood transfusion in hospital patients who
have no evidence of predisposing illness.[54] Administration of both drugs simultaneously is likely to increase this hazard.

Anticholinesterase Drugs   A combination of corticosteroids with anticholinesterase preparations in the treatment of myasthenia gravis aggravates myas-
thenic symptoms.[16] It has been postulated that the corticosteroid molecule
binds to acetylcholine receptors and interferes with neuromuscular transmission.[85]

Antidiabetic Agents   The diabetogenic properties of corticosteroids have been
described. Introduction of antidiabetic therapy may be necessary in latent
diabetics who start corticosteroids, and readjustment of insulin or oral hypoglycaemic therapy may be necessary in established diabetics.

Diuretics Hypokalaemia due to diuretic therapy may be enhanced by the potassium-losing effect of corticosteroids which have residual mineralocorticoid activity (for example, cortisol, prednisolone). The serum potassium concentration should be monitored regularly when these two types of preparation are given simultaneously, and supplementary potassium should be administered if necessary.

CORTICOSTEROID THERAPY IN CLINICAL PRACTICE

General Principles

Because of the high risk of complications, systemic corticosteroids should only be used when there is a positive indication and when alternative forms of treatment have proved ineffective. For example, intravenous hydrocortisone should *not* be used in the treatment of an acute exacerbation of chronic obstructive pulmonary disease unless there is positive clinical evidence of an asthmatic aetiology; and oral prednisolone should *not* be prescribed for chronic asthma until a reasonable trial of alternative bronchodilators has been carried out. If corticosteroid therapy takes the form of a clinical trial, as it often does in the management of fibrosing or granulomatous lung disease, the response to therapy must be determined on *objective* grounds and treatment discontinued if the outcome is neutral or negative.

Supervision of Therapy It is particularly important that the patient understands the nature and objective of the treatment regimen from the start so that he can make an intelligent contribution in controlling symptoms and avoiding complications. It is essential that the dosage of systemic corticosteroids should be minimised and that the drug be discontinued if the illness goes into remission; but it is equally important that the dose be increased promptly in an exacerbation or whenever the patient is subjected to serious infection or to severe surgical or accidental trauma which may precipitate adrenal insufficiency. For the latter purpose, all patients on corticosteroid therapy (including aerosols) should carry a card giving details of current therapy so that health personnel can be forewarned in an emergency.

Regular surveillance is necessary for patients on systemic corticosteroids, and this nearly always means regular measurements of lung function. For asthmatics it is usually enough to record FEV_1 or PEFR from time to time, but during periods of instability or changing therapy it is invaluable if the patient keeps a diary of symptoms and a twice-daily record of PEFR so that short-term progress can be assessed objectively. For patients with pulmonary fibrosis a full series of pulmonary function tests (of which measurements of transfer factor

[TLCO] and lung volumes are the most important) are necessary every 3 months to determine the efficacy of treatment.

Avoidance of Unwanted Effects   The management of any patient on long-term corticosteroids is a continuous tug-of-war between adequate dosage to control the disease and minimum dosage to avoid unwanted effects. A dynamic situation of this sort requires regular medical supervision and intelligent cooperation on the patient's part. Assuming that all other alternative or accessory forms of therapy have been utilised, there are three ways of reducing the suppressive influence of corticosteroids on the hypothalamo-pituitary-adrenocortical axis: (1) aerosol therapy, (2) intermittent oral therapy, and (3) alternate-day oral therapy. There is a good deal of evidence to show that the aerosol corticosteroids enable oral treatment of asthma to be reduced and often discontinued,[15,29] with return of normal HPA function in those who can be maintained on aerosol therapy alone.[64] This form of treatment is remarkably well accepted in children down to 5 years of age and sometimes even younger,[48] and in Britain it is the preferred method of corticosteroid therapy in all age groups—provided that the recipient can administer the aerosol effectively. Wyatt and his colleagues[119] in the United States have recently expressed doubts about the freedom from side-effects of aerosol corticosteroids in childhood asthma, compared with alternate-day oral therapy—which they contend is easier to administer to children. Intermittent oral corticosteroid therapy for asthma is inevitably associated with long-term aerosol therapy because patients who experience exacerbations during the course of aerosol treatment must resort to a short course of systemic corticosteroids in order to control bronchospasm. The initiation and management of aerosol and intermittent oral corticosteroid therapy for asthma is described in Chapter 7.

Long-term oral corticosteroids are required for asthmatics and patients with chronic widespread pulmonary fibrosis who are disabled without them. Alternate-day therapy enables the total corticosteroid dosage to be reduced and so diminishes the level of HPA suppression[52]; it is based on the premise that the therapeutic effects of corticosteroids persist longer than their metabolic effects so that the oral administration of just over double the total daily requirement of an intermediate-acting corticosteroid such as prednisolone on the morning of day 1 will produce a therapeutic effect for 2 days but a metabolic effect for only 1 day, allowing the natural circadian rhythm of adrenocortical activity to reassert itself on day 2 and so maintain a certain degree of function in the HPA axis. Alternate-day oral corticosteroid therapy seems to be as effective as daily therapy in asthma with less effect on growth in children[97] and on adrenal function.[1]

If alternate-day therapy is contemplated it should be introduced when adequate control of symptoms has been obtained by regular daily therapy but before HPA function has been entirely suppressed. The transition from alternate-day therapy is achieved gradually over several weeks using an intermediate-acting corticosteroid such as prednisolone with the objective of eliminating it altogether on the "off" days.[106] There is no advantage in maintaining different doses on alternate days if the "off" day dosage has to remain above 7.5 mg, since this is high enough to suppress HPA function.

Problems of Withdrawal Pathological studies have shown histological changes and atrophy of the adrenals in some individuals within 5 days of starting high-dose corticosteroid therapy.[99] Withdrawal of systemic corticosteroids should therefore be gradual and systematic in any patient who has been treated for more than a few days and should be more gradual the longer the duration and the higher the dosage, because HPA suppression tends to be greater.[61] A suggested withdrawal protocol is described by Byyny.[17] A flare-up of the underlying disease or the development of withdrawal symptoms indicates the need for a temporary return to higher dosage followed by more gradual dosage reduction.

While the HPA is suppressed, plasma cortisol and ACTH levels remain low, but during recovery ACTH levels first rise to normal or even above normal while plasma cortisol remains depressed; subsequently plasma cortisol returns to normal.[49] It is not helpful to administer exogenous ACTH to hasten recovery since this merely stimulates the adrenal cortex temporarily but delays recovery of hypothalamic-pituitary function.[42] Return of normal function can be assessed by means of an ACTH stimulation test[56]; patients who have to undergo major pre-emptive surgery within a year of discontinuation of therapy should have a precautionary ACTH stimulation test and supplementary hydrocortisone should be administered to cover the operation if residual HPA suppression is apparent. Emergency surgery, severe trauma, and serious infections should be similarly treated.

Treatment of Reversible Airway Obstruction

Asthma Treatment of asthma commonly involves the use of several different drugs in series or in parallel, including various bronchodilator preparations, cromolyn sodium, and corticosteroids. Treatment regimens for asthma which include the administration of corticosteroid preparations are discussed in Chapter 7.

Chronic Obstructive Lung Disease The reversibility of airway obstruction in patients with chronic obstructive bronchitis is very variable because bronchial narrowing is due to several factors which differ in importance from one patient to the next, and from time to time in the same patient. For example, in one case bronchial obstruction results from expiratory airway collapse due to widespread panacinar emphysema, in another case from mucous gland hypertrophy and excessive mucus production by the bronchial epithelium, and in a third case from a combination of these factors associated with inflammatory exudate due to recurring infections. The contribution which corticosteroid therapy can make in this type of chronic lung disease is usually very small, presumably because an allergic bronchoconstrictor element plays only a small part in pathogenesis in a great majority of cases. Nevertheless the syndrome of chronic productive cough, breathlessness, and wheeze may occur in people with long-standing asthma and is a not uncommon feature of intrinsic asthma coming on later in life,[58] so that among a heterogeneous group of patients with chronic obstructive bronchitis there is likely to be a minority with a substantial element of reversible bronchospasm who may show a useful specific bronchodilator response to corticosteroids.[8]

The identification of the responder is a difficult problem because many patients with chronic lung disease will show a non-specific response to systemic corticosteroids, such as an increase in appetite, weight, energy, or general well-being. A controlled trial is therefore necessary to avoid the serious error of attributing corticosteroid-responsiveness (implying the need for corticosteroid therapy with all its hazards) to a patient whose response is in fact only minimal or subjective. Webb, Clarke, and Chilvers[114] recently showed that 12 out of 13 patients with chronic airflow obstruction who responded to 40 mg oral prednisolone per day did so within 8 days, while Harding and Freedman[51] carried out a double-blind controlled trial giving prednisolone 30 mg by mouth for 10 days, showing that 5 out of 36 patients with apparently irreversible airway obstruction had a clear measured improvement in ventilatory capacity. More work is needed to devise and standardise appropriate tests for making a positive identification of those patients with chronic obstructive lung disease who respond significantly to corticosteroids. At present it seems most rational to consider all patients with chronic obstructive bronchitis as possible responders to corticosteroids; to seek for any indicator such as a family or personal history of allergy, blood and sputum eosinophilia, or marked variation in airflow obstruction from day to day which might indicate an asthmatic basis and strengthen the argument for trying out corticosteroid therapy; and, in selected cases, to perform an objective controlled trial of oral prednisolone in substantial dosage (30–40 mg per day) for at least 8 days of active therapy. What constitutes a "positive" response warranting an extended application of corticosteroid therapy, and whether by mouth or by aerosol, still needs to be determined.

Lung Parenchymal Disease Due to Known Allergens

Pulmonary Infiltration with Eosinophilia   There is a small group of conditions characterised by eosinophilia in blood and sputum associated with a variable degree of asthma and patchy infiltration of the lung parenchyma, usually transient but progressing in chronic cases to pulmonary fibrosis. The commonest of these is bronchopulmonary aspergillosis which is associated with Type I and Type III skin reactions and specific IgE antibody[66]; this condition tends to follow a rather chronic and relapsing course, and short-term oral corticosteroid treatment is sometimes necessary to relieve bronchial obstruction and prevent fibrosis and bronchiectasis.[113] A very similar syndrome of pulmonary infiltration with eosinophilia unassociated with *Aspergillus fumigatus* or any other recognised antigen has been designated cryptogenic pulmonary eosinophilia.[67] An association between this condition and polyarteritis nodosa has been noticed.[95] The symptoms and radiological abnormalities often resolve spontaneously, but short-term oral corticosteroids may be necessary to control asthmatic symptoms and to hasten resolution of the radiological and mild functional changes. Eosinophilic pulmonary infiltrations may also be due to parasitic worm infestations, such as filariasis, which respond to specific chemotherapy; and to a number of drugs of which nitrofurantoin is a well-known example. Withdrawal of the drug usually leads to prompt resolution of symptoms and of the pulmonary infiltrate, but a short course of systemic corticosteroid therapy is indicated if symptoms are troublesome or if radiological changes are slow to resolve.

Extrinsic Allergic Alveolitis   The widespread granulomatous inflammatory reaction of the lung which occurs in extrinsic allergic alveolitis is caused by a Type III allergic response to a variety of antigens derived from thermophilic actinomycetes, fungal spores, and material from animals or birds. Well-known examples include Farmer's Lung due to the fungus *Micropolyspora faeni* which flourishes in mouldy hay, Bird Fancier's Lung due to antigenic material from feathers and bird droppings, and hypersensitivity pneumonitis due to contamination of heating or air-conditioning systems by thermophilic actinomycetes. These conditions usually resolve when the patient avoids further exposure to the relevant antigen but a short course of corticosteroids may be necessary to control the fever and other acute manifestations of the reaction, and more prolonged therapy may be indicated if there is evidence of impaired pulmonary function which persists or progresses. Careful serial observation of the patient's clinical, radiological, and functional status is therefore necessary to determine the need for corticosteroid therapy, and these observations are continued during the course of therapy to monitor the response. It is usual to start with a high dosage of 40–60 mg prednisolone daily for 2 to 4 weeks, reducing dosage gradually thereafter over a period of 2 or 3 months. Long-term corticosteroid treatment is not indicated but it is obviously most important that all further exposure to the antigen is strictly avoided.

Other Conditions Causing Widespread Pulmonary Fibrosis

Corticosteroids are used with varying success in the treatment of a number of conditions which lead to diffuse or widespread fibrous thickening of the alveolar walls which goes on to more extensive scarring and shrinkage of the lung. The main physiological effects of these changes are loss of lung volume, reduced compliance, impairment of gas transfer, and disturbance of ventilation/perfusion ratios. Ultimately hypoxic respiratory failure and cor pulmonale occur. Generally speaking the progression of these changes is slow, and it is sometimes interrupted by long periods of apparent stability or even spontaneous remission.

Experience has shown that corticosteroids in diffuse fibrosing lung conditions are a crude form of therapy, because they have to be used in high dosage, at least initially, their side-effects are troublesome, and their clinical efficacy is often doubtful. Biopsy of the lung may provide an indication of the potential reversibility of the lesion,[18,100] but in practice the therapeutic responsiveness can only be determined by a clinical trial. Corticosteroid therapy should therefore be introduced with reluctance unless there is good histological evidence of potential reversibility or the patient is deteriorating rapidly. The decision to start treatment is based on clinical and radiological evidence of disease progression and on objective measurements of pulmonary function obtained serially over a period of several weeks or months. Clinical, radiological, and physiological monitoring is necessary throughout treatment which requires scrupulous surveillance in order to limit dosage and avoid side-effects.

Pulmonary sarcoidosis provides an example which illustrates the doubts and difficulties of corticosteroid treatment in diffuse fibrosing lung conditions. It consists of a granulomatous inflammatory reaction which often resolves spontaneously but sometimes progresses to widespread pulmonary fibrosis.[102] Surveillance entails regular monthly or bi-monthly clinical examinations, chest radiographs, and pulmonary function tests to determine progress; if there is deteriorating function over a period of several months a point is eventually reached at which the physician decides that the need to try and prevent further deterioration is greater than the hazards of systemic corticosteroid therapy, and treatment is instituted with oral prednisolone. No strict criteria have been established for determining the point at which treatment should start, and some evidence suggests that corticosteroids do not prevent functional deterioration in sarcoidosis.[53,121] However many physicians accept that progressive functional deterioration warrants a careful trial of corticosteroid therapy[25] using an initial regimen of 30–40 mg of prednisolone daily for two months, reducing to

20 mg daily for 4 to 8 months, and then decreasing the dose by decrements of 5 mg every 3 to 6 weeks. Relapse is not uncommon during or soon after withdrawal, requiring reintroduction of therapy at a higher dose. Alternate-day therapy starting with 40 mg in a single morning dose has also been recommended as a means of reducing the incidence of side-effects.[33]

These principles of carefully supervised corticosteroid therapy, using serial measurements of lung function to monitor the response, can be applied to the management of other fibrosing lung conditions in which the probability of success is doubtful, such as diffuse interstitial fibrosis, that is, cryptogenic fibrosing alveolitis,[103] chronic berylliosis,[105] and possibly idiopathic pulmonary haemosiderosis and Goodpasture's syndrome.[91] If a reasonable trial of therapy for 1 to 2 months in adequate dosage of 30–60 mg per day fails to produce objective improvement then corticosteroids should be withdrawn in the usual way, but if a useful response is obtained the dosage should be reduced very slowly to establish the maintenance level at which symptoms can be tolerated without unacceptable side-effects.

Pulmonary Oedema Due to Diffuse Lung Injury

There is a large heterogeneous group of clinical conditions in which the major abnormality is pulmonary oedema, that is, excessive accumulation of liquid and solute in the extravascular tissues and spaces of the lung.[93] One mechanism of pulmonary oedema is an alteration in permeability of the alveolar epithelium or capillary endothelium due to diffuse physical or chemical damage which may have acute or chronic effects on the morphology and function of the lungs. The acute reaction, which used to be known as the "adult respiratory distress syndrome,"[79] leads to alveolar collapse, stiff lungs, and gross disturbance of alveolar-capillary gas exchange, while recurrent or chronic reactions may produce persistent disability from pulmonary fibrosis (Table 8-2).

The treatment of pulmonary insufficiency due to the acute type of reaction may require fluid restriction, diuretics, controlled oxygen administration, and mechanically assisted ventilation with positive end-expiratory pressure (PEEP). High dosage corticosteroid therapy has also been recommended in the treatment of many of these conditions, largely on the theoretical grounds that it diminishes the exudative reaction by reducing capillary permeability and maintaining the integrity of the alveolar epithelium; for example, in trauma and shock,[118] in fat embolism,[89] and in direct chemical injuries to the lung.[84] On the other hand, these recommendations have often been based on uncontrolled clinical observations, and where attempts have been made to assess the value of corticosteroids carefully, for example, in the treatment of aspiration pneumonia,[120] paraquat poisoning,[38] or near-drowning[75] the results of treatment have appeared inconclusive. If a decision to treat a critically ill patient with

Table 8-2 / Pulmonary Oedema Due to Altered Alveolar or Capillary Permeability

Acute Reactions

Inhaled toxins	Smoke
	Toxic fumes and gases (such as oxides of nitrogen; cadmium; phosgene)
	Prolonged O_2 therapy at high inspired concentration
Aspiration	Stomach contents
	Drowning or near-drowning
Infection	Viral pneumonia
	Septicaemia
Trauma and shock	Severe haemorrhage
	Severe tissue injury
	Fat embolism
	Massive transfusion
Circulating toxins	Paraquat

Chronic Reactions

Cytotoxic drugs	Bleomycin
	Busulphan
	Cyclophosphamide
	Chlorambucil
	Methotrexate
Other drugs	Hexamethonium
	Nitrofurantoin
	Practolol
	Pindolol
Irradiation	

corticosteroids is reached on empirical grounds it is usual to give intravenous hydrocortisone in a dosage of 1 g or more over each 24-hour period for 2 or 3 days, although longer acting methylprednisolone is preferred by some because it has little sodium-retaining action.

The use of prednisolone in treating chronic fibrosing reactions, which are largely due to drug toxicity, seems to be effective in quite a high proportion of cases, although this impression is based on case reports rather than on controlled investigations, such as interstitial pulmonary fibrosis due to busulphan,[82] methotrexate,[117] chlorambucil,[23] and nitrofurantoin.[9] Treatment is given for 2 or 3 weeks in high dosage followed by fairly rapid dosage reductions. Pneumonitis due to irradiation may be helped symptomatically by corticosteroids, but long-term fibrosis is not prevented.[21]

REFERENCES

1. ACKERMAN GL, NOLAN CM: Adrenocortical responsiveness after alternate-day corticosteroid therapy. N Engl J Med 278: 405–409, 1968.
2. ALAVI IA, SHARMA BK, PILLARY VKG: Steroid-induced diabetic ketoacidosis. Am J
   Med Sci 262: 15–23, 1971.
3. ATKINSON JP, FRANK MM: Effect of cortisone therapy on serum complement
   components. J Immunol 111: 1061–1066, 1973.
4. BAGDADE JD, PORTE D, BIERMAN EL: Steroid-induced lipemia. A complication of
   high-dosage corticosteroid therapy. Arch Intern Med 125: 129–134, 1970.
5. BALLARD PL, CARTER JP, GRAHAM BS, BAXTER JD: A radioreceptor assay for evaluation of the plasma glucocorticoid activity of natural and synthetic steroids in man.
   J Clin Endocrinol Metab 41: 290–304, 1975.
6. BALOW JE, ROSENTHAL AS: Glucocorticoid suppression of macrophage migration
   inhibiting factor. J Exp Med 137: 1031–1041, 1973.
7. BAXTER JD, FORSHAM PH: Tissue effects of glucocorticoids. Am J Med 53: 573–
   589, 1972.
8. BEEREL F, JICK H, TYLER MD: A controlled study of the effect of prednisone on
   air-flow obstruction in severe pulmonary emphysema. N Engl J Med 268: 226–
   230, 1963.
9. BONE RC, WOLFE J, SOBONYA RE, KERBY GR, STECHSCHULTE D, RUTH WE, WELCH
   M: Desquamative interstitial pneumonia following chronic nitrofurantoin therapy.
   Chest 69 (Suppl 2): 296–297, 1976.
10. BOSTON COLLABORATIVE DRUG SURVEILLANCE PROGRAM Acute adverse reactions to
    prednisone in relation to dosage. Clin Pharmacol Ther 13: 694–698, 1972.
11. BRITTON MG, COLLINS JV, BROWN D, FAIRHURST NPA, LAMBERT RG: High-dose
    corticosteroids in severe acute asthma. Br Med J 2: 73–74, 1976.
12. BROMPTON HOSPITAL/MEDICAL RESEARCH COUNCIL COLLABORATIVE TRIAL: Double-
    blind trial comparing two dosage schedules of beclomethasone dipropionate
    aerosol in the treatment of chronic bronchial asthma. Lancet 2: 303–307, 1974.
13. BROOKS SM, WERK EE, ACKERMAN SJ, SULLIVAN I, THRASHER K: Adverse effects of
    phenobarbital on corticosteroid metabolism in patients with bronchial asthma. N
    Engl J Med 286: 1125–1128, 1972.
14. BROOKS SM, SHOLITON LJ, WERK EE, ALTENAU P: The effects of ephedrine and
    theophylline on dexamethasone metabolism in bronchial asthma. J Clin Pharma-
    col 17: 308–318, 1977.
15. BROWN HM, STOREY G, JACKSON FA: Beclomethasone dipropionate aerosol in
    long-term treatment of perennial and seasonal asthma in children and adults: a
    report of five-and-half years' experience in 600 asthmatic patients. Br J Clin
    Pharmacol 4: 2593–2675, 1977.
16. BRUNNER NB, NAMBA T, GROB D: Corticosteroids in management of severe gener-
    alised myasthenia gravis. Neurology 22: 603–610, 1972.
17. BYYNY RL: Withdrawal from glucocorticoid therapy. N Engl J Med 295: 30–32,
    1976.
18. CARRINGTON CE, GAENSLER EA, COUTU RE, FITZGERALD MX, GUPTA RG: Natural

history and treated course of usual and desquamative interstitial pneumonia. N Engl J Med 298: 801–809, 1978.

19. Cayton RM, Howard P: Adrenal failure in bronchial asthma. Br Med J 2: 547, 1973.

20. Choo-Kang YFJ, Cooper EJ, Tribe AE, Grant IWB: Beclomethasone dipropionate by inhalation in the treatment of airways obstruction. Br J Dis Chest 66: 101–106, 1972.

21. Chu FCH, Nickson JJ, Uzel AR: Effect of ACTH and cortisone on radiation pneumonitis. Am J Roentgenol 75: 530–541, 1956.

22. Clark TJH, Costello JF, Soutar CA: The effects of beclomethasone dipropionate aerosol given in high doses to patients with asthma. Postgrad Med J 51 (Suppl 4): 72–75, 1975.

23. Cole SR, Myers TJ, Klatsky AU: Pulmonary disease with chlorambucil therapy. Cancer 41: 455–459, 1978.

24. Collins JV, Clark TJH, Brown D, Townsend J: The use of corticosteroids in the treatment of acute asthma. Q J Med 44: 259–73, 1975.

25. Colp C: Sarcoidosis. Cause and treatment. Med Clin North Am 61: 1267–1278, 1977.

26. Cooke AR: Drugs and gastric damage. Drugs 11: 36–44, 1976.

27. Cooke NJ, Cameron SJ, Crompton GK, Grant IWB: Adrenal failure in bronchial asthma. Br Med J 4: 49, 1973.

28. Coombs RRA, Gell PAH: Classification of allergic reactions responsible for clinical hypersensitivity and disease. Clinical Aspects of Immunology, 3rd Edn, Gell PGH, Coombs RRA, Lachmann PJ (eds). Ch.25, pp. 761–781. Oxford: Blackwell, 1975.

29. Cooper EJ, Grant IWB: Beclomethasone dipropionate aerosol in treatment of chronic asthma. Q J Med 46: 295–308, 1977.

30. Coutts II, Jegarajah S, Stark JE: Tuberculosis in renal transplant recipients. Br J Dis Chest 73: 141–148, 1979.

31. Dale DC, Petersdorf RG: Corticosteroids and infectious diseases. in Steroid Therapy, Azarnoff DL (ed). Ch. 3, pp. 209–222, Philadelphia: Saunders, 1976.

32. David DS, Griece MH, Cushman P: Adrenal glucocorticoids after 20 years: a review of their clinically relevant consequences. J Chronic Dis 22: 637–711, 1970.

33. Deremee RA: The present status of treatment of pulmonary sarcoidosis: A house divided. Chest 71: 388–93, 1977.

34. Dreisin RR, Schwarz MI, Theofilopoulos AN, Stanford RE: Circulating immune complexes in the idiopathic interstitial pneumonias. N Engl J Med 298: 353–357, 1978.

35. Dujovne CA, Azarnoff DL: Clinical complications of corticosteroid therapy: A selected review. in Steroid Therapy. Azarnoff DL (ed). Ch. 3, pp. 27–41. Philadelphia: Saunders, 1976.

36. Edwards UM, Courtenay-Evans RJ, Galley JM, Hunter J, Tait AD: Changes in cortisol metabolism following rifampicin therapy. Lancet 2: 549–551, 1974.

37. Ellul-Micallef R, Fenech FF: Effect of intravenous prednisolone in asthmatics with diminished adrenergic responsiveness. Lancet 2: 1269–1271, 1975.

38. FAIRSHTER RD, WILSON AP: Paraquot poisoning. Manifestations and therapy. Am J Med 59: 751–753, 1975.

39. FAUCI AS, DALE DC: The effect of in vivo hydrocortisone on subpopulations of human lymphocytes. J Clin Invest 53: 240–246, 1974.

40. FAUCI AS, DALE DC: Alternate-day prednisone therapy and human lymphocyte subpopulations. J Clin Invest 55: 22–32, 1975.

41. FAUCI A, DALE DC, BALOW JE: Glucocorticosteroid therapy: mechanisms of action and clinical considerations. Ann Intern Med 84: 304–315, 1976.

42. FLEISCHER N, ABE K, LIDDLE GW, ORTH DN, NICHOLSON WE: ACTH antibodies in patients receiving depot porcine ACTH to hasten recovery from pituitary-adrenal supression. J Clin Invest 46: 196–204, 1967.

43. FRENKEL M: Blindness due to steroid induced glaucoma. Ill Med J 135: 160–163, 1969.

44. FRIEDMAN M, FLETCHER J, HINTON JM, LENNARD-JONES JE, MISIEWICZ JJ, PARRISH JA: Observations on the absorption of oral betamethasone 17- valerate and its therapeutic value in ulcerative colitis. Br Med J 1: 335–337, 1967.

45. GADDIE J, PETRIE GR, REED IW, SINCLAIR DJM, SKINNER C, PALMER KNV: Aerosol beclomethasone dipropionate: A dose-response study in chronic bronchial asthma. Lancet 2: 280–281, 1973.

46. GERMUTH FG, VALDES AJ, SENTERFIT LB, POLLACK AD: A unique influence of cortisone on transit of specific macromolecules across vascular walls in immune complex disease. Johns Hopkins Med J 122: 137–153, 1968.

47. GLASER GH: Psychotic reactions induced by corticotrophin (ACTH) and cortisone. Pychosomat Med 15: 280–291, 1953.

48. GODFREY S: Childhood asthma. in Asthma, Clark TJH, Godfrey S (eds). Ch. 17, pp. 324–366. London: Chapman and Hall, 1977.

49. GRABER AL, NEY RL, NICHOLSON WE, ISLAND DP, LIDDLE AW: Natural history of pituitary-adrenal recovery following long-term suppression with corticosteroids. J Clin Endocrinol Metab 25: 11–16, 1965.

50. GRAHAM GG, CHAMPION GD, DAY RD, PAULL PD: Patterns of plasma concentrations and urinary excretion of salicylate in rheumatoid arthritis. Clin Pharmacol Ther 22: 410–420, 1977.

51. HARDING SM, FREEDMAN S: A comparison of oral and inhaled steroids in patients with chronic airways obstruction: Features determining response. Thorax 33: 214–218, 1978.

52. HARTER JG, REDDY WJ, THORN GW: Studies on an intermittent corticosteroid dosage regimen. N Engl J Med 269: 591–596, 1963.

53. ISRAEL L, FOUTS DW, BEGGS RA: A controlled trial of prednisone treatment of sarcoidosis. Am Rev Resp Dis 107: 609–614, 1973.

54. JICK H, PORTER J: Drug-induced gastrointestinal bleeding. Lancet 2: 87–89, 1978.

55. JUBIZ W, MEIKLE AW: Alterations of glucocorticoid actions by other drugs and disease states. Drugs 18: 113–121, 1979.

56. KEHLET H, BINDER C: Value of an ACTH test in assessing hypothalmic-pituitary-adrenocortical function in glucocorticoid-treated patients. Br Med J 2: 147–149, 1973.

57. KLINENBERG JR, MILLER F: Effects of corticosteroids on blood salicylate concentration. JAMA 194: 601–604, 1965.

58. LEE HY, STRETTON TB: Asthma in the elderly. Br Med J 4: 93–95, 1972.

59. LEWIS GP, JUSKO WJ, BURKE CW, GRAVES L: Prednisone side effects and serum protein levels. Lancet 2: 778–781, 1971.

60. LIEBERMAN P, PATTERSON R, KUNSKE R: Complications of long-term steroid treatment for asthma. J Allergy Clin Immunol 49: 329, 1972.

61. LIVANOU T, FERRIMAN D, JAMES VHT: Recovery of hypothalamo-pituitary-adrenal function after corticosteroid therapy. Lancet 2: 856–859, 1967.

62. LOGSDON PJ, MIDDLETON E, COFFEE RG: Stimulation of leukocyte adrenyl cyclase by hydrocortisone and isoproterenol in asthmatic and non-asthmatic subjects. J Allergy Clin Immunol 50: 45–56, 1972.

63. LORENZEN I: The effects of glucocorticoids on connective tissue Acta Med Scand (Suppl 500): 17–21, 1969.

64. MABERLY DJ, GIBSON GJ, BUTLER AG: Recovery of adrenal function after substitution of beclomethasone dipropionate for oral corticosteroids. Br Med J 1: 778–782, 1973.

65. MCALLEN MK, KOCHANOWSKI SJ, SHAW KM: Steroid aerosols in asthma: an assessment of betamethasone valerate and a 12-month study of patients on maintenance treatment. Br Med J 1: 171–175, 1974.

66. MCCARTHY DS, PEPYS J: Allergic bronchopulmonary aspergillosis. Clinical immunology: (1) Clinical features; (2) Skin, nasal and bronchial tests. Clin Allergy 1: 261–286, 415–432, 1971.

67. MCCARTHY DS, PEPYS J: Cryptogenic pulmonary eosinophilia. Clin Allergy 3: 339–351, 1973.

68. MCCOMBS RP: Diseases due to immunologic reactions in the lungs. N Engl J Med 286: 1186–1194, 1245–1252, 1972.

69. MALO JL, HAWKINS R, PEPYS J: Studies in chronic bronchopulmonary aspergillosis. 1. Clinical and physiological findings. Thorax 32: 254–261, 1977.

70. MANGANIELLO V, VAUGHAN M: An effect of dexamethasone on adenosine 3', 5'-mono-phosphate content and adenosine 3', 5'-mono-phosphate phosphodiesterase activity of cultured hepatoma cells. J Clin Invest 51: 2763–2767, 1972.

71. MARTIN LE, TANNER RJN, CLARK TJH, COCHRANE GM: Absorption and metabolism of orally administered beclomethasone dipropionate. Clin Pharmacol Ther 15: 267–275, 1973.

72. MEIKLE AW, TYLER FH: Potency and duration of action of glucocorticoids. Effects of hydrocortisone, prednisone and dexamethasone on human pituitary-adrenal function. Am J Med 63: 200–207, 1977.

73. MELBY JC: Adrenocorticosteroids in medical emergencies. Med Clin North Am 45: 875–876, 1961.

74. MELBY JC: Systemic corticosteroid therapy: pharmacology and endocrinologic considerations. Ann Intern Med 81: 505–512, 1974.

75. MODELL JH, GRAVES SA, KETOVER A: Clinical cause of 91 consecutive near-drowning victims. Chest 70: 231–238, 1976.

76. MONCADA S, FERREIRA SH, VANE JR: Prostaglandins, aspirin-like drugs and the oedema of inflammation. Nature 246: 217–219, 1973.
77. MUE S, ISE T, SHIBAHARA S, TAKAHASHI M, ONO Y, TAKISHIMA T: Leucocyte cyclic 3', 5' - nucleotide phosphodiesterase activity in human bronchial asthma. Ann Allergy 37: 201–207, 1976.
78. MUNCK A, LEUNG K: Glucocorticoid receptors and mechanisms of action, in Receptors and Mechanisms of Action of Steroid Hormones, Part 2, Pasqualini J.R (ed). pp. 311–397. New York: Marcel Dekker, 1977.
79. MURRAY JF: The adult respiratory distress syndrome (may it rest in peace) Am Rev Resp Dis 111: 716–718, 1975.
80. NAKAGAWA H, FUKUHARA M, TSURUFUJU S: Effect of a single injection of betamethasone disodium phosphate on the synthesis of collagen and non-collagen protein of carrageenin granuloma in rats. Biochem Pharmacol 20: 2253–2261, 1971.
81. NELP WB: Acute pancreatitis associated with steroid therapy. Arch Intern Med 108: 702–710, 1961.
82. OLINER H, SCHWARTZ R, RUBIO F, DAMASHEK W: Interstitial pulmonary fibrosis following busulfan therapy. Am J Med 31: 134–139, 1961.
83. PARKER CW, SMITH JW: Alterations in cyclic adenosine mono-phosphate metabolism in human bronchial asthma. 1. Leucocyte responsiveness to β-adrenergic agents. J Clin Invest 52: 48–59, 1973.
84. PARKES WR: in Occupational Lung Disorders, Ch. 12, pp. 450–502, London: Butterworths, 1974.
85. PATTEN BM, OLIVER KL, ENGEL WK: Adverse interaction between steroid hormones and anticholinesterase drugs. Neurology 24: 442–449, 1974.
86. PEPYS J: Immunopathology of allergic lung disease. Clin Allergy 3: 1–22, 1973.
87. PERSELLIN RH, KU LC: Effects of steroid hormones on human polymorphonuclear leucocyte lysosomes. J Clin Invest 54: 919–925, 1974.
88. PETEREIT LB, MEIKLE AW: Effectiveness of prednisolone during phenytoin therapy. Clin Pharmacol Ther 22: 912–916, 1977.
89. PETTY TL, ASHBAUGH DG: The adult respiratory distress syndrome. Clinical features, factors influencing prognosis and principles of management. Chest 60: 233–239, 1971.
90. PRATT WB: The mechanism of glucocorticoid effects in fibroblasts. J Invest Dermatol 71: 24–35, 1978.
91. PROSKEY AJ, WEATHERBEE L, EASTERLING RE, GREENE JA, WELLER JM: Goodpasture's syndrome. A report of five cases and review of the literature. Am J Med 48: 162–173, 1970.
92. RAMER SJ, YU TY: Effect of corticosteroids on committed lymphocytes. Clin Exp Immunol 32: 545–553, 1978.
93. ROBIN ED, CROSS CE, ZELIS R: Pulmonary edema. N Engl J Med 288: 239–246, 292–304, 1973.
94. ROSCOE P, CHOO-KANG YFJ, HORNE NW: Betamethasone valerate in corticosteroid-dependent asthmatics. Br J Dis Chest 69: 240–246, 1975.
95. ROSE GA, SPENCER H. Polyarteritis nodosa. Q J Med 26: 43–81, 1957.
96. RYAN GB, MAJNO G: Acute inflammation. Am J Pathol 86: 185–276, 1977.

97. SADGHI-NEJAD A, SENIOR B: Adrenal function, growth, and insulin in patients treated with corticoids on alternate days. Pediatrics 43: 277–283, 1969.

98. SAHN SA, LAKSHMINARAYAN S: Tuberculosis after corticosteroid therapy. Br J Dis Chest 70: 195–205, 1976.

99. SALASSA RM, BENNETT WA, KEATING FR: Postoperative adrenal cortical insufficiency: occurrence in patients previously treated with cortisone. JAMA 152: 1509–1515, 1953.

100. SCADDING JG, HINSON KFW: Diffuse fibrosing alveolitis (diffuse interstitial fibrosis of the lungs). Thorax 22: 291–304, 1967.

101. SCHATZ M, PATTERSON R, KLONER R, FALK J: Prevalance of tuberculosis and positive tuberculin skin tests in a steroid-treated asthmatic population. Ann Intern Med 84: 261–265, 1976.

102. SMELLIE H, HOYLE C: The natural history of pulmonary sarcoidosis. Q J Med 29: 539–559, 1960.

103. STACK BHR, CHOO-KANG YFJ, HEARD BE: The prognosis of cryptogenic fibrosing alveolitis. Thorax 27: 535–542, 1972.

104. STERIOFF S, ORINGER MG, CAMERON JL: Colon perforation associated with steroid therapy. Surgery 75: 56–58, 1974.

105. STOECKLE JD, HARDY HL, WEBER AL: Chronic beryllium disease. Long-term follow-up of sixty cases and selective review of the literature. Am J Med 46: 545–561, 1969.

106. SWARTZ SL, DLUHY RG: Corticosteroids: Clinical pharmacology and therapeutic use. Drugs 16: 238–255, 1978.

107. SYMPOSIUM: Inflammation. Ann R Coll Surg Engl 60: 192–218, 1978.

108. THOMPSON EB, LIPPMAN ME: Mechanism of action of glucocorticoids. Metabolism 23: 159–202, 1974.

109. TURK JL: Mechanisms in delayed hypersensitivity. Ann R Coll Surg Engl 60: 207–211, 1978.

110. TURNER-WARWICK M: A perspective view on widespread pulmonary fibrosis. Br Med J 1: 371–376, 1974.

111. URIBE M, GO VLW: Corticosteroid pharmacokinetics in liver disease. Clin Pharmacokinet 4: 233–240, 1979.

112. VAN METRE TE, PINKERTON HL: Growth suppression in asthmatic children receiving prolonged therapy with prednisone and methylprednisolone. J Allergy Clin Immunol 30: 103–113, 1959.

113. WANG JLF, PATTERSON R, ROBERTS M, GHORY AC: The management of allergic bronchopulmonary asthma. Am Rev Resp Dis 120: 87–92, 1979.

114. WEBB J, CLARK TJH, CHILVERS C: Corticosteroid trials in patients with chronic airflow obstruction. Thorax 34: 419, 1979.

115. WEISSMANN G, THOMAS L: Studies on lysosomes. 2. The effect of cortisone on the release of acid hydrolases from a large granule fraction of rabbit liver induced by an excess of vitamin A. J Clin Invest 42: 661–669, 1963.

116. WESTON WL, CLAMAN HN, KRUEGER CG: Site of action of cortisol in cellular immunity. J Immunol 110: 880–883, 1973.

117. WHITCOMB ME, SCHWARZ MI, TORMEY DC: Methotrexate pneumonitis: case report and review of the literature. Thorax 27: 636–639, 1972.

118. WILSON JW: Treatment or prevention of pulmonary cellular damage with pharmacologic doses of corticosteroid. Surg Gynecol Obstet 134: 675–681, 1972.
119. WYATT R, WASCHEK J, WEINBERGER M, SHERMAN B: Effects of inhaled beclomethasone dipropionate and alternate-day prednisolone on pituitary-adrenal function in children with chronic asthma. N Engl J Med 299: 1387–1392, 1978.
120. WYNNE JW, MODELL JH: Respiratory aspiration of stomach contents. Ann Intern Med 87: 466–474, 1977.
121. YOUNG RL, HARKLEROAD LE, LORDON RE, WEG JG: Pulmonary sarcoidosis: a prospective evaluation of glucocorticoid therapy. Ann Intern Med 73: 207–212, 1970.
122. YU DTY, CLEMENTS PJ, PAULUS HE, PETER JB, LEVY J, BARNETT EV: Human lymphocyte subpopulations. Effect of coricosteroids. J Clin Invest 53: 565–571, 1974.
123. ZURIER RB, WEISSMANN G: Anti-immunologic and anti-inflammatory effects of steroid therapy. Med Clin North Am 57: 1295–1307, 1973.

9

Respiratory Failure

The primary function of the lungs is to maintain pulmonary gas exchange at a level which provides adequate tissue oxygenation at all times, and the simplest way of estimating the adequacy of pulmonary gas exchange is by blood gas measurements. Inability to maintain normal arterial blood gas tensions is the accepted criterion of respiratory failure, which in practice is usually taken to mean an arterial oxygen tension of less than 60 mm Hg (8.0 kPa) with or without an arterial carbon dioxide tension greater than 47 mm Hg (6.3 kPa). These abnormalities are clearly non-specific and can be produced by many different types of respiratory disturbance such as impaired control of ventilation (for example, in overdose with hypnotic drugs), disordered airway function (such as in acute bronchial asthma), and by increased right-to-left shunting (such as in shock lung). The treatment of acute respiratory failure therefore depends upon understanding and correcting its cause, and successful management may include a variety of specific measures such as physiotherapy, antibiotics, bronchodilators, corticosteroids, and diuretics, which together are intended to restore respiratory function to normal or at least to a condition of relative stability. While these therapeutic measures are taking effect it is usually necessary to maintain pulmonary gas exchange for a limited period by taking additional supportive steps, such as by administering oxygen or respiratory stimulants, by endotracheal intubation and bronchial lavage, or by resorting to controlled ventilation.

Two of these supportive measures come within the scope of this book: the use of oxygen and the administration of respiratory stimulant drugs in acute respiratory failure. The account is extended to include the applications of long-term oxygen therapy in chronic respiratory failure.

253

PATHOPHYSIOLOGY

In clinical practice hypoxaemia is caused by disturbance of ventilation/perfusion balance in the lungs or by overall ventilatory insufficiency. Both abnormalities lead to decreased alveolar gas exchange so that arterial oxygen tension begins to fall and arterial carbon dioxide tension to rise, stimulating an increase in total ventilation through the regulatory mechanisms of the respiratory centre which responds to chemoreceptor activity of the carotid bodies and to changes in the tension of carbon dioxide and the concentration of hydrogen ions in the region of the respiratory reticular formation of the medulla. Most patients with impaired alveolar gas exchange compensate for the abnormality by an increase in ventilation—initially on exertion but subsequently also at rest—so maintaining the arterial tensions of oxygen and carbon dioxide within the normal physiological range at the cost of increased ventilatory effort and diminished exercise tolerance. Further progression of the pathological disturbance to gas exchange may result in failure to maintain normal arterial blood gas tensions despite hyperventilation.

Acute Respiratory Failure

Ventilation/Perfusion Imbalance   In the absence of ventilatory insufficiency ventilation/perfusion imbalance leads to arterial hypoxaemia but with normal or low arterial carbon dioxide tension. The reason for this lies in the difference between the haemoglobin dissociation curves for oxygen and carbon dioxide depicted in Figure 9-1, which shows that the curve for carbon dioxide is steeper and straighter than that for oxygen, so that increased ventilation effectively "washes out" carbon dioxide from well-ventilated alveoli and compensates for the reduced excretion of carbon dioxide from poorly ventilated regions. In contrast, hyperventilation does not have a similar compensatory effect for hypoxaemia because it cannot increase the oxygen *content* of pulmonary capillary blood significantly, even in the well-ventilated regions of the lung, due to the flatness of the upper part of the haemoglobin dissociation curve for oxygen. Thus, unless there is complicating ventilatory insufficiency, hypoxaemia without hypercapnia is the typical finding in severe ventilation/perfusion imbalance of many causes, whether due to primary disturbance of pulmonary blood flow, unevenness of pulmonary ventilation, or a combination of the two (Table 9-1). In this context it is worth recalling that right-to-left shunt, whether due to a congenital cardiopulmonary defect or to perfusion of unventilated lung tissue, can be considered as an extreme case of ventilation/perfusion imbalance in which ventilation is zero, and it characteristically produces hypoxaemia without hypercapnia.

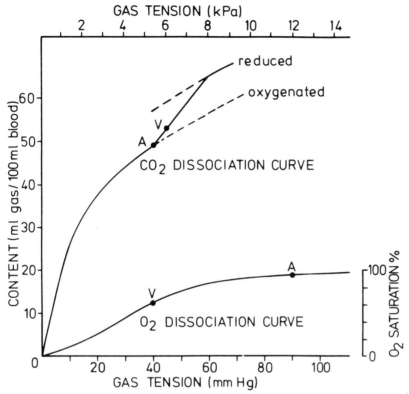

Figure 9-1   *The dissociation curves of blood for oxygen and carbon dioxide drawn on the same scale for comparison, assuming normal values for bicarbonate and haemoglobin concentration, illustrating the different shapes of the two curves. Since the amount of carbon dioxide that can be carried by the blood depends on the degree of reduction of haemoglobin, the "physiologic" carbon dioxide curve follows a course which lies between the curves for fully oxygenated and fully reduced haemoglobin. A and V mark the normal values for arterial and mixed venous blood, respectively. (From Clinical Physiology, 4th edition, edited by E.J.M. Campbell, C.J. Dickinson and J.D.H. Slater, 1974, Oxford: Blackwell; by permission).*

If there is no evidence of overall ventilatory insufficiency patients with acute respiratory failure due to ventilation/perfusion imbalance can usually be given oxygen freely without risk of developing hypercapnia. However this statement requires the important qualification that alveolar hypoventilation may develop during the course of the acute illness, or may have been present but unrecognised from the outset, so that close surveillance of oxygen therapy is always necessary in order to avoid the insidious development of hypercapnia.

Table 9-1 / Common Causes of Respiratory Failure

Pathophysiology	Clinical Examples
Ventilation/perfusion disturbance (hypoxaemia without hypercapnia)	Obstructive lung disease [such as acute asthma (mild to moderate severity), chronic obstructive pulmonary disease (COPD) in its early stages, kyphoscoliosis]
	Diffuse pulmonary fibrosis
	Shock lung
	Respiratory distress syndrome of the newborn
	Pulmonary thromboembolism
	Left ventricular failure
	Right-to-left cardiac or pulmonary shunt
Ventilatory insufficiency (hypoxaemia with hypercapnia)	Acute ventilatory obstruction (such as blocked airway, laryngeal spasm, sleep apnoea)
	Respiratory centre depression (such as brain stem lesion, hypnotic or sedative drugs, inappropriate O_2 therapy)
	Neuromuscular disorders (such as polyneuritis, myasthenia gravis, acute anterior poliomyelitis, tetanus)
	Thoracic cage injury, "flail chest"
	Obesity and the Pickwickian syndrome
Ventilatory insufficiency superimposed on ventilation/perfusion disturbance	Acute pulmonary infection superimposed on severe COPD
	Use of hypnotic or sedative drugs in COPD or asthma or kyphoscoliosis
	Incautious use of oxygen in severe asthma or COPD
	Mucous plugging and respiratory fatigue in severe asthma
	Atelectasis and failing compliance in shock lung

Ventilatory Insufficiency Ventilatory insufficiency affects the alveolar exchange of oxygen and carbon dioxide equally and leads to hypercapnia as well as hypoxaemia. Hypercapnic respiratory failure is seen in individuals with normal lungs whose ventilation is depressed by conditions such as overdosage with hypnotic drugs or neuromuscular disease affecting the respiratory muscles, but it occurs even more commonly in clinical practice when alveolar hypoventilation is aggravated by acute bronchial infection, injudicious sedation, or uncontrolled oxygen administration in patients with severe chronic obstructive pulmonary disease (Table 9-1). A typical instance of progressive respiratory failure of this sort sometimes occurs in a severe attack of asthma in which the initial ventilation/perfusion imbalance caused by widespread bronchospasm leads to arterial hypoxaemia with a low arterial carbon dioxide tension due to the patient's increased ventilatory efforts, but if bronchospasm is unrelieved the respiratory failure subsequently progresses to further hypoxaemia and hypercapnia as alveolar ventilation becomes increasingly jeopardised by mucous plugging of the airways and fatigue of the respiratory muscles.[73]

A rise in arterial carbon dioxide tension results in respiratory acidosis, which is compensated for by the excretion of an acid urine associated with a rise in bicarbonate concentration of the blood and an increase in the buffering capacity of blood and cerebrospinal fluid. Thereafter any further rise in carbon dioxide tension causes a smaller increase in hydrogen ion concentration and hence a smaller stimulus to respiration, leading to a progressive reduction in the responsiveness of the respiratory centre to increasing hypercapnia. The respiratory drive is then maintained by the stimulus of hypoxaemia to the peripheral chemoreceptors, and removal of this stimulus by the administration of oxygen in too high a concentration may aggravate the underlying hypoventilation and cause an additional rise in arterial carbon dioxide tension—which further depresses the respiratory centre. This unstable situation lies at the heart of the problem of treating hypercapnic respiratory failure with supplementary oxygen and necessitates the administration of oxygen in such a way as to improve tissue oxygenation without depressing ventilation sufficiently to cause intolerable hypercapnia.[14]

It has long been recognised that the withdrawal of supplementary oxygen from patients in acute hypercapnic respiratory failure may lead temporarily to a more intense degree of hypoxaemia than if oxygen had never been administered at all[25,55] and this has been variously attributed to persistent hypoventilation induced during the period of oxygen breathing or to the different storage capacity of the tissues for oxygen and carbon dioxide.[11] These explanations have been challenged on the basis of recent evidence obtained in admittedly stable respiratory failure patients, which suggests that the exacerbation of hypoxaemia is attributable to a change in ventilation/perfusion relationships induced by oxygen breathing.[74] Whatever its cause, this increase in hypoxia may be dangerous in seriously ill patients, and interruptions in oxygen administration for longer than a few minutes should be avoided.[13] If a trial of oxygen therapy, even at carefully controlled concentrations, leads to carbon dioxide narcosis, it is important not to withdraw the oxygen but to initiate other measures which will help to maintain ventilation, by either physically rousing the patient, using respiratory stimulant drugs, or resorting to mechanical ventilation.

Chronic Respiratory Failure

Patients with chronic obstructive pulmonary disease often tolerate moderate degrees of hypoxaemia and hypercapnia for long periods as a result of various adaptive mechanisms which help to maintain adequate tissue oxygenation, such as increased erythropoiesis and augmentation of cardiac output. Nevertheless gas exchange in such cases is often taking place on the steep part of the

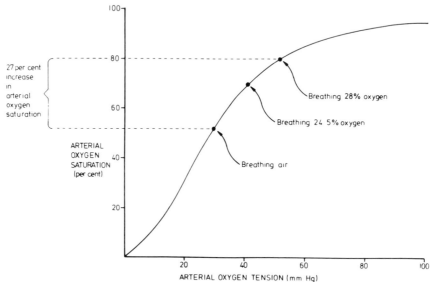

Figure 9-2 *The oxyhaemoglobin dissociation curve in respiratory failure. This diagram illustrates the relatively large increase in oxygen saturation of arterial blood which results from small increases in inspired oxygen concentration produced by breathing 24.5 percent and 28 percent oxygen instead of air in patients with severe hypoxaemic respiratory failure, whose gas exchange takes place on the steep part of the curve. Values for arterial oxygen tension are those given by Warrel et al.[82]*
The oxyhaemoglobin dissociation curve is derived from the charts published by Rahn and Fenn[67] assuming an arterial carbon dioxide tension of 64 mmHg, 8.53 kPa.

haemoglobin dissociation curve (Figure 9-2) where a small fall in oxygen tension due to a slight reduction in ventilation may lead to a relatively large fall in oxygen saturation. In addition, the respiratory centre in these patients is often relatively insensitive to a small rise in carbon dioxide tension so that any factor which adversely affects alveolar ventilation is likely to precipitate acute respiratory failure. Most commonly this arises from an infection such as acute bronchitis or pneumonia, but it may also follow the administration of a central depressant drug such as codeine given for cough or diarrhoea, a mild sedative such as diazepam, or a beta-blocking drug which may aggravate bronchospasm.

Patients in chronic respiratory failure may survive for many months or even years in this highly precarious state with periodic relapses into acute respiratory failure which recur with increasing frequency. Although chronic obstructive pulmonary disease is the commonest underlying pathology, chronic respiratory failure also develops at a late stage in emphysema and in widespread pulmonary fibrosis when mechanical factors eventually prevent adequate ventilation despite a well maintained respiratory drive, in severe ankylosing spondylitis and kyphoscoliosis, and in patients with slowly progressive neurological or muscular disorders who gradually develop ventilatory insufficiency.

Pulmonary Hypertension and Cor Pulmonale

Chronic hypoxaemia due to impaired pulmonary gas exchange has important effects on cardiac function which lead to the type of congestive cardiac failure known as cor pulmonale. In part these effects are due to hypoxia of cardiac muscle, affecting left as well as right ventricular function,[32] to an increase in cardiac output, and to impairment of renal function with a tendency to retain sodium. However it is the increase in pulmonary vascular resistance brought about by alveolar hypoxia which is the main cause of heart failure. In acute respiratory failure alveolar hypoventilation leads to transient pulmonary vasoconstriction which can be largely relieved by increasing the inspired oxygen concentration,[2] while chronic hypoxia causes hypertrophy of the smooth muscle of small pulmonary arterioles and contributes significantly to the development of pulmonary hypertension.[3] These vascular changes can be reversed in some patients with chronic obstructive lung disease by long-term treatment with supplementary oxygen.[1,52] There has also been some recent evidence to suggest that transient hypoxaemia occurring during sleep in some patients with chronic bronchitis and emphysema may contribute to the development of pulmonary hypertension.[8,29]

Although there is no doubt that pulmonary hypertension resulting from hypoxia is due to contraction of pulmonary vascular smooth muscle and conversely, that relief of hypoxia by oxygen administration leads to its relaxation, it is not at all clear what causes the hypoxic contraction. Bohr[6] argues that the trigger which turns on the contractile protein in the sarcoplasm is an increase in the intracellular concentration of ionised calcium, and that an excitatory process which causes an increase in membrane permeability to calcium may allow sufficient calcium influx to initiate a contraction. A number of observations support the view that hypoxic contraction of pulmonary vascular smooth muscle correlates with an increase in plasma membrane permeability to calcium,[40,56] and studies of the effect of hypoxia in other types of smooth muscle are consistent with this hypothesis.[17,27] It is suggested that an elevation in oxygen tension rapidly reverses the change in membrane permeability and leads to relaxation. Other possible mechanisms have been proposed to explain the pulmonary vascular effect of hypoxia, such as inhibition of oxidative phosphorylation which generates ATP, or a direct effect on the contractile protein itself. The involvement of various mediators in the process has been investigated, including histamine, serotonin, cyclic nucleotides and others, without as yet providing a satisfactory coherent explanation for the pulmonary vascular hypoxic response.[24]

Despite the current uncertainty about its precise mechanism of action, it is now widely accepted that oxygen is of practical value in the long-term treatment of pulmonary hypertension due to chronic respiratory failure,[65,77] in addition to its accustomed use for relieving tissue hypoxia in the acute illness.

OXYGEN

Availability of Oxygen

In hospitals oxygen is usually piped to the patient's bedside from a central bank of gas cylinders or a liquid oxygen reservoir, or is provided from a compressed gas cylinder at the bedside. Standard oxygen cylinders are available for home and hospital use in a wide range of sizes, varying in capacity from 75 to 6,907 litres in the United States and from 170 to 6,800 litres in Britain. For domiciliary supply on prescription in Britain the 1,360 litres cylinder (size F) is used, fitted with a contents gauge or pressure gauge, a reducing valve, and a flow meter. Lightweight portable oxygen cylinders can be used to allow the patient greater mobility for short periods, being recharged either from large gas cylinders (such as the Portogen [B.O.C., Britain]) or from liquid oxygen tanks (such as the Linde Walker [Union Carbide, United States]).

The alternative to compressed gas or liquid oxygen systems for domiciliary oxygen supplies are oxygen concentrators which use air as the source of ox-

ygen by separating molecular nitrogen from oxygen either with a semiperme-
able membrane or by using the principle of the molecular sieve. The one
membrane device available provides a fractional oxygen concentration of
approximately 40 percent and consequently requires a rather high flow of gas
to produce the necessary inspired oxygen concentration,[65] while the molecular
sieve devices provide oxygen fractions of 0.9 or slightly more at 2 l/min.[9,65]
Both can be run on domestic electricity and their use precludes the need for
maintaining a supply system for cylinders or liquid oxygen, except in the rare
instance of the patient who is totally dependent upon a continuous oxygen
supply, for whom a reserve system of compressed gas is required.

Methods of Oxygen Administration

A low concentration of inspired oxygen (24–30 percent) is required for patients
with carbon dioxide retention in whom removal of the hypoxic respiratory
drive may cause carbon dioxide narcosis, while for those whose respiratory
function is impaired by ventilation/perfusion imbalance without ventilatory
insufficiency, higher oxygen concentrations can be given (40–60 percent). The
choice of device depends primarily on the level and accuracy of the inspired
concentration required; ease of administration and the patient's comfort are
important but secondary considerations.

Predictable Administration of 24 Percent Oxygen   In patients with hypercapnic respiratory failure it is often necessary to start oxygen administration very
cautiously with a device which can be confidently relied on to provide an
inspired oxygen concentration of 24 percent. In my experience the only masks
which are sufficiently reliable for this purpose act on the Venturi principle,
whereby a jet of oxygen entrains air from holes around the oxygen inlet to
produce an inspired oxygen concentration which is constant and relatively
independent of the patient's rate or depth of breathing,[12,37] although some
variation between the actual and claimed performance occurs.[36] Carbon dioxide does not accumulate because of the high flow rate of air and oxygen
through the mask. A fixed performance Venturi mask providing 24 percent
oxygen is the preferred method of oxygen administration in this clinical situation, but has the disadvantages that it is sometimes poorly tolerated by the
patient because it is uncomfortable and it interferes with the vital activities of
coughing, drinking, and eating. It is therefore important to keep the patient
under observation to ensure that the mask is not surreptitiously removed.

Administration of 24–30 Percent Oxygen   For patients who can tolerate inspired oxygen concentrations slightly higher than 24 percent without develop-

ing carbon dioxide narcosis there is a wider range of equipment. Venturi-type masks are available as fixed performance devices—such as the Ventimask or Mix-o-Mask, providing 28 and 35 percent oxygen concentrations which are relatively independent of flow rate within a rage of 1–4 l/min—or alternatively as variable performance masks supplying an inspired oxygen concentration which can be altered by varying the oxygen flow rate—such as the "Edinburgh" mask which provides 25–29 percent oxygen at a flow rate of 1 l/min and 31–35 percent oxygen at a flow rate of 2 l/min but which is sensitive to changes in the patient's ventilation.[33] The latter type of mask is more comfortable to wear than the Ventimask, but it suffers from similar disadvantages because it covers the patient's nose and mouth, and its use may be more prone to error because the oxygen flow rate may be set incorrectly or changed inadvertently.

A better solution for these patients is to use a nasal cannula to provide an inspired oxygen concentration of about 30 percent, because of its much greater acceptability to the patient and the ease with which nursing procedures and physiotherapy can be carried out. The concentration of oxygen administered will vary by 2 or 3 percent about a mean of 30 percent if oxygen is given by nasal cannula at a flow rate of 2 l/min,[37] but in my experience it is not necessary to deliver 30 percent oxygen with the same degree of accuracy as it is when 24 percent oxygen is needed. The main discomfort of a nasal cannula comes from irritation of the anterior nares by the prongs which should have smooth round-ed ends, and by drying of the nasal mucosa. Mouth breathing may produce a 1–2 percent fall in the inspired oxygen concentration.[37]

The administration of oxygen by nasal cannula at flow rates of about 2 l/min has proved to be a practicable way of providing long-term domiciliary oxygen therapy for treating pulmonary hypertension and cor pulmonale in patients with chronic respiratory failure due to chronic obstructive pulmonary disease,[64,78] and it is effective when given for 15 hours per day or longer.[77] Such a regimen can be readily tolerated in the home, and it enables some patients to undertake regular work free from the constraints of an oxygen supply.

Higher Concentrations of Inspired Oxygen   Oxygen concentrations ranging up to 60–70 percent are required in situations of acute emergency when there is any form of anoxia and should be administered for a limited period without concern for the precise inspired oxygen concentration, but there are certain conditions of impaired ventilation/perfusion imbalance such as left ventricular failure and shock lung where high oxygen concentrations are needed for many hours. Variable performance masks are available in which the inspired oxygen concentration is determined by the oxygen flow rate and the patient's ventilation (such as the M.C. mask, the Hudson See-Thru mask, or the Polymask). During quiet breathing oxygen flow rates of 8–10 l/min will provide an inspired oxygen concentration of 60–80 percent, but if the patient is hyperventilating much higher flow rates of 25–30 l/min may be required to obtain this concentration of inspired oxygen.[18] At low flow rates significant rebreathing may occur with this type of mask and its use is obviously inappropriate in patients who are liable to develop hypercapnia.

There is probably little danger of causing oxygen toxicity (see below) by providing too high a level of inspired oxygen using a face mask in the conscious patient because it is difficult to achieve a sufficiently close fit for long enough to maintain a concentration higher than 60 percent, but it is easy to administer oxygen at less than the desired concentration unwittingly with a variable performance mask. It is also difficult to interpret the patient's response to treatment, or lack of it, if the inspired concentration of oxygen is uncertain.[51]

There are therefore good practical reasons for using a system of oxygen delivery which can be confidently expected to provide an inspired concentration at or close to the desired level; and if oxygen therapy in high concentrations has to be given for more than 2 or 3 hours, it is preferable to use a fixed performance mask working on the Venturi principle (for example, 40 percent and 60 percent Ventimasks) which are relatively independent of the patient's rate and pattern of breathing but require a higher flow rate of oxygen.[16]

Oxygen tents are now rarely used in the treatment of adults unless the patient is unable to tolerate a mask or nasal cannula. They have the disadvantage that they make nursing and observation difficult, represent an increased fire risk, and require high gas flows of up to 20 l/min to produce inspired oxygen concentrations of 40–50 percent which can only be maintained if the canopy is left undisturbed. The Venturi Head Tent[15] is a possible alternative, although patients find it uncomfortably warm and it has not achieved widespread use. Oxygen tents have a greater application in the management of acute lower respiratory tract infections in infants for whom an inspired oxygen concentration of 40 percent or more may be necessary to maintain a normal arterial oxygen tension.[76]

Adverse Effects of Oxygen Therapy

The most frequently encountered adverse effect of oxygen is its depressant action on the respiratory centre in hypercapnic respiratory failure, which has been discussed earlier in this chapter, and which can usually be avoided by careful administration of controlled oxygen therapy at inspired concentrations of between 24 and 30 percent according to the precepts of Campbell.[14] It is generally considered that the risks of oxygen toxicity are negligible at inspired concentrations of less than 50 percent even if given continuously for many hours or days,[23] but in principle the longer oxygen is administered and the higher its concentration the more likely is the occurrence of serious toxic effects on the lung and on certain other tissues; these factors impose severe limitations on its prolonged use at high concentrations.

Pulmonary Atelectasis   In alveoli which are perfused but very poorly venti-lated, the effect of breathing pure oxygen is to reduce expired ventilation in relation to inspired ventilation so that the alveoli take in less oxygen than is removed by their blood flow in the same period of time, leading to absorption atelectasis.[26] The tendency for such lung units to collapse increases the closer the inspired oxygen concentration approaches 100 percent, and is most likely to occur in diseased lungs where there is a greater degree of ventilation/perfusion imbalance. The effect of these changes is to increase the size of the arteriovenous shunt and aggravate the tendency toward hypoxaemia. The risk of absorption atelectasis may be reduced by maintaining a significant propor-tion of nitrogen in the inspired gas, and hence an inspired oxygen concentra-tion of 80 percent is the highest that should be used for more than a few hours. It is very difficult to achieve this level of inspired oxygen concentration for long using a face mask, and in practice absorption atelectasis is only likely to occur in patients who are being artificially ventilated.

Pulmonary Oxygen Toxicity   Prolonged exposure to oxygen at high concen-tration in patients on artificial ventilation leads to severe pathological lesions of the lung parenchyma. These consist of acute exudative lesions characterised by alveolar oedema, haemorrhages, and the formation of fibrinous hyaline membranes in the alveoli; and proliferative lesions which appear after longer exposure and take the form of interstitial tissue proliferation, hyperplasia of the alveolar lining cells, and desquamation of the cells lining the bronchioles and some alveoli.[61] Experimental studies in animals have shown that it is the oxygen tension in the structures of the gas exchanging regions of the lung which determines the development of toxic changes, rather than the level of oxygen in the arterial blood.[4]

The actual mechanism whereby oxygen produces these toxic effects in the lung is thought to be due to the formation of superoxide anion (O_2^-), a highly reactive free radical with cytotoxic actions which is also capable of further intracellular reactions to form singlet oxygen $(^1O_2)$ and the extremely toxic hydroxyl radical $(HO\cdot)$.[35,60] These short-lived oxygen metabolites have various cytotoxic effects which include the alteration of the structure of DNA, inactiva-tion of sulphydryl enzymes, and lipid peroxidation of cellular membranes with loss of membrane integrity. The normal defence mechanism against these destructive reactions is a system of antioxidant enzymes which serves to prevent free radical injury; these include superoxide dismutase, catalase, and glutathione peroxidase. This protective enzyme system seems to be adequate at tissue levels of oxygen which occur during air breathing and up to 40 percent oxygen breathing at normal atmospheric pressure, but begins to fail at higher oxygen concentrations.[80] There is considerable variation in individual susceptibility to oxygen toxicity but at present there is no method of identifying relative resistance to toxicity in individual patients, and no specific treatment is available to counter its effects.

Retrolental Fibroplasia   Retrolental fibroplasia is an abnormal proliferation of the vasculature of the immature retina following exposure to high tensions of oxygen which may resolve with time or progress to fibrosis and lead to partial or total blindness.[43] The initial phase of the process is constriction of developing retinal vessels with suppression of retinal vascularisation and destruction of endothelial cells. After removal from oxygen exposure, a disorganised vascular proliferation occurs from the remaining endothelial cells.[63] Susceptibility is highly variable, but the condition occurs most commonly in infants who weigh less than 1,500 g or who have a gestational age of less than 32 weeks at birth. Although it has been described mainly in premature infants requiring prolonged oxygen therapy because of cardiorespiratory disease it may also occur after exposure to hyperoxia for only 2 or 3 hours in infants receiving oxygen during the course of neonatal surgical procedures.[66]

Hyperbaric Oxygen Toxicity   The use of oxygen at high pressure is limited by the availability of hyperbaric chambers—which are very expensive in capital outlay and personnel—and by its toxicity. Pressures over 2.5 atmospheres are usually avoided because of the rapid onset of toxic effects, but even below this level gradual deterioration in lung function is observed, similar to that resulting from oxygen toxicity at atmospheric pressure but of earlier onset. The other important toxic effect of hyperbaric oxygen therapy is on the central nervous system,[28] causing paraesthesiae, muscle twitching, convulsions, and coma.

Clinical Uses

In developed countries oxygen is widely available for medical use in hospitals, clinics, and health centres, and it forms part of the basic resuscitative equipment of ambulancemen, first aid workers, hospital emergency teams, and other professional rescuers. It can be readily provided for domiciliary therapy although in many cases it is made use of in such a casual way that the benefit to be obtained from it seems unlikely to be commensurate with the cost of its supply.[44] As with all other drugs, oxygen should be administered with a definite purpose in mind and the effects of treatment should be evaluated as objectively as possible to determine whether this aim is being achieved, taking account of the patient's adherence to the regimen, the incidence of adverse effects, and the cost in deciding how long treatment should be continued. If critical criteria such as these are applied the indications for oxygen therapy in clinical cardiorespiratory problems can be limited to the following:

1. Maintenance of adequate tissue oxygenation during resuscitation in an acute emergency such as cardiac arrest, electrocution, haemorrhagic and traumatic shock, carbon monoxide poisoning, and near-drowning, using high concentrations of inspired oxygen.
2. Treatment of hypoxic respiratory failure in conditions such as pneumonia, bronchial asthma, left ventricular failure, shock lung, and respiratory disease of the newborn, using inspired oxygen concentrations of 40–60 percent but with adequate supervision against the possible development of hypercapnia.
3. Treatment of hypoxic and hypercapnic respiratory failure, which occurs most commonly in acute exacerbations of chronic obstructive pulmonary disease, but also in conditions such as hypnotic drug overdosage and neuromuscular disease affecting the respiratory muscles, using controlled inspired oxygen concentrations of 24–30 percent with stringent monitoring of blood gas tensions.
4. Long-term domiciliary oxygen therapy given for at least 15 hours per day by nasal cannula at a concentration of approximately 30 percent for treating pulmonary hypertension and cor pulmonale due to chronic respiratory failure.
5. Hyperbaric oxygen therapy has been advocated for a variety of conditions[48] and has a well-established place in the treatment of carbon monoxide poisoning and gas gangrene, and possibly as an adjuvant to radiotherapy in malignant disease.[47]

Other uses for oxygen therapy in chronic respiratory disease have been recommended,[34] but the indications are not clearly defined. Secondary polycythaemia due to chronic hypoxia can be alleviated by continuous oxygen therapy,[19] but this can probably be treated as effectively by venesection. Improvement in neuropsychiatric function has been described in patients with chronic obstructive pulmonary disease given continuous oxygen,[46] but more work is needed to establish the practical value of this therapeutic approach. Exercise intolerance can be improved in severely dyspnoeic patients with chronic obstructive pulmonary disease who develop arterial hypoxaemia on exertion,[50] and the provision of a wheeled oxygen supply may benefit these grossly incapacitated patients.

RESPIRATORY STIMULANTS

It has been stressed earlier in this chapter that the management of an episode of respiratory failure entails the maintenance of tissue oxygenation for long enough to allow specific therapeutic measures such as physiotherapy, antibiotics, or corticosteroids to rectify the immediate cause of the acute illness. This strategy is also applied in sustaining ventilation until the effects of respiratory depressant drugs have worn off, or until the patient has made a natural recovery from a neuromuscular disorder affecting respiration, such as polyneuritis. If the patient is unable to maintain adequate ventilation unaided, experience has shown that mechanical ventilation is the safest and most effective way of providing temporary respiratory support.

The only circumstances in which the respiratory physician hesitates to use mechanical means to sustain ventilation is when he fears that the patient has become too crippled to be weaned successfully from the respirator after the acute illness is over, or when the risks of intubation and mechanical ventilation appear to be excessive; this may be because the patient is too ill to withstand the manipulations and hazards involved in establishing mechanical ventilation, or because the available facilities are inadequate. In such situations respiratory stimulant drugs provide a possible alternative for maintaining gas exchange until the acute cause of respiratory failure has subsided.

With this end in view, analeptic agents have been used to stimulate respiration in two different ways. A non-specific CNS stimulant drug such as nikethamide has been used to arouse semi-comatose patients at intervals so that they can be persuaded to breathe deeply, cough, and expectorate secretions[22,57]; alternatively a stimulant such as doxapram, which is thought to have a more selective effect on the central and peripheral chemoreceptors, is sometimes used continuously with the object of providing sustained ventilatory stimulation over a period of hours or days.[42,70] There are considerable limitations to the value of respiratory stimulants used in this way because stimulation of ventilation of itself is unlikely to improve the underlying ventilation/perfusion imbalance, and the increase in muscular activity resulting from analeptic stimulation leads to an increase in oxygen consumption and carbon dioxide output which may offset any improvement in blood gas tensions resulting from the increased ventilation,[20,72] particularly if the work of breathing is increased by airway obstruction or the mechanical inefficiency of a hyperinflated chest.[69] For example, it is clear that respiratory stimulants should never be used in the treatment of asthma.

Apart from these theoretical limitations, all respiratory stimulants have a general stimulatory action on the entire central nervous system, and unwanted effects such as vomiting, bronchospasm, and convulsions are likely to occur at doses close to those needed to produce a significant increase in ventilation. Their use therefore requires constant vigilance to avoid serious or even lethal side-effects and this, combined with doubt of their clinical efficacy has led to the virtual abandonment of drugs such as dimefline, ethamivan, and prethcamide for the treatment of ventilatory failure.[5,54] Further discussion of respiratory stimulants is therefore restricted to nikethamide, which has a very limited place as a general analeptic in respiratory failure, and doxapram which appears to have a greater degree of respiratory selectivity and can be used with somewhat greater confidence, although it is no substitute for properly supervised controlled oxygen therapy, or for mechanical ventilation where this is possible.

Nikethamide

Nikethamide (N, N-diethylnicotinamide) is a non-specific analeptic which produces widespread excitation of the CNS. Respiratory stimulation may be due to excitation of the peripheral chemoreceptors or of the respiratory centre in the medulla,[41] and other medullary centres are also stimulated, producing increases in heart rate, blood pressure, and cardiac output. Its major action is cortical stimulation which can produce arousal in the therapeutic dose range, and in this respect it is of similar potency to doxapram and ethamivan.[84]

The drug is available as a 25 percent aqueous solution in sterile ampoules, and is administered intravenously by intermittent injections in a sufficient dose (usually 2–5 ml) to arouse the patient. This dose can then be repeated every 30 minutes, enabling verbal stimulation and physiotherapy to promote expectoration and improve ventilation in the severely hypercapnic, near-comatose patient.[22] It has also been administered by continuous intravenous infusion for a 15-minute period every 2 hours,[85] or for longer periods up to 2–3 hours,[30] but the risk of causing convulsions is much greater than with doxapram,[84] and in my view continuous infusion of nikethamide should be avoided.

In a comparative trial of several analeptic preparations,[84] the incidence of side-effects with nikethamide appeared to be high, but most of these were minor, consisting of coughing, sneezing, breath-holding, and itching. The most serious side-effects are bronchospasm, vomiting, and convulsions which may be lethal in the seriously hypoxic patient, and it must be recognised that adverse reactions are difficult to avoid altogether because of marked and unpredictable variations in individual sensitivity.

Nikethamide has only a very minor role as an arousal agent in the management of a limited group of acute respiratory failure patients who are unsuitable for treatment by mechanical ventilation. Doxapram is preferable because it has a wider margin of safety.

Doxapram

Doxapram (1-ethyl-4-(2-morpholinoethyl)-3, 3-diphenyl-2-pyrrolidinone) is a short-acting CNS stimulant which has been shown not only to have a direct effect on the respiratory centre but also to act on the peripheral chemoreceptors, both in animals[45,58] and in humans.[75] In normal subjects anaesthetised with thiopental, doxapram was shown to be by far the most powerful respiratory stimulant of all the analeptic agents studied, and to be one of the most effective in arousing patients from anaesthesia.[84] It appears on rather slender evidence to be more effective and less toxic than other analeptic agents.[31,84]

Administration   In acute respiratory failure doxapram is usually administered by prolonged intravenous infusion, but it has also been given as an intravenous bolus injection or as a short-duration infusion for post-operative respiratory depression associated with narcotic analgesia and for respiratory depression in the newborn. The drug is available as a sterile solution of doxapram hydrochloride in water containing 20 mg/ml, or as a solution containing 2 mg/ml in 5 percent dextrose for intravenous infusion (the latter preparation is not available in the United States). The usual dosage for the treatment of ventilatory depression in acute respiratory failure is 2–3 mg/min,[59,70] and a similar dosage schedule of 1.5–2.5 mg/min has been used for a prolonged 18-day infusion given to a patient with obesity and hypoventilation.[42] To hasten arousal after anaesthesia, a dose of 1 mg/kg body weight may be given as a bolus injection over a period of 1 minute.[38] Doxapram has also been used as a single injection in a dose of 0.5–3.0 mg/kg for the treatment of respiratory depression in the newborn.[39]

Clinical Pharmacology[71]   After a single injection of doxapram in a dose of 1.5 mg/kg body weight a mean peak concentration of 3 μg/ml was obtained in healthy subjects, falling rapidly in the first hour and then more slowly over the following 24 hours, suggesting that distribution is a major factor in lowering plasma concentration following an intravenous bolus or brief infusion. The plasma half-life was 2.5–4.5 hours during the phase of linear decline in log concentration which was observed 4–12 hours after the injection. Following intravenous infusion a steady-state plasma concentration is not reached for many hours with the usual constant rate infusion regimen. Doxapram is extensively metabolised, less than 5 percent being excreted unchanged in the urine during the first 24 hours.

Toxic Effects   Following intravenous injection unpleasant sensations may be experienced which include a metallic taste, light-headedness, warmth and "an alarming sensation of extreme perineal heat."[71] During infusions of doxapram nausea, vomiting, tremulousness, headache, and feelings of apprehension or agitation may occur.[79] In one patient hallucinations and frank psychosis were encountered.[59]

MANAGEMENT OF RESPIRATORY FAILURE IN CHRONIC OBSTRUCTIVE PULMONARY DISEASE

Treatment of Acute Hypercapnic Respiratory Failure

The most difficult form of respiratory failure is that which occurs in patients with chronic obstructive pulmonary disease who develop hypercapnia, and the physiological principles which form the basis of controlled oxygen therapy in this condition have been described in the classical papers by Campbell.[13,14] The essential steps in management are (1) to initiate specific treatment which will rectify the precipitating cause of respiratory failure; (2) to relieve dangerous hypoxia without causing excessive hypercapnia; and (3) to maintain ventilation in patients who become comatose during oxygen therapy.

Treatment of the Precipitating Cause   Most patients who present with acute hypercapnic respiratory failure have serious underlying lung disease such as bronchitis and emphysema, long-standing asthma, or gross kyphoscoliosis which is responsible for severe ventilation/perfusion imbalance but which is largely not amenable to correction. Superimposed on this is bronchial obstruction due to secretions, inflammatory exudate, impacted mucus, and bronchospasm—which has aggravated the ventilation/perfusion disturbance and added to alveolar hypoventilation; this is the usual precipitating cause of the acute illness, and it is this element in the pathogenesis of the respiratory failure which needs to be identified and treated.

In most cases infection plays an important part and the institution of treatment with the appropriate antibiotic in adequate dosage, usually parenterally, is an essential first step; ampicillin or trimethoprim-sulfamethoxazole (cotrimoxazole) are often chosen because they are effective against the two most common micro-organisms in this context, *Streptococcus pneumoniae* and *Haemophilus influenzae*. Physiotherapy is the next most important form of intervention, patients with bronchial infection requiring active encouragement by nursing or medical staff to cough and expectorate every 15 or 30 minutes during the first 24–36 hours of hospital care in order to improve ventilation.[13] Bronchodilators are essential in the severe asthmatic with an acute exacerbation but are less effective in those with chronic bronchitis and emphysema; nevertheless a bronchodilator such as aminophylline or salbutamol should always be given by intravenous infusion, and hydrocortisone should be added if the history suggests that there is an asthmatic element to the patient's illness. Inhaled aerosol bronchodilators are not as effective as intravenous preparations in the acute illness, presumably because they fail to penetrate the obstructed bronchial tree.[83]

Other corrective measures may be necessary in certain circumstances where the onset of respiratory failure can be attributed to a specific cause—for example, pleural intubation if there is a pneumothorax, or bronchial lavage when mucus plugging is obstructing the bronchial tree in the severe asthmatic. Fluid replacement is nearly always necessary in this type of patient because his breathlessness interferes with drinking and extra fluid is lost because of tachypnoea and sweating. Diuretics are necessary for the treatment of congestive heart failure particularly if impaired left ventricular function is a contributory factor.

Controlled Oxygen Administration   The first few hours of oxygen therapy for acute hypercapnic respiratory failure are critically important because it is all too easy to suppress the hypoxaemic ventilatory drive by administering oxygen in too high a concentration and so precipitate coma due to excessive hypercapnia. The first step is to obtain base-line blood gas measurements and to begin controlled oxygen therapy using a Venturi mask which provides 24 percent oxygen. This small increment in the inspired oxygen concentration is often sufficient to provide a substantial improvement in arterial oxygen saturation,[82] since in these seriously hypoxaemic patients oxygen uptake is occurring on the steep part of the hamoglobin dissociation curve (Figure 9-2). Campbell[14] estimates that increasing the inspired oxygen concentration by 4–7 percent increases the arterial oxygen saturation from 40–70 percent and may double the oxygen supply to the tissues. Although this increase in arterial oxygen tension will probably produce slight reduction of ventilation and some increase in hypercapnia which may cause some neurologic depression, the effect is usually not enough to cause serious narcosis; a rise in arterial carbon dioxide tension of up to 10 mm Hg (1.3 kPa) commonly occurs, but this is not in itself sufficient reason for resorting to other methods of maintaining ventilation, unless the patient becomes drowsy and unresponsive to physiotherapy. Serial measurements of arterial carbon dioxide tension are necessary at intervals of half an hour during the first 2 hours of oxygen therapy, and then at longer intervals as a new equilibrium becomes established, while frequent assessments of the patient's ability to cough and respond to questioning should be carried out to monitor the clinical response. Withdrawal of oxygen causes a profound exacerbation of hypoxaemia and uncooperative patients should therefore be kept under surveillance to ensure that the oxygen mask is not removed except briefly for drinking and expectoration.

In the critically ill patient it is a mistake to attempt to raise the arterial oxygen tension to some arbitrary "satisfactory" level, for example, greater than 50 mm Hg (6.3 kPa), since some patients will not tolerate so large an increment in oxygen tension without severe ventilatory depression. Instead, supplementary oxygen should be introduced simply by adding a small increment to the inspired oxygen concentration, and thereafter it is necessary to judge from the clinical response and blood carbon dioxide tension when further oxygen can be added. It is safest always to start with 24 percent oxygen although as a general rule moderately ill patients whose arterial carbon dioxide tension is below 50 mm Hg (6.7 kPa) at the outset of treatment can usually be started with 28 percent oxygen by Venturi mask or nasal cannula without aggravating carbon dioxide retention seriously. Attempts have been made to predict which patients are likely to tolerate oxygen therapy poorly,[7] but although it was shown that the best predictors of severe hypercapnia proved to be the initial arterial oxygen tension and pH values rather than arterial carbon dioxide tension, it was not possible to forecast the need for mechanical ventilation on this basis in the individual case.

Some clinicians have combined controlled oxygen therapy with the infusion of doxapram during the first few hours of treatment in an effort to prevent the suppressant effect of oxygen on ventilation. Although the rise in arterial carbon dioxide tension may be prevented or reduced in some patients,[70] the evidence suggests that the use of doxapram in this way fails to reduce the incidence of carbon dioxide narcosis.[59]

Treatment of Impending Carbon Dioxide Narcosis   If the patient fails to respond in spite of the treatment described above, the only methods available for maintaining adequate tissue oxygenation are by using respiratory stimulant drugs or by resorting to mechanical ventilation. Provided that there seems to be a reasonable chance that the acute ventilatory disturbance is remediable and that the blood gases can be re-established at a level which can subsequently be maintained by normal respiration, the most effective way of tiding the patient over the acute illness is by using a ventilator. Before ventilation is started endotracheal intubation and bronchial lavage may be carried out in an attempt to improve alveolar ventilation and arrest the deterioration.

Knowledge of the patient's previous state of health is an important factor in deciding whether mechanical ventilation is justifiable, and many clinicians reserve it for those who are well enough to be at work or to undertake equivalent activity before the onset of the acute illness which precipitated respiratory failure.[57] Nikethamide or doxapram are used when the case is unsuitable for mechanical ventilation because the patient's respiratory reserve is so reduced that the chances of ultimate recovery or independence are poor. Nikethamide can be given in this type of patient with reasonable safety, and some expectation of success, using 2–5 ml of 25 percent solution injected intravenously every 30 minutes. Each time the patient can be aroused and encouraged to cough and expectorate during the lucid interval.[22] Alternatively a bolus injection of doxapram can be administered in a similar way in a dose of 1–1.5 mg/kg body weight.

Long-term Oxygen in Chronic Respiratory Failure

Patients with chronic obstructive pulmonary disease who develop pulmonary hypertension and cor pulmonale have a poor prognosis, with a mortality of 73 percent within 4 years.[68] A comparable figure has been found in Britain.[81] Experimental studies in this type of patient have shown that pulmonary hypertension can be relieved by continuous oxygen therapy at low concentrations (30 percent) for 4 to 8 weeks,[1,52] and subsequent investigation has demonstrated that this effect can be obtained by administering oxygen by nasal cannula at a flow rate of 2 l/min for 15 hours daily,[78] a regimen which is compatible with a modified working day in some cases. The major benefits to be obtained from this type of therapy include a reduction in the amount of time spent by the patient in hospital[49]; a striking clinical improvement in terms of appetite, mood, and exercise tolerance[64]; and in a few cases a return to work.[78] Earlier results suggested that mortality was decreased in the first 2½ years among those who received continuous oxygen,[62] but subsequent follow-up has shown that long-term survival is poor in spite of oxygen therapy,[65] and lung function is not improved. Nevertheless, sufficient advantage can be gained by some patients to warrant 15-hour-per-day therapy in selected cases provided that they are hypoxaemic at rest (arterial oxygen tension less than 60 mm Hg, 8.0 kPa) and have had at least one episode of cor pulmonale.[9] There is little evidence that patients with hypoxaemia alone gain any benefit from continuous oxygen therapy,[53] but nocturnal oxygen therapy may have a place in the prevention of pulmonary hypertension and cor pulmonale in patients with chronic obstructive pulmonary disease who are shown to become hypoxaemic during sleep,[8] and it has been shown to be effective in a patient with primary alveolar hypoventilation.[10]

The organisation of long-term oxygen therapy even limited to 15 hours per day is a formidable and expensive exercise which may become easier with the introduction of oxygen concentrators currently being evaluated for domiciliary use.[9,21,65] Large-scale studies are needed to discover the most cost-effective way of providing domiciliary oxygen and to determine the criteria for prescribing this expensive form of treatment.

REFERENCES

1. ABRAHAM AS, COLE RB, BISHOP JM: Reversal of pulmonary hypertension by pro-longed oxygen administration. Circ Res 23: 147–157, 1968.
2. ABRAHAM AS, COLE RB, GREEN ID, HEDWORTH-WHITTY RB, CLARKE SW, BISHOP JM: Factors contributing to the reversible pulmonary hypertension of patients with acute respiratory failure studied by serial observations during recovery. Circ Res 24: 51–60, 1969.
3. ABRAHAM AS, KAY JM, COLE RB, PINCOCK AC: Haemodynamic and pathological study of the effect of chronic hypoxia and subsequent recovery of the heart and pulmonary vasculature of the rat. Cardiovasc Res 5: 95–102, 1971.
4. ASHBAUGH DG: Oxygen toxicity in normal and hypoxemic dogs. J Appl Physiol 31: 664–668, 1971.
5. BADER ME, BADER TA: Respiratory stimulants in obstructive lung disease. Am J Med 38: 165–171, 1965.
6. BOHR DF: The pulmonary hypoxic response. Chest 71: 244–246, 1977.
7. BONE RC, PIERCE AK, JOHNSON RL: Controlled oxygen administration in acute respiratory failure in chronic obstructive pulmonary disease: A reappraisal. Am J Med 65: 896–902, 1978.
8. BOYSEN PG, BLOCK AJ, WYNNE JW, HUNT LA, FLICK MR: Nocturnal pulmonary hypertension in patients with chronic obstructive pulmonary disease. Chest 76: 536–542, 1979.
9. BRITISH MEDICAL JOURNAL: Domiciliary oxygen. Br Med J 2: 77–78, 1977.
10. BUBIS MJ, ANTHONISEN NR: Primary alveolar hypoventilation treated by nocturnal administration of O_2. Am Rev Resp Dis 118: 947–953, 1978.
11. CAMPBELL EJM: Respiratory failure: the relation between oxygen concentrations of inspired air and arterial blood. Lancet 2: 10–11, 1960.
12. CAMPBELL EJM: A method of controlled oxygen administration which reduces the risk of carbon-dioxide retention. Lancet 2: 12–14, 1960.
13. CAMPBELL EJM: Respiratory failure. Br Med J 1: 1451–1460, 1965.
14. CAMPBELL EJM: The management of acute respiratory failure in chronic bronchitis and emphysema. Am Rev Resp Dis 96: 626–639, 1967.
15. CAMPBELL EJM, GEBBIE T: Masks and tent for providing controlled oxygen concentrations. Lancet 1: 468–469, 1966.
16. CAMPBELL EJM, MINTY KB: Controlled oxygen therapy at 60% Concentration: why and how. Lancet 1: 1199–1203, 1976.
17. CASTEELS R, RAEYMAEKERS L, GOFFIN J, WUYTACK F: A study of factors affecting the cellular calcium content of smooth muscle cells. Arch Int Pharmacodyn Ther 201: 191–192, 1973.
18. CATTERALL M, KAZANTZIS G, HODGES M: The performance of nasal catheters and a face mask in oxygen therapy. Lancet 1: 415–417, 1967.
19. CHAMBERLAIN DA, MILLARD FJC: The treatment of polycythaemia secondary to hypoxic lung disease by continuous oxygen administration Q J Med 32: 341–350, 1963.
20. CHERNIAK RM, YOUNG G: An evaluation of ethamivan as a respiratory stimulant in

barbiturate intoxication and alveolar hypoventilation in emphysema and obesity. Ann Intern Med 60: 631–640, 1964.

21. CHUSID EL, LIBROT M, UTZURRUM F, BICKERMAN HA: Treatment of hypoxemia with an oxygen enricher. Chest 76: 278–282, 1979.

22. CLARK TJH: Respiratory failure. Br J Hosp Med 7: 692–696, 1972.

23. CLARK JM, LAMBERTSON CJ: Pulmonary oxygen toxicity: A review. Pharmacol Rev 23: 37–133, 1971.

24. CONFERENCE: 19th Aspen Lung Conference: The pulmonary Circulation. Chest 71: 243–316, 1977.

25. CULLEN JH, KAEMMERLEN JT: Effect of oxygen administration at low rates of flow in hypercapnic patients. Am Rev Resp Dis 95: 116–120, 1967.

26. DANTZKER DR, WAGNER PD, WEST JB: Instability of lung units with low $\bar{V}A/\bar{Q}$ ratios during O_2 breathing. J Appl Physiol 38: 886–895, 1975.

27. DETAR R, BOHR DF: Contractile responses of isolated vacular smooth muscle during prolonged exposure to anoxia. Am J Physiol 222: 1269–1277, 1972.

28. DONALD KW: Oxygen poisoning in man. Br Med J 1: 712–717, 1947.

29. DOUGLAS NJ, CALVERLEY PMA, LEGGETT RJE, BRASH HM, FLENLEY DC, BREZINOVA V: Transient hypoxaemia during sleep in chronic bronchitis and emphysema. Lancet 1: 1–4, 1979.

30. DULFANO MJ, SEGAL MS: Nikethamide as a respiratory analeptic. JAMA 185: 69–74, 1963.

31. EDWARDS G, LESZCYZYNSKI SO: A double-blind trial of five respiratory stimulants in patients in acute ventilatory failure. Lancet 2: 226–229, 1967.

32. FISHMAN A: The left ventricle in "chronic bronchitis and emphysema". N Engl J Med 285: 402–404, 1971.

33. FLENLEY DC, HUTCHISON DCS, DONALD KW: Behaviour of apparatus for oxygen administration. Br Med J 2: 1081–1088, 1963.

34. FOX MJ, SNIDER GL: Respiratory therapy. Current practice in ambulatory patients with chronic airflow obstruction. JAMA 241: 937–940, 1979.

35. FRANK L, MASSARO D: The lung and oxygen toxicity. Arch Intern Med 139: 347–350, 1979.

36. FRIEDMAN SA, WEBER, B, BRISCOE WA, SMITH JP, KING TKC: Oxygen therapy: evaluation of various air-entraining masks. JAMA 228: 474–478, 1974.

37. GREEN ID: Choice of method for administration of oxygen. Br Med J 3: 593–596, 1967.

38. GUPTA PK, DUNDEE JW: Hastening of arousal after general anaesthesia with doxapram hydrochloride. Br J Anaesth 45: 493–496, 1973.

39. GUPTA PK, MOORE J: The use of doxapram in the newborn. J Obset Gynecol 80: 1002–1006, 1973.

40. HAACK DW, ABEL JH, JAENKE RS: Effects of hypoxia on the distribution of calcium in arterial smooth muscle cells of rats and swine. Cell Tiss Res 157: 125–140, 1975.

41. HAHN F: Analeptics. Pharmacol Rev 12: 447–530, 1960.

42. HOUSER WC, SCHLUETER DP: Prolonged doxapram infusion in obesity-hypoventilation syndrome. JAMA 239: 340–41, 1978.

43. JAMES LS, LANMAN JT: (eds): History of oxygen therapy and retrolental fibroplasia. Pediatrics 57 (Suppl): 591–642, 1976.

44. JONES MM, HARVEY JE, TATTERSFIELD AE: How patients use domiciliary oxygen. Br Med J 1: 1397–1400, 1978.

45. KATO H, BUCKLEY JP: Possible sites of action of the respiratory stimulant effect of doxapram hydrochloride. J Pharmacol Exp Ther 144: 260–264, 1964.

46. KROP HD, BLOCK AJ, COHEN E: Neuropyschiatric effects of continuous oxygen therapy in chronic obstructive pulmonary disease. Chest 64: 317–322, 1973.

47. KYLSTRA JA: Hyperbaric oxygen. in Advances in Respiratory Care and Physiology, Caldwell TB, Moya F (eds). Ch. 15, p. 162–167, Springfield Ill,: Charles C Thomas, 1973.

48. LEDINGHAM IM: Hyperbaric oxygen. in Recent Advances in Surgery, 7th Ed. Taylor S, (ed), Ch. 10, p. 295–338. London: J. and A. Churchill, 1969.

49. LEGGETT RJ, COOKE NJ, CLANCY L, LEITCH AG, KIRBY BJ, FLENLEY DC: Long-term domiciliary oxygen therapy in cor pulmonale complicating chronic bronchitis and emphysema. Thorax 31: 414–418, 1976.

50. LEGGETT RJE, FLENLEY DC: Portable oxygen and exercise tolerance in patients with chronic hypoxic cor pulmonale. Br Med J 2: 84–86, 1977.

51. LEIGH JM: Ideas and anomalies in the evolution of modern oxygen therapy. Anaesthesia 29: 335–348, 1974.

52. LEVINE BE, BIGELOW DB, HAMSTRA RD, BECKWITT HJ, MITCHELL RS, NETT LM, STEPHEN TA, PETTY TL: The role of long-term continuous oxygen administration in patients with chronic airway obstruction with hypoxemia. Ann Intern Med 66: 639–650, 1967.

53. LILKER ES, KARNICK A, LERNER L: Portable oxygen in chronic obstructive lung disease with hypoxemia and cor pulmonale. A controlled double-blind crossover study. Chest 68: 236–241, 1975.

54. MARK LC: Analeptics: changing concepts, declining status. Am J Med Sci 254: 296–302, 1967.

55. MASSARO DJ, KATZ S, LUCHSINGER PC: Effect of various modes of O_2 administration on the arterial gas values in patients with respiratory acidosis. Br Med J 2: 627–629, 1962.

56. McMURTRY IF, DAVIDSON AB, REEVES JT, GROVER RF: Inhibition of hypoxic pulmonary vasoconstriction by calcium antagonists in isolated rat lungs. Circ Res 38: 99–104, 1976.

57. McNICOL MW: The management of respiratory failure. Hosp Med 1: 601–610, 1967.

58. MITCHELL RA, HERBERT DA: Potencies of doxapram and hypoxia in stimulating carotid-body chemoreceptors and ventilation in anaesthetised cats. Anasthesiology 42: 559–566, 1975.

59. MOSER KM, LUCHSINGER PC, ADAMSON JS, McMAHON SM, SCHLUETER DP, SPIVACK M, WEG JG: Respiratory stimulation with intravenous doxapram in respiratory failure: A double-blind co-operative study. N Engl J Med 288: 427–431, 1973.

60. MUSTAFA MG, TIERNEY DF: Biochemical and metabolic changes in the lung with oxygen, ozone and nitrogen dioxide toxicity. Am Rev Resp Dis 188: 1061–1090, 1978.

61. Nash G, Blennerhassett JB, Pontoppidan H: Pulmonary lesions associated with oxygen therapy and artificial ventilation. N Engl J Med 276: 368–374, 1967.

62. Neff TA, Petty TL: Long-term continuous oxygen therapy in chronic airway obstruction. Ann Intern Med 72: 621–626, 1970.

63. Patz A: The effect of oxygen on immature retinal vessels. Invest Ophthalmol 4: 988–999, 1965.

64. Petty TL, Finigan MM: Clinical evaluation of prolonged ambulatory oxygen therapy in chronic airway obstruction. Am J Med 45: 242–252, 1968.

65. Petty TL, Neff TA, Creagh CE, Sutton FD, Nett LM, Bailey D, Fernandez E: Outpatient oxygen therapy in chronic obstructive pulmonary disease. A review of 13 years' experience and an evaluation of modes of therapy. Arch Intern Med 139: 28–32, 1979.

66. Phibbs RH: Oxygen therapy: A continuing hazard to the premature infant. Anesthesiology 47: 486–487, 1977.

67. Rahn H, Fenn WO: A graphical analysis of the respiratory gas exchange. The O_2-CO_2 diagram. Washington, D.C.: American Physiological Society, 1955.

68. Renzetti AD, McClement JH, Litt BD: The Veterans Administration co-operative study of pulmonary function. III. Mortality in relation to respiratory function in chronic obstructive pulmonary disease. Am J Med 41: 115–129, 1966.

69. Riley RL: The work of breathing and its relation to respiratory acidosis. Ann Intern Med 41: 172–176, 1954.

70. Riordan JF, Sillett RW, McNicol MW: A controlled trial of doxapram in acute respiratory failure. Br J Dis Chest 69: 57–62, 1975.

71. Robson RH, Prescott LF: A pharmacokinetic study of doxapram in patients and volunteers. Br J Clin Pharmacol 7: 81–87, 1978.

72. Rodman T, Fennelly JF, Kraft AJ, Close HP: Effect of ethamivan on alveolar ventilation in patients with chronic lung disease. N Engl J Med 267: 1279–1285, 1962.

73. Roussos CS, Macklem PT: Diaphragmatic fatigue in man. J Appl Physiol 43: 189–197, 1977.

74. Rudolf M, Turner JAM, Harrison BDW, Riordan JF, Saunders KB: Changes in arterial blood gases during and after a period of oxygen breathing in patients with chronic hypercapnic respiratory failure and in patients with asthma. Clin Sci 57: 389–396, 1979.

75. Scott RM, Whitwam JG, Chakrabarti MK: Evidence of a role for the peripheral chemoreceptors in the ventilatory response to doxapram in man. Br J Anaesth 49: 227–231, 1977.

76. Simpson H, Flenley DC: Arterial blood-gas tensions and pH in acute lower-respiratory tract infections in infancy and childhood. Lancet 1: 7–12, 1967.

77. Stark RD, Finnegan P, Bishop JM: Daily requirement of oxygen to reverse pulmonary hypertension in patients with chronic bronchitis. Br Med J 3: 724–728, 1972.

78. Stark RD, Finnegan P, Bishop JM: Long-term domiciliary oxygen in chronic bronchitis with pulmonary hypertension. Br Med J 3: 467–470, 1973.

79. Steele AD, Rodman R: The effect of a new analeptic agent on arterial blood gases and minute ventilation in adult males. Am Rev Resp Dis 94: 600–607, 1966.

80. TIERNEY DF, AYERS L, KASUYAMA RS: Altered sensitivity to oxygen toxicity. Am Rev Resp Dis 115 (Suppl 2): 59–65, 1977.
81. UDE AC, HOWARD P: Controlled oxygen therapy and pulmonary heart failure. Thorax 26: 572–578, 1971.
82. WARRELL DA, EDWARDS RHT, GODFREY S, JONES NL: Effect of controlled oxygen therapy on arterial blood gases in acute respiratory failure. Br Med J 2: 452–455, 1970.
83. WILLIAMS S, SEATON A: Intravenous or inhaled salbutamol in severe acute asthamma? Thorax 32: 555–558, 1977.
84. WINNIE AP: Chemical respirogenesis: a comparative study. Acta Anaesthesiol (Suppl 51): 1–32, 1973.
85. WOOLF CR: The use of "respiratory stimulant" drugs. Chest 58: 49–53, 1970.

10

Anticoagulant and Thrombolytic Agents

There must be few clinicians who have not at some time felt distressed and frustrated by the unexpected death due to pulmonary embolism of a patient who was recovering from some other illness or surgical operation and whose long-term prognosis appeared to be excellent. Dalen and Alpert[23] have estimated that pulmonary embolism is the third commonest cause of death in the United States, leading to 200,000 deaths per annum, in about half of which it is the sole cause. The same authors have calculated that the total number of symptomatic episodes of pulmonary embolism per year is 630,000, making the disease about half as common as acute myocardial infarction and 3 times as common as strokes. It is widely accepted that the treatment of symptomatic pulmonary embolism with antithrombotic drugs prevents recurrence and reduces mortality,[8] and it is also established that prophylactic administration of anticoagulants can prevent venous thrombosis and pulmonary embolism in high risk patients,[19,65] although the criteria for selecting patients and choosing a regimen for this type of preventive therapy are still a matter for debate.[146]

By its very nature antithrombotic therapy carries a high risk of serious unwanted effects due to bleeding, and the aim of this chapter is to describe the mode of action and pharmacological characteristics of anticoagulant and thrombolytic drugs so that they may be used to greatest effect in the treatment and prevention of pulmonary embolism.

PATHOGENESIS AND NATURAL HISTORY OF PULMONARY EMBOLISM

There are very few clear-cut answers to the questions which worry the clinician contemplating treatment with antithrombotic drugs for a patient at risk from deep venous thrombosis or pulmonary embolism: for example, when should thrombolytic therapy be employed in preference to anticoagulants? Which type of patient is likely to benefit from prophylactic therapy with low-dose heparin? How long should anticoagulant therapy be continued? In the present state of knowledge many of the questions have to be answered empirically on the basis of our understanding of the pathogenesis and natural history of the disease.

Venous Thrombosis

The venous thrombi from which most pulmonary emboli originate begin to form in the veins of the calf and thigh and they may extend forward by propagation and backward after venous obstruction. About three-fourths of major pulmonary emboli come from the iliofemoral segment,[82] although some may originate from the veins of the calf[16] or less frequently from the pelvic veins, the vessels of the arms, and the right side of the heart. The precise mechanism which initiates the formation of venous thrombi is unknown, but three factors are thought to have an important influence:

1. Structural changes in the vessel wall.
2. Decreased venous blood flow.
3. Increased coagulability of the blood.

Current theories of how these factors may interact in the genesis of venous thrombosis are reviewed by Morris and Mitchell.[91]

Changes in the Vessel Wall Experiments *in vitro* have shown that platelets aggregate when exposed to constituents of the vessel wall which lie beneath the endothelium, such as collagen, basement membrane, and microfibrils,[94] and in the process of aggregation various substances are released which may further promote platelet adhesion and thrombus formation. It has therefore been suggested that vessel wall injury provides a starting-point for the accumulation of platelets which form the "head" of a thrombus. Conventional histological studies have failed to show any change in the vessel wall in association with venous thrombosis in humans,[104] but some studies in experimental animals suggest that ultramicroscopic changes in blood vessels due to vasodilatation[131] or to leucocyte migration through the vessel wall[127] might allow platelets to reach subendothelial tissues through gaps in the endothelium which are not visible by light microscopy. Nevertheless, current experience suggests that substances which impede the aggregation of platelets such as aspirin and dipyridamole are not very effective in preventing venous thrombosis,[92,119,139] possibly because platelets only play a minor role in the genesis of venous thrombi.

Decreased Blood Flow   Thrombosis can be produced in isolated venous segments in animals following injection with substances such as autologous serum,[144] thrombin, or activated factor X,[148] suggesting that stasis combined with a trigger mechanism may initiate thrombosis. However, the blood clots so formed do not have the characteristic features of *in vivo* thrombi, suggesting that these experiments may not be relevant to the natural origination of venous thrombosis in human disease. The main reason for supposing that venous stasis is important comes from clinical and post mortem observations which demonstrate a correlation between deep venous thrombosis and clinical states characterised by diminished venous blood flow. Such evidence shows the following:

1. The incidence of venous thrombosis is high among people who are immobilised by injury.[122]
2. Known predisposing factors to deep venous thrombosis such as surgical operations are associated with diminished venous flow in the legs.[96]
3. The frequency of venous thrombosis in patients immobilised by surgical operations or bedrest can be reduced by mechanical and electrical methods of stimulating venous blood flow.[30]

Altered Blood Coagulability   Certain conditions which are known to cause changes in blood coagulation mechanisms also predispose to venous thrombosis. They include *surgical operations and injury* which lead to an increase in platelet count and platelet adhesiveness,[153] enhanced platelet aggregation,[34] raised fibrinogen and factor VIII levels,[3] and alterations in fibrinolytic activity[58]; *pregnancy and the puerperium* which are associated with raised platelet counts and increased platelet adhesiveness,[153] with an increase in fibrinogen and factors VII, VIII, and X and depression of fibrinolytic activity[55]; the use of *oral contraceptive agents* containing oestrogens which produce similar changes in coagulation factors[32,109]; and *malignant disease* which is sometimes associated with raised factor VIII levels, accelerated *in vitro* coagulation tests, and elevated platelet counts.[3,17,73]

According to current concepts, venous thrombosis is triggered by an undefined mechanism which may sometimes be related to local injury or inflamma-

Table 10-1 / Conditions Predisposing to Venous Thromboembolism

Immobilisation
Increasing age
Surgical operations, trauma or burns
Pregnancy and parturition
Oral contraceptive therapy
Obesity
Varicose veins
Previous venous thromboembolism
Heart disease, notably congestive cardiac failure and atrial fibrillation
Cancer, especially pancreas, stomach, and lung

tion causing platelet adhesion, or to hypercoagulability of the blood. Evolution of the incipient thrombus is influenced by local blood flow, being greatly enhanced by venous stasis. This simple picture of the beginnings of venous thrombus formation, although incomplete, provides a model which helps to explain why certain conditions predispose to venous thromboembolic disease.

Conditions Predisposing to Venous Thrombosis   These are listed in Table 10-1 from which it can be inferred that in any individual several predisposing factors may coexist and can therefore be presumed to have an additive effect in increasing the liability to deep venous thrombosis and embolism. In some high risk groups such as elderly patients who have suffered a hip fracture and who are thus subject to the combined predisposing factors of age, injury, often a surgical operation, and immobilisation, a highly significant reduction in the incidence of pulmonary embolism has been demonstrated by the use of prophylactic anticoagulation.[90,121] On the other hand, in many medical patients in whom a high risk of venous thrombosis can be presumed because of a similar combination of predisposing factors there are no specific studies to show the value of antithrombotic prophylaxis in reducing mortality or morbidity, and a decision whether or not to give prophylactic treatment to such patients depends on an empirical assessment of the risk factors weighed against the possibility of haemorrhagic complications.

Evolution of Pulmonary Embolism

Studies using ^{125}I-fibrinogen and phlebography in surgical patients have shown that the majority of thrombi begin in the calf veins,[66] possibly starting from small aggregations of platelets and fibrin which form in areas of turbulence or silting behind the cusps of venous valves.[57] Whatever the initiating process, there appears to be some degree of platelet-fibrin deposition at the head of the thrombus where it is attached to the vein wall[103]; but the major part of the thrombus consists of a "tail" of blood cells and platelets intermeshed with fibrin strands which often floats freely in the lumen and is liable to propagate proximally along the deep veins without necessarily obstructing venous flow completely. Many such thrombi undergo spontaneous lysis,[66] and only about 20 percent extend into the popliteal, femoral, and iliac veins which constitute the source of the great majority of pulmonary emboli.

Death has been estimated to occur in 11 percent of all cases of pulmonary embolism within 1 hour,[23] in many without premonitory signs of minor emboli or clinical evidence of deep venous thrombosis. Survival of the acute pulmonary arterial obstruction is often followed by clinical improvement as the embolus fragments and re-embolises to more peripheral parts of the lungs where the cross-sectional area of the pulmonary vascular bed is greater. Some patients may remain in a highly critical state for several hours before succumbing to the effects of circulatory obstruction, which is often aggravated by further embolism, and it is this group of patients which is most likely to benefit from early thrombolytic therapy. Survival after the first few hours is followed by resolution of the emboli due to physiological fibrinolysis, and studies in untreated animals have shown that there is striking clearance of emboli from the pulmonary circulation occurring from a few hours to a week after the acute episode.[145] Serial angiographic studies of patients treated with heparin and/or venous ligation showed slight evidence of resolution after 7 days which became more apparent during the following 2 weeks although haemodynamic and angiographic abnormalities were found to persist in some patients for many weeks longer.[24] Similar rates of resolution were shown with serial lung scans, two-thirds of the patients studied having improved or returned to normal within 4 months, irrespective of the severity of the initial embolism.[130]

Long-term follow-up of patients who have survived massive pulmonary embolism for up to 9 years has shown that the eventual prognosis is good, none of the patients studied having evidence of pulmonary hypertension and only 6 percent experiencing a possible non-fatal recurrence.[47] Chronic thromboembolic pulmonary hypertension is a rare complication of recurrent pulmonary embolism, but it is preventable by giving long-term prophylactic anticoagulant therapy to patients who have repeated episodes.[28]

It is important to appreciate that pulmonary emboli are commonly multiple, the main objective of anticoagulant therapy being to prevent the propagation of new thrombus, which may be a source of recurrent embolism, while allowing time for natural fibrinolysis of thrombus which is already causing circulatory obstruction. Thrombolytic agents have the additional theoretical advantage of increasing the rate of dissolution of thrombi in patients whose haemodynamic status is critically balanced in the first few hours after acute embolism.[41]

Mechanisms of Coagulation and Fibrinolysis

Anticoagulants and thrombolytic agents exert their therapeutic effects by interfering with the normal blood coagulation mechanism and fibrinolytic enzyme system, which are described below.

Coagulation Mechanisms   Blood coagulation occurs by two pathways in
which activation of specific plasma proteins starts a cascade of reactions which
eventually lead to the deposition of an insoluble fibrin clot: The first pathway
(intrinsic system) begins with injury to the endothelium, exposing collagen or
other subintimal components which activate factor XII. Activated factor XII
activates factor XI, which in turn activates factor IX. Together with Ca^{++}, a
platelet phospholipid and a cofactor (factor VIII), activated factor IX then activates factor X.

In the second pathway (extrinsic system) tissue injury leads to the release
of tissue thromboplastin which reacts with factor VII to activate factor X directly. Once it is formed by either pathway, activated factor X in association with
factor V and platelet phospholipid transforms prothrombin to thrombin. Finally
thrombin converts fibrinogen to fibrin which polymerises to form a clot (Figure
10-1).

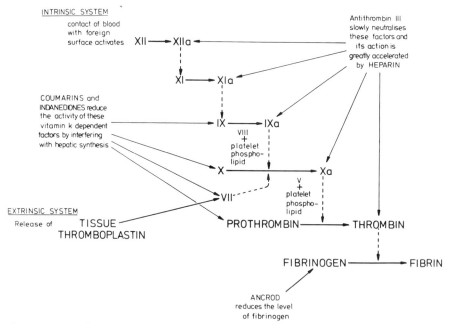

Figure 10-1   *The coagulation mechanisms, showing the sites of action of anticoagulant drugs.*

Antithrombin III, an α_2-globulin, is a naturally occurring inhibitor of several activated clotting factors, which all have a reactive serine residue at their enzymatically active centre, namely XIIa, XIa, IXa, Xa, and thrombin. Antithrombin III slowly and progressively inactivates these activated clotting factors by forming stable inhibitor-enzyme complexes; but in the presence of heparin, inactivation is almost instantaneous.[115] The oral anticoagulants—coumarins and indanediones—exert their effect by interfering with the hepatic synthesis of factors IX, X, VII, and prothrombin, which is dependent on vitamin K. Ancrod is a defibrinating enzyme derived from snake venom that produces its anticoagulant effect by converting fibrinogen into an unstable form of fibrin which is then promptly removed from the circulation.

Physiological Fibrinolysis The fibrinolytic enzyme system depends on the enzyme plasmin, which digests fibrin and fibrin products (Figure 10-2). Body fluids which contain fibrinogen, the precursor of fibrin, also contain plasminogen, the precursor of plasmin. Plasminogen is converted to plasmin by the action of enzymes which are widespread in body fluids and tissues, known as plasminogen activators.

Plasmin is a rather non-specific protease which is capable of digesting many different proteins, an action which is prevented in plasma by the presence of an excess of antiplasmins, particularly α_2-antiplasmin. The rather specific *in vivo* activity of plasmin against fibrin is due to the fact that the

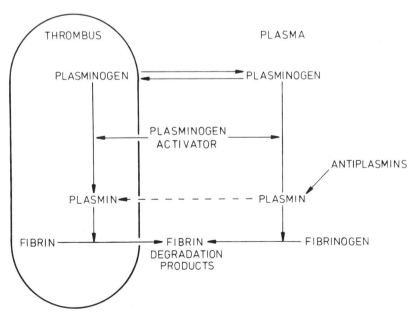

Figure 10-2 *The fibrinolytic enzyme system.*

generation of plasmin takes place within the fibrin clot because both plasmin-ogen and plasminogen activators have a very high affinity for fibrin and are adsorbed onto the fibrin surface. Thus the biological specificity of plasmin for fibrin is conferred by the activator's site of action,[151] so that plasmin formed within the clot digests fibrin, while plasmin formed in plasma is neutralised by antiplasmins.

The thrombolytic agents which have been used most successfully in the treatment of venous thrombosis and pulmonary embolism are both plasmin-ogen activators: streptokinase and urokinase. Other agents have been shown to increase the amount of plasma activator and produce a minor stimulus to fibrinolysis which might have a role in the prophylaxis of deep venous thrombosis[138]; they include the combination of a biguanide (phenformin) with an anabolic steroid (ethyloestrenol), and another anabolic steroid (stanozolol) given alone. Further work is needed to determine whether this form of oral prophylactic thrombolytic therapy, which is safe and requires no laboratory control, is of clinical value.

Summary

This brief survey of the pathogenesis of venous thromboembolism shows that pulmonary emboli commonly arise from thrombi lying in the femoral and iliac veins and emphasises that the current objectives of antithrombotic therapy are largely preventive ones, such as the following:

1. Prophylaxis against venous thrombosis in predisposed individuals.
2. Prevention of the propagation of thrombus which has already formed.
3. Prevention of repeated pulmonary embolism in patients who survive the first episode.

Drugs which interfere with platelet aggregation (antiplatelet agents) have a possible role in prophylaxis, although their effectiveness against venous throm-bosis has yet to be established.[19,93,139] The anticoagulant drugs, particularly heparin and the vitamin K antagonists, are widely used both in prophylaxis and in the treatment of established deep-vein thrombosis and pulmonary em-bolism, while thrombolytic agents are at present mainly reserved for the early treatment of serious pulmonary embolism when rapid dissolution of the ob-structing thrombus is considered to be essential.

ANTICOAGULANTS

Heparin

Heparin is a complex mixture of sulphated mucopolysaccharides with molecu-lar weights ranging from 4,000 to 30,000 daltons; it is found in many different animal tissues. The commercially available product is extracted from bovine lung tissue or from the intestinal mucosa of pigs and cattle. The properties of heparin and its clinical use are reviewed in detail by Gallus and Hirsh,[38] and by Wessler and Gitel.[147]

Mode of Action Heparin exerts its anticoagulant action by accelerating the rate at which the α_2-globulin antithrombin III neutralises the actions of several activated clotting factors which take part in the normal sequence of coagulation, notably factors Xa and thrombin but also XIIa, XIa, and IXa (Figure 10-1). Thus it inhibits the intrinsic clotting system and also the common pathway, which lead to the formation of fibrin. It appears to act as a catalyst either by binding reversibly to antithrombin III and producing a conformational change in the inhibitor, which greatly increases its reactivity toward its substrates,[115] or by binding reversibly to thrombin and thereby increasing the reactivity of thrombin to antithrombin III, or by a combination of these processes.

To achieve effective anticoagulation, higher dosage of heparin must be given for the treatment of established venous thrombosis than is needed for prophylactic therapy, because thrombin, once formed, accelerates its own production through its aggregating effect on platelets, which leads to the liberation of phospholipid (platelet factor 3), so facilitating the coagulation cascade mechanism.[64] The success of prophylactic low-dose heparin depends on the prompt neutralisation of factor Xa, which is generated in increased amounts following surgical operations, thus preventing the formation of thrombin and the augmentation of the coagulation mechanism.[48]

Clinical Pharmacokinetics Heparin is not absorbed from the gastrointestinal tract and must therefore be given by parenteral injection. It exerts its anticoagulant effect immediately. The biological half-life in normals appears to be $1\frac{1}{2}$–2 hours,[36] but considerable variations have been reported which seem to depend partly on the methods of measurement[83] and partly on the dose, the half-life being increased when larger doses are used. It is also altered by certain clinical conditions: for instance, pulmonary embolism (but not venous thrombosis alone) decreases it significantly,[54,124] while different investigators have observed varying effects on half-life patients with impaired renal or hepatic function.[146] Heparin does not cross the placenta and is not secreted in milk.

Administration and Dosage Most heparin is used in the form of the sodium salt, although calcium heparin is also available. Neither preparation appears to have any particular advantage. It is prescribed on a unit basis and is available in the United States as Heparin Sodium Injection U.S.P. in solutions containing varying strengths ranging from 200–40,000 U.S.P. units/ml. In Britain it is available as Heparin Injection B.P. in multidose 5 ml vials containing 1,000, 5,000, or 25,000 International Units (IU)/ml or in single-dosage ampoules containing 5,000 IU/0.2 ml for low-dose prophylactic use. For the treatment of established venous thrombosis or pulmonary embolism, heparin is administered intravenously, either by intermittent injection or continuous infusion; both dextrose-in-water solution or normal saline can be used as diluents without significant loss of activity over 48 hours.[87] For prophylactic therapy, it is given subcutaneously in concentrated aqueous solution containing 5,000 units in 0.2 ml; great care must be taken to avoid local bleeding due to the trauma of the injection. Administration of heparin by inhaling a nebulised aerosol has been described,[61] but its clinical usefulness has yet to be established.

For the treatment of *established venous thrombosis* heparin is started with a loading dose of 5,000 units by bolus injection and is continued with a maintenance dose of 30,000–40,000 units/24 hours, either by intermittent injection or by continuous infusion. If it is given by continuous infusion, heparin should be administered using a constant rate infusion pump to avoid fluctuations in dosage, and it requires careful nursing and laboratory surveillance. The activated partial thromboplastin time (APTT)[128] or the clotting time (CT)[72] should be measured before treatment is started, again 6 hours after the initial bolus injection and thereafter at daily intervals, the dose of heparin being adjusted to keep the APTT between 1½–2 times the control value or the CT between 25 and 30 minutes. For patients who are at greater risk of bleeding such as those with hepatic or renal disease, or in the immediate post-operative period, the initial loading dose and maintenance dose should be halved and the APTT or CT measured more often, with the aim of keeping them at the lower end of the therapeutic range. Although spontaneous haemorrhage is rare during the first 48 hours of therapy using the above dosage schedule,[79] it then becomes a real risk which can be aggravated by antiplatelet drugs such as aspirin, by surgical procedures, and by minor trauma. It is therefore advisable to reduce the dose of heparin to 20,000–25,000 units/day after the first 48 hours of therapy. Heparin therapy should be given for at least 7 days.[147]

Intermittent intravenous therapy should be given every 4 hours, either in a standard dosage of 5,000 units or by regulating dosage according to daily measurements of CT in order to reduce the risk of bleeding,[150] the aim being to keep the CT between 25 and 30 minutes when measured 15–30 minutes before the next heparin dose. The APTT does not seem to be very helpful in controlling intermittent intravenous heparin therapy.[79,117] On the basis of present evidence, it is difficult to say whether intermittent or continuous therapy is more likely to cause bleeding, and it must be appreciated that either technique will cause haemorrhagic complications in a proportion of patients.

There is no firm agreement about the dosage of heparin to be used in *acute pulmonary embolism* but it is common practice to use about 40,000 units of heparin per 24 hours as described above. For massive embolism some authorities recommend an initial loading dose of 15,000 units of heparin[85] followed by as much as 100,000 units over the first 24 hours, in order to antagonise possible serotonin-induced pulmonary vasoconstrictor and bronchoconstrictor effects,[21] rather than primarily for its anticoagulant effect. The significance of the serotonin-mediated effects is controversial,[88,112] and in the absence of guidance from clinical trials these large dose schedules should only be used for patients in shock, and should be reduced to the usual dose range within 12–24 hours.

When heparin is used in the *prophylaxis of venous thrombosis,* it is given subcutaneously in a dose of 5,000 units every 8 or 12 hours. In an International Multicentre Trial,[59] 5,000 units of heparin were administered 2 hours before surgery and 8-hourly after surgery for at least 7 days, but it is not known whether a twice-daily or thrice-daily regimen is preferable, since both appear to be equally effective in most patients. Judging from the absence of serious bleeding complications in clinical trials of low-dose heparin, it appears to be unnecessary to monitor this type of treatment with laboratory tests.[39,56]

Unwanted Effects   The commonest unwanted effect of heparin therapy is bleeding, which may sometimes be catastophic.[75] Spontaneous bleeding may even occur when the CT or APTT are within the therapeutic range, especially in elderly women,[62,141] in patients with an underlying haemostatic defect,[107] or in the early post-operative period.[9] It is not unusual for patients to have a gradual fall in haematocrit over several days without any definite site of bleeding being revealed. Other unwanted effects include the following:

1. Thrombocytopenia, an uncommon occurrence[111] which may be due to the production of heparin-dependent antiplatelet antibodies.[132] When heparin therapy is discontinued the platelet count returns to normal within a few days.[42]
2. Osteoporosis, which is said to occur in patients receiving heparin for more than 6 months in high dosage.[43]
3. Hypersensitivity reactions, including acute anaphylaxis.[11,22]
4. Arterial thrombosis and skin necrosis.[149]

Because of the possibility of thrombocytopenia it is prudent to monitor the platelet count in patients receiving heparin.

Drug Interactions   The addition of erythromycin, cephaloridine, gentamicin, kanamycin, or tetracyclines to solutions of heparin in sodium chloride or dextrose produces cloudiness or visible precipitation,[60] and it is better avoided, although the clinical significance of this observation is unknown.

Inhibitors of platelet function such as aspirin should be avoided during heparin therapy because they enhance the risk of bleeding. It is also important to enquire into the use of aspirin-containing preparations during the 5 days prior to starting prophylactic low-dose heparin therapy, since they can increase the likelihood of postoperative bleeding.[154]

Neutralisation of Heparin   The anticoagulant effect of heparin can be rapidly neutralised with intravenous protamine sulphate. The appropriate dose of protamine depends on the dose of heparin, 1 mg of protamine being sufficient to neutralise about 100 units of heparin. Because of the rapid clearance of heparin from the circulation, only half this dose is needed if 1 hour has elapsed since the heparin was administered, and only a quarter after two hours. After subcutaneous heparin, protamine sulphate should be given in a dose equivalent to half of the last heparin dose.

Oral Anticoagulants

There are two groups of oral anticoagulants, the coumarin and indanedione compounds. Warfarin sodium is by far the most extensively used of the coumarin group which also includes phenprocoumon, ethyl biscoumacetate, and bishydroxycoumarin. Of the indanediones, phenindione has had the widest use, but it has been largely superseded by warfarin because of its liability to cause hypersensitivity reactions. The chemical structure of these oral anticoagulants is illustrated in Figure 10-3. The main differences between individual compounds lies in their pharmacokinetic properties and in the patterns of unwanted effects; this account is limited mainly to the properties of warfarin sodium.

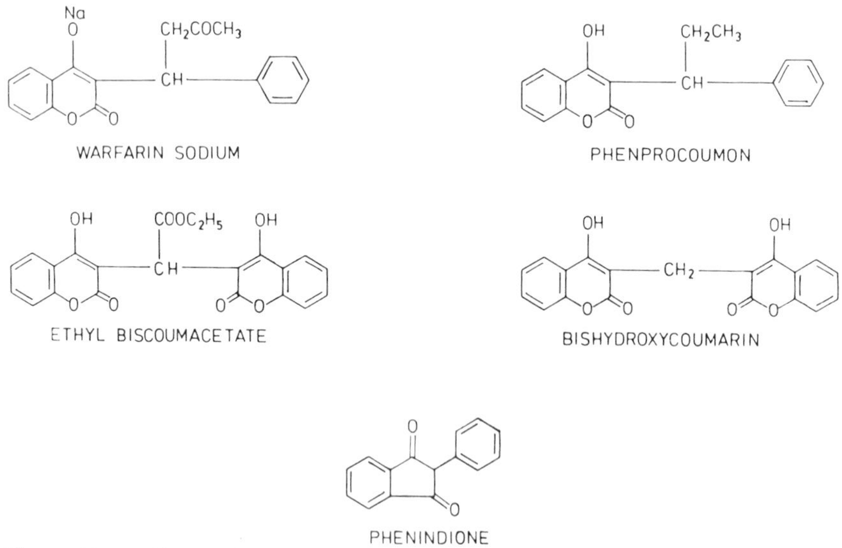

WARFARIN SODIUM

PHENPROCOUMON

ETHYL BISCOUMACETATE

BISHYDROXYCOUMARIN

PHENINDIONE

Figure 10-3   *Chemical structure of some oral anticoagulants.*

Mode of Action   Fat-soluble vitamin K is present in the diet and is also synthesized by Gram-positive intestinal bacteria. It is essential for the hepatic synthesis and release of clotting factors II, VII, IX, and X (see Figure 10-1), but their synthesis is interfered with by the oral anticoagulants which cause the production of biologically inactive forms of these proteins.[35] The anticoagulant effect of these drugs is delayed until the level of the normal clotting factors has been reduced by metabolism, usually from 18–72 hours after administration of an oral loading dose.

Clinical Pharmacokinetics   With the exception of bishydroxycoumarin, the oral anticoagulants are well absorbed from the gastrointestinal tract. They are 90–99 percent bound to plasma albumin and are mainly metabolised by hydroxylation in the liver to inactive compounds which are excreted in the urine.[71] Oral anticoagulants cross the placenta and are secreted into milk. Because of the extensive protein-binding only a small fraction of these drugs is pharmacologically active or available for metabolism and excretion at any time, but a small change in the concentration of unbound drug due to displacement from the protein binding site by another agent will lead temporarily to an augmentation of the anticoagulant effect until a new equilibrium is established. In effect the plasma proteins act as a reservoir for bound drug which is gradually released as the concentration of free drug is lowered by biotransformation, the high level of albumin-binding being an important factor in the prolonged half-life of oral anticoagulants (Table 10-2). Because of their long plasma half-life, some of the coumarins show only a slow change in steady-state concentration after an adjustment to the maintenance dose; for example, after a change in the dose of warfarin it takes 6 days to complete 90 percent and 12 days to complete 99 percent of the change to a new steady-state plasma concentration.[71]

Warfarin (and also phenprocoumon) contains an asymmetric carbon atom and is therefore optically active. The two enantiomers (R and S forms) have different pharmacokinetic properties because their metabolic pathways differ[12]; and they also differ in their anticoagulant potential, S warfarin being about 4 times as potent as R warfarin. Commercial warfarin is a racemic mixture of the two forms and some drug interactions with warfarin have a stereo-chemical basis, notably that of phenylbutazone which inhibits the rate of metabolism of the more potent S isomer and may thereby help to potentiate the anticoagulant effect.[74] A stereospecific interaction also occurs between metronidazole and racemic or S warfarin (but not R warfarin) leading to prolongation of the prothrombin time.[98]

Administration and Dosage   Warfarin sodium U.S.P. is available in tablets containing 2, 2.5, 5, 7.5, 10, and 25 mg of the drug and also as a preparation for injection. Warfarin tablets B.P. are available in 1, 3, 5, and 10 mg tablets. Oral anticoagulant therapy is usually started with a modest loading dose of 10

Table 10-2 / Pharmacokinetics and Usual Dose Requirements of Some Oral Anticoagulants

	Percentage Bound to Plasma Protein	Plasma Half-Life (hours)	Gastrointestinal Tract Absorption	Usual Dosage Initial Dosage (mg)	Usual Dosage Daily Maintenance (mg)
COUMARINS					
Warfarin sodium	97	44	rapid and complete	10 daily for the first 3 days	1–15
Phenprocoumon	99	150	complete	21 on first day 9 on second day	0.75–4.5
Ethyl biscoumacetate	90	2	rapid and complete	1200 daily in divided doses for the first 2 days	150–900
Bishydroxycoumarin (Dicumarol)	99	24	slow and variable	300 on first day 200 on second day	25–150
INDANEDIONE					
Phenindione	unknown	5	rapid and complete	200 on first day 100 on second day	25–150

mg on 3 successive days to avoid a possible increased risk of haemorrhage which may arise if a single large initial loading dose is used.[99] Thereafter a daily maintenance dose is given, based on measurements of the one-stage prothrombin time (PT) which are made daily initially, and then at longer intervals, as the patient's maintenance dose is stabilised, to produce a PT of between 2 and 2½ times the normal control value. Alternatively, the Thrombotest[102] may be used to measure anticoagulant control, maintaining it between 8 and 15 percent of the control value. There is wide individual variation in the dose of warfarin required to achieve appropriate anticoagulation, the maintenance dose usually lying somewhere between 1 mg and 15 mg daily. The usual loading and maintenance dose requirements for other oral anticoagulants are shown in Table 10-2.

Unwanted Effects   The most important undesirable effect of oral anticoagulant therapy is bleeding, most commonly presenting in the form of microscopic haematuria which is often overlooked or disregarded but which may be associated with an underlying urinary tract infection or neoplasm. Apart from this, the cause of bleeding when tht PT is in the therapeutic range is usually surgical or related to other trauma, or sometimes is related to an unsuspected peptic ulcer. Bleeding may occur spontaneously and from more than one site when the PT is seriously prolonged due to overdosage.

If bleeding occurs and neutralisation of the anticoagulant effect seems necessary the specific antidote is vitamin K_1, which is best given intravenously in a dose of 10–20 mg by slow injection at a rate of 5 mg/min. It will probably restore the PT to a safe level within 6–12 hours.

Other important side-effects of the oral anticoagulants are the following:

1. Hypersensitivity reactions[31] which occur most commonly with phenindione and include rashes, fever, leucopenia, hepatitis, nephropathy, and diarrhoea. They tend to occur within a few days but may arise as late as 6 weeks after starting therapy and they can affect as much as 3 percent of patients treated with phenindione.
2. Skin necrosis, often symmetrically distributed and affecting the breast or the lower limbs, is a rare complication of coumarin therapy, particularly with bishydroxycoumarin and phenprocoumon.[95] It may be due to a vasculitis.
3. A red discolouration of the urine due to indanediones. This is important clinically because it may be confused with haematuria.
4. A saddle-nose deformity may occur in the infants of mothers treated with warfarin during the first 3 months of pregnancy.[106]

Drug Interactions   It is of the greatest importance for clinicians to be aware of the interactions which other drugs may have with the oral anticoagulants since the control of anticoagulation may be profoundly affected (for reviews see references 71 and 77). Other drugs may affect the action of the oral anticoagulants in a number of different ways (Table 10-3):

1. Alteration in the absorption of coumarins, particularly the effect of tricyclic antidepressants which increase the absorption of bishydroxy-coumarin, and of cholestyramine which reduces warfarin absorption.
2. Displacement of anticoagulants from the albumin binding site, leading to a transient increase in the concentration of unbound, pharmacologically active drug. This is an important cause of drug interaction with phenylbutazone and possibly chloral hydrate.
3. Alteration in the rate of anticoagulant metabolism due to enzyme induction by drugs such as barbiturates, glutethimide, dichloralphenazone and rifampin, which increase it; or due to enzyme inhibition by drugs such as phenylbutazone, phenyramidol, and chloramphenicol which reduce it.[71] The rate of elimination of bishydroxycoumarin, but not warfarin, is also decreased by allopurinol in some individuals.[110]
4. Reduction in the absorption of vitamin K and thereby potentiation of anticoagulant effect. Although a drug such as cholestyramine, which binds bile salts and therefore interferes with fat absorption, is potentially capable of affecting the absorption of fat soluble vitamin K, this type of interaction seems to be of little clinical significance. However, in surgical patients a combination of reduced dietary intake of vitamin K plus treatment with a broad-spectrum antibiotic (such as neomycin, tetracycline) may cause prolongation of the PT or even spontaneous bleeding,[5] and it should be considered as a possible cause of anticoagulation instability in severely malnourished individuals.[133]
5. Production of a combined defect in haemostasis by drugs such as aspirin which impair platelet function and increase the likelihood of haemorrhage.

It is important to appreciate that the untoward effects of the drugs which alter the pharmacokinetics of oral anticoagulants are most likely to occur when a *change* is made in the dosage of the interacting drug. For example a patient taking regular barbiturates for nocturnal sedation may be satisfactorily stabilised on warfarin until the barbiturate is discontinued, whereupon there will be a prolongation of PT due to the removal of the enzyme inducing effect of the barbiturate. Accordingly, when any drug therapy is initiated or discontinued in a patient on anticoagulant medication, careful laboratory control should follow the change, and the anticoagulant dosage should be adjusted appropriately.

Clinical Use   The oral anticoagulants, mainly warfarin sodium, are commonly used in respiratory medicine to maintain anticoagulation in ambulant patients

Table 10-3 / Some Important Drug Interactions With the Oral Anticoagulants

Mechanism of Interaction	Anticoagulant Drug	Interacting Drug	Effect of Anticoagulation	References
Altered coumarin pharmacokinetics				
(i) Increased absorption	Bishydroxycoumarin	Tricyclic antidepressants	Potentiation	140
(ii) Decreased absorption	Coumarins	Cholestyramine	Inhibition	37
(iii) Displacement from albumin binding sites	Coumarins	Phenylbutazone Oxyphenbutazone (?) Chloral hydrate Triclofos Clofibrate	Transient potentiation	1, 44, 120
(iv) Increased rate of metabolism due to enzyme induction	Coumarins	Barbiturates Glutethimide Dichloralphenazone Rifampin Phenytoin Carbamazepine	Inhibition	76, 114, 116
(v) Decreased rate of metabolism due to enzyme inhibition	Bishydroxycoumarin Coumarins	Allopurinol Metronidazole Phenylbutazone Dextropropoxyphene Phenyramidol Chloramphenicol	Potentiation	18, 74, 98, 100, 110
Decreased vitamin K absorption	Coumarins and indanediones	Broad-spectrum antibiotics, (for example, neomycin, tetracyclines)	Potentiation if there is associated malnutrition	133
Combined defect in haemostasis	Coumarins and indanediones	Aspirin	Potentiation	126
(?) Increased metabolism of clotting factors	Coumarins	D-thyroxine	Potentiation	71

who have suffered deep venous thrombosis or pulmonary embolism. Treatment with warfarin is usually initiated while the patient is already anticoagulated with heparin, which has been given to achieve a rapid effect in the acute stages of the illness, and is continued on an out-patient basis for a period of 2–4 months or until reversible causative factors such as injury or immobilisation have been corrected. Patients with recurrent pulmonary emboli may be maintained on warfarin anticoagulation indefinitely in order to prevent chronic thromboembolic pulmonary hypertension.

Oral anticoagulant therapy with warfarin or phenindione is the only method of prophylactic therapy which has been shown beyond reasonable doubt to prevent venous thrombosis and fatal pulmonary embolism even in high risk groups such as elderly patients with hip fracture.[93] But this form of prophylaxis is relatively unpopular because of the risk of bleeding during surgical procedures and the need for regular laboratory supervision of anticoagulation control. The place of oral anticoagulant drugs in the prevention and management of venous thromboembolic disease, and the practical problems of managing oral anticoagulant therapy effectively are discussed in the final section of this chapter.

Ancrod

Ancrod is the partially purified fraction of the venom of the Malayan pit viper. It acts by converting plasma fibrinogen into an unstable form of fibrin which is susceptible to fibrinolysis and is rapidly removed from the circulation, leading to hypofibrinogenaemia.[108] After intravenous injection the plasma half-life of ancrod is 3–5 hours.

Administration and Dosage   The drug is normally infused intravenously, initially in a dose of 2–3 unit/kg body weight over 6–8 hours and then 2 unit/kg every 12 hours to produce a sustained hypofibrinogenaemia of approximately 50 mg/100 ml.[7]

Unwanted Effects   As with all anticoagulants the major side-effect of ancrod is bleeding, but this appears to be uncommon even when hypofibrinogenaemia is marked.[123] If bleeding occurs it is often sufficient simply to stop administration of the drug; but if it is excessive, antivenom should be given to neutralise ancrod, and the fibrinogen level should be restored by an infusion of reconstituted freeze-dried fibrinogen. Urticaria and microangiopathic haemolytic anaemia have been described.

Clinical Uses   There are a few clinical studies which compare the effect of ancrod in the treatment of venous thrombosis with that of heparin and streptokinase.[25,67,129] According to these, ancrod, like heparin, prevented extension of thrombosis, as judged by repeated venographic examinations, but failed to produce significant thrombolysis. There is little evidence to show that the drug is useful as a prophylactic agent for preventing postoperative venous thrombosis or pulmonary embolism.[7] On the basis of present data ancrod seems to have no advantage over heparin and is much more expensive. It is not available for general use in the United States.

THROMBOLYTIC AGENTS

Although heparin is widely used in the early treatment of acute deep venous thrombosis and pulmonary embolism, its use is only preventive since it fails to relieve pulmonary vascular obstruction caused by emboli which have already impacted in the lungs, or to eliminate thrombus which has already formed in the deep veins and threatens further embolisation or chronic venous damage. It would be much more rational to use a drug which would lyse thrombi and emboli with the aim of restoring the circulation to normal as rapidly as possible, but fear of bleeding complications and lack of experience with thrombolytic agents have tended to limit their widespread use. With all forms of antithrombotic therapy the clinician has to weigh the benefits of alternative methods of treatment against the possible risks of haemorrhage, and many prefer to use heparin because they are better acquainted with it. Nevertheless the theoretical arguments for using thrombolytic therapy are compelling, and further developments aimed at improving its efficacy and reducing the risk of bleeding could make this the preferred form of initial treatment in acute venous thrombosis and pulmonary embolism.[97]

The thrombolytic drugs which are currently employed are streptokinase and urokinase; their properties and clinical uses are the subject of several recent reviews.[10,38,41]

Streptokinase

Streptokinase is a protein produced by the beta-haemolytic streptococcus. It is antigenic, and immune antibodies to streptokinase are present in all individuals, presumably as a result of previous streptococcal infections. An initial intravenous infusion of streptokinase leads to the formation of streptokinase-antibody complexes which are rapidly cleared from the circulation. After neutralisation of antibodies streptokinase has a half-life of 83 minutes in the circulation.

Mode of Action   Streptokinase combines with plasminogen to form a complex which then converts free plasminogen to plasmin. If the dose of streptokinase is small, only limited quantities of the activator complex are formed and most of the remaining plasminogen is converted to plasmin, whereas a large dose of streptokinase converts most of the circulating plasmin to the activator complex, leaving relatively small amounts of free plasminogen available for activation to plasmin.[14] Thus the amount of plasmin generated depends on the relative amounts of streptokinase and plasminogen present. In thrombolytic therapy large doses of streptokinase are given with the aim of producing levels which will facilitate the diffusion of the activator complex into thrombus where it can activate local plasminogen to produce fibrinolysis, but with relatively little plasmin activity in the circulating blood to avoid bleeding from recent wounds.

Administration and Dosage   It is usual to adopt a fixed dosage schedule for streptokinase administration which produces sufficient activation of plasmin in the great majority of patients.[137] The drug is available as a lyophilised powder in vials containing 250,000 International Units. An initial antibody-neutralising dose of 250,000 IU is administered intravenously in normal saline or 5 percent dextrose solution over 30 minutes, followed by 100,000 IU per hour for 24–72 hours, using a constant rate infusion pump. Higher initial doses of streptokinase up to 600,000 IU have been used in the past but have been shown to cause a higher mortality,[2] and the standard initial dose of 250,000 IU is now widely accepted. Following a period of treatment with streptokinase heparin therapy is introduced as soon as the thrombin time has returned to less than twice the control value (see below).

Urokinase

Urokinase is a β-globulin consisting of a single polypeptide chain which is actively secreted by the kidney and appears in the urine. It is expensive to produce, being obtained by purification of human urine or from human embryonic kidney-cell culture. It is nonantigenic in man. Like streptokinase it is not absorbed from the gastrointestinal tract and is therefore administered by intravenous infusion, being rapidly cleared from the circulation, with a half-life of about 15 minutes. Urokinase differs from streptokinase in that it is a direct activator of plasminogen.[70]

Administration and Dosage   In the treatment of pulmonary embolism urokinase has been given successfully in a fixed dose regimen by means of a 12-hour intravenous infusion, starting with an initial loading dose of 4,400 IU (or CTA units) per kg body weight over 10 minutes followed by maintenance therapy consisting of the same dosage per hour for a total of 12 hours.[135] The ideal dosage regimen for urokinase is still not established and alternative dosage schemes are reviewed by Barlow.[6] There appears to be no additional benefit in prolonging the infusion beyond 12 hours.[137] As with streptokinase, heparin therapy is introduced after the urokinase infusion has been terminated.

Monitoring Thrombolytic Therapy

Before beginning thrombolytic therapy the platelet count, thrombin time, prothrombin time, and partial thromboplastin time should be determined to exclude the presence of any underlying coagulation disorder. The aim of therapy should be to prolong the thrombin time between 2 and 5 times the control value, and this can be checked by measuring the thrombin time 4 hours after starting treatment. With urokinase Bell and Meek[10] advise a further check of thrombin time 4 hours later and with streptokinase, every 12 hours; if the thrombin time on any occasion is less than twice the control value it is likely that there is insufficient plasminogen substrate, indicating the need to replace thrombolytic therapy with conventional heparin anticoagulant treatment. If at any time the thrombin time is greater than 7–8 times the control value the infusion of urokinase or streptokinase should be stopped, and restarted only when the thrombin time has returned to less than 5 times the control value. The danger of continued thrombolytic infusion when the thrombin time is unduly prolonged is the risk of severe hypofibrinogenaemia and excessive quantities of fibrinogen degradation products which are conducive to haemorrhage. Although measurement of thrombin time is necessary to confirm that thrombolysis is established, it is rather unhelpful in predicting the extent of clot lysis[81] or the likelihood of haemorrhagic complications.[136]

Unwanted Effects, Contraindications, and Antidotes

The main risk of thrombolytic therapy is bleeding which usually occurs after surgery or as a result of trauma or invasive procedures such as venous or arterial puncture. With this danger in mind, the physician should select patients for thrombolytic therapy on the basis of a carefully taken history and clinical examination, and on laboratory tests for any coagulation defect. The following groups of patients should be excluded:

1. Patients who have had a surgical procedure within the previous ten days, including arterial puncture, invasive biopsy, pleural aspiration, or the like.
2. Those with active peptic ulcer or other causes of gastrointestinal bleeding, such as colitis or diverticulitis.
3. Those with severe hypertension, recent stroke, or conditions predisposing to embolisation such as subacute bacterial endocarditis.
4. Patients with metastatic malignancy, cavitating lung disease, or ulcerative lesions of the skin or mucous membranes.
5. Pregnant women and those in the first 10 days after childbirth.
6. Patients with any coagulation disorder or bleeding diathesis, and those who have shown previous hypersensitivity to any thrombolytic agent.

During thrombolytic therapy, all invasive procedures should be avoided except for careful venepuncture with a small needle. Care must be taken not to handle the patient roughly or unnecessarily, and any treatment with drugs which influence coagulation such as antiplatelet agents should be strictly avoided. Anticoagulants must be discontinued before thrombolytic therapy is started, and heparin should not be recommenced at the end of thrombolytic therapy until the thrombin time has returned to less than twice the control value.

Minor bleeding at cutaneous puncture sites can be controlled with pressure dressing but if bleeding is excessive or an emergency operation necessary, thrombolysis can be terminated more rapidly after stopping the thrombolytic agent by administering epsilon-aminocaproic acid intravenously in a loading dose of 5 g followed by 1 g per hour for 2–4 hours.[84]

The other adverse effects consist of mild allergic reactions including fever, headache, urticaria, nausea, and muscle pains, with occasional instances of asthma or angioneurotic oedema. They are more common with streptokinase than with urokinase and may be treated with antihistamines or, when necessary, with corticosteroids. Streptokinase can also occasionally produce more severe systemic reactions such as vomiting, diarrhoea, jaundice, and cardiac arrhythmias.

Clinical Use of Thrombolytic Agents

The indications for thrombolytic agents are not clearly established because most comparative studies have shown that although streptokinase and urokinase are more effective than heparin in promoting the dissolution of pulmonary emboli or deep venous thrombi, they do not improve mortality and are more likely than heparin to cause serious bleeding.[136,137] Some reports suggest that the postphlebitic syndrome due to deep venous thrombosis is less frequent after thrombolytic therapy than after heparin[33,68]; but the increased risk of haemorrhage and allergic reactions offsets this advantage. For these reasons the theoretical enthusiasm of many clinicians for thrombolytic agents is tempered with caution, and the strongest indication for their use arises in patients who suffer prolonged cardiac or pulmonary decompensation following serious pulmonary embolism, who need rapid relief of the vascular obstruction if they are to survive.

CLINICAL MANAGEMENT

Although there is a wide variety of antithrombotic drugs to choose from, they all increase the risk of haemorrhage and should therefore be avoided unless there is good experimental clinical evidence that the benefits of their use in a given clinical situation outweigh the dangers. If this premise is accepted, it means that clinicians who prescribe anticoagulant or thrombolytic agents should be aware of the current "state of the art" for this form of therapy, and their choice of treatment regimen should either be based on a critical appraisal of currently available data or, if unconventional, should constitute an explicit attempt to broaden our knowledge of this type of treatment by carrying out a controlled, ethically-acceptable trial of the chosen regimen. A number of recent critical reviews have questioned the value of some widely-used prophylactic or therapeutic regimens which on the evidence available do not entirely justify the optimistic assessment of their advocates, and these provide salutary reading for the enthusiastic anticoagulator.[86,93,113] In this final section of the chapter, I have tried to present the current orthodox views of antithrombotic therapy.

Prophylaxis

Oral Anticoagulants The usefulness of prophylactic antithrombotic therapy has been tested most extensively among high-risk surgical patients and in medical patients with congestive heart failure, and it is generally conceded that oral anticoagulant therapy is effective both in preventing deep venous thrombosis and in reducing mortality from pulmonary embolism in such patients.[4,52,118] However, fear of bleeding and the problems of laboratory control have prejudiced many clinicians against the application of this method of prophylactic therapy.[89] Nevertheless it has been emphasized that oral anticoagulant therapy is safe, provided that certain contraindications to its use are recognised (Table 10-4).[19] It is the prophylactic method of choice in elderly patients with hip fractures, and in other high-risk surgical and medical patients (see Table 10-1).[93]

Low-dose Heparin The main alternative form of prophylactic anticoagulant therapy in surgical patients is low-dose heparin, which is given to prevent surgical trauma from activating the clotting mechanisms and is therefore most effective when begun before the operation. Given in this way, low-dose heparin has been shown to reduce the incidence of deep venous thrombosis detected by ^{125}I-fibrinogen limb scans in patients over the age of 40 years undergoing major elective surgery,[59] but the investigation failed to show convincingly that treatment reduced mortality due to pulmonary embolism,[86] and ongoing studies by Immelman and his colleagues[45] have so far failed to show that low-dose heparin prophylaxis reduces the incidence of proximal deep vein thrombosis or pulmonary embolism in patients undergoing abdominal opera-

Table 10-4 / Contraindications to Oral Anticoagulant Therapy

Malignant hypertension
Recent stroke
Active peptic ulceration
Bleeding diathesis
Gastrointestinal bleeding
Alcoholism

tions. There is therefore some uncertainty about the value of this form of treatment at the present time and it is recognised that in some types of surgical patients low-dose heparin is of little value, notably in elderly patients with hip fractures[92] and in patients undergoing emergency and elective hip operations.[40,51]

Among medical patients low-dose heparin has been tested in those with myocardial infarction and has been shown to reduce the incidence of venous thromboembolism as judged by radioisotope studies.[50,143] However, at present there is insufficient data on mortality rates to recommend it as a routine in patients with heart disease or respiratory failure,[78,147] and a decision to use low-dose heparin in medical patients still depends upon an assessment of the risk factors in each case.

Dextran and Antiplatelet Agents Dextran and agents which inhibit platelet aggregation such as aspirin and dipyridamole have been advocated for prophylaxis of venous thromboembolism, but the evidence of their effectiveness is inconsistent and insufficient to warrant their routine use. The subject is discussed in several recent reviews.[19,93,119,139]

Routine Treatment of Venous Thromboembolism

Once the diagnosis of deep venous thrombosis or pulmonary embolism has been made on clinical grounds and confirmed if possible by radiographic and radioisotope studies, it is usual to start anticoagulant treatment with intravenous heparin, which may be administered either by 4-hourly intermittent injection or by continuous infusion. If heparin is to be administered by continuous infusion the dosage should be adjusted according to measurements of APTT or CT, but if laboratory monitoring is not possible then intermittent injections are the preferred method of administration. Heparin is continued for about 7 days, and during this time oral anticoagulant treatment is started with warfarin sodium, using a modest loading dose of 10 mg per day on 3 successive days. Thereafter the maintenance dose of warfarin is determined by daily measurements of prothrombin time, and heparin therapy is discontinued. The patient is usually gently mobilised as soon as the pain or swelling of the affected leg has settled down or the acute symptoms of embolism have resolved, and discharged from hospital on warfarin therapy which is continued for 2 to 4 months or until the underlying precipitating factor for venous thrombosis has been corrected.

Extensive venous thrombosis involving the iliofemoral segment, especially when the proximal end of the thrombus floats freely in the lumen of the vein, is considered by some to be an indication for thrombolytic therapy.[10,15,80] It is usual to adopt a fixed dose schedule as previously described, and to treat with streptokinase for 24–72 hours. When fibrinolytic therapy is discontinued and the thrombin time has returned to less than twice the control value, heparin is restarted and anticoagulation eventually maintained with warfarin as indicated above. The aim of using thrombolytic agents in the initial treatment of extensive deep vein thrombosis is to prevent permanent damage to the venous circulation of the legs which may result in the post-phlebitic syndrome, characterised by oedema, eczema, ulceration, and occasionally venous claudication.[81] There is some evidence to suggest that the long-term incidence of post-phlebitic complications is less with streptokinase-treated patients than with those given heparin,[33,63,68] but the frequency and severity of haemorrhagic complications are greater than with heparin and impose a serious limitation on the use of thrombolytic agents in patients who have recently undergone a surgical operation. There is also some doubt about their value if the thrombus is more than 5 days old.[2] These constraints tend to restrict the use of thrombolytic therapy to younger patients with a high risk of post-phlebitic disability and no contraindications to this form of treatment.

Management of Anticoagulation in Outpatients   Long-term treatment of patients with oral anticoagulants presupposes an efficient system of surveillance which will minimise the likelihood of unwanted effects. The requirements for providing such a service in a hospital setting have been described by Deykin,[29] and have been recently reviewed by Davis et al.,[26] who emphasised the following guidelines:

1. Careful selection of patients, taking account of medical contraindications to oral anticoagulant therapy (see Table 10-4) and personal or social contraindications such as uncooperativeness or unreliability, inability to attend hospital regularly, or serious alcohol abuse.
2. Continuing education of the patient in the causes and avoidance of haemorrhagic complications throughout the course of treatment, with particular regard to drug interactions.
3. Discontinuation of anticoagulant therapy if control is unsatisfactory.
4. Regular laboratory and clinical surveillance.
5. Effective communication between the hospital doctor and the primary care physician.

It is important that continuity of surveillance is maintained throughout the full duration of anticoagulation, both by keeping effective records of the results of laboratory tests, anticoagulant dosage, other drug therapy and side-effects, and by continued personal contact between the clinic personnel and the patients. Junior hospital doctors in training are often unsuitable for this type of patient care because they change jobs so frequently, and we have found that anti-coagulant clinics organised jointly by hospital pharmacists and senior medical staff are highly effective, the patient being interviewed routinely by the pharmacist and the dosage recommendations being confirmed on each occasion by the physician. Similar successful schemes have been reported elsewhere.[27,69] Whatever organisation is provided for supervising oral anti-coagulant therapy, it is vital that tight control be kept over laboratory results, drug prescribing, and attendance so that any deviation is recognised and corrected immediately.

Anticoagulation in Pregnancy   Anticoagulant therapy is indicated if venous thrombosis or pulmonary embolism occurs during pregnancy or in the puerperium, since pulmonary embolism is an important though rare cause of maternal death,[49] and anticoagulants are effective in reducing this source of mortality.[142] Because coumarin derivatives cross the placenta and are liable to cause congenital malformations if given during the first trimester,[105] and to cause foetal haemorrhage due to the trauma of delivery if used near term,[53] it is generally held that warfarin and the other oral anticoagulants should only be used after the first trimester and should be discontinued before the onset of labour.[13] Heparin is considered the safer alternative because it does not cross the placental barrier, although Hall and her colleagues[46] suggest that the outcome is hardly better than with coumarins. A reasonable compromise is to begin treatment with intravenous heparin, which is changed to maintenance therapy with warfarin from the 12th to the 36th week, and then to change back to heparin until term.[53] Anticoagulant treatment is continued for 6 weeks after delivery, recent evidence suggesting that warfarin may be safely used because the amount secreted into breast milk is insufficient to affect the infant.[101] An alternative to the combined heparin-oral anticoagulant regimen outlined above is long-term self-administered subcutaneous heparin,[125] but heparin-induced osteoporosis is a possible complication of this form of therapy.[152]

Massive Pulmonary Embolism

Acute pulmonary embolism which obstructs more than half of the pulmonary vascular bed causes a severe haemodynamic disturbance with right ventricular failure and a dramatic fall in cardiac output. A similar effect may be produced by a lesser degree of pulmonary vascular obstruction in patients already suffering from cardiopulmonary disease. Fifty percent of those who die from pulmonary embolism do so within 15 minutes,[20] and the prime consideration is to institute emergency resuscitative measures[85]:

1. Apply external cardiac massage, which may help to fragment the embolus and force the particles to more distal pulmonary arterial branches.
2. Administer oxygen in high concentration by mask or endotracheal tube.
3. Inject 15,000 units of heparin intravenously.
4. Correct acidosis with intravenous sodium bicarbonate.

Patients who survive the immediate catastrophe may be continued on anticoagulant therapy with heparin in doses of up to 100,000 IU in the first 24 hours, but those who remain in shock may be treated with streptokinase or urokinase—which have been shown to produce early physiological improvement in massive pulmonary embolism.[134,137] It has been reasonably suggested that thrombolytic therapy should be used in the following groups of patients[38]:

1. Those who are critically ill from the haemodynamic disturbance of pulmonary artery obstruction when first seen.
2. Those who survive the acute episode for over 24 hours but who do not make the usual recovery on heparin treatment.
3. Those with underlying cardiopulmonary disease.

REFERENCES

1. AGGELER PM, O'REILLY RA, LEONG L, AND KOWITZ PE: Potentiation of anticoagulant effect of warfarin by phenylbutazone. N Eng J Med 276: 496–501, 1967.
2. AMERY A, DELOOF W, VERMYLEN J, AND VERSTRAETE, M: Outcome of recent thromboembolic occlusions of limb arteries treated with streptokinase. Br Med J 4: 639–644, 1970.
3. AMUNDSEN MA, SPITTELL JA, THOMPSON JH, AND OWEN CA: Hypercoagulability associated with malignant disease and with the post-operative state. Ann Intern Med 58: 608–616, 1963.
4. ANDERSON GM, AND HULL, E: The effect of dicumarol upon the mortality and incidence of thromboembolic complications in congestive heart failure. Am Heart J 39: 697–702, 1950.
5. ANSELL JE, KUMAR R, AND DEYKIN D: The spectrum of vitamin K deficiency. JAMA 238: 40–42, 1977.
6. BARLOW GH: Pharmacology of fibrinolytic agents. Prog Cardiovasc. Dis. 21: 315–326, 1979.
7. BARRIE WW, WOOD, EH, CRUMLISH P, FORBES CD, AND PRENTICE CRM: Low-

dosage ancrod for prevention of thrombotic complications after surgery for fractured neck of femur. Br Med J 4:130–133, 1974.

8. BARRITT DW, AND JORDAN SC: Anticoagulant drugs in the treatment of pulmonary embolism: A controlled trial. Lancet 1: 1309–1312, 1960.

9. BASU D, GALLUS A, HIRSH J, AND CADE, J: A prospective study of the value of monitoring heparin treatment with the activated partial thromboplastin time. N Engl J Med 287: 324–327, 1972.

10. BELL WR, AND MEEK AG: Guidelines for the use of thrombolytic agents. N Engl J Med 301: 1266–1270, 1979.

11. BERNSTEIN IL: Anaphylaxis to heparin. JAMA 161: 1379–1381, 1956.

12. BRECKENRIDGE A, ORME M, WESSELING H, LEWIS RJ, GIBBONS R: Pharmacokinetics and pharmacodynamics of the enantiomers of warfarin in man. Clin Pharmacol Ther 15: 424–430, 1974.

13. BRITISH MEDICAL JOURNAL: Thromboembolism in pregnancy. Br Med J 1: 1661, 1979.

14. BROGDEN RN, SPEIGHT TM, AVERY GS: Streptokinase: A review of its clinical pharmacology, mechanism of action and therapeutic uses. Drugs 5: 357–445, 1973.

15. BROWSE NL: Personal view on published facts. What should I do about deep vein thrombosis and pulmonary embolism? Ann R Coll Surg Engl 59: 138–142, 1977.

16. BROWSE NL, CLEMENSON G, CROFT DN: Fibrinogen-detectable thrombosis in the legs and pulmonary embolism. Br Med J 1: 603–604, 1974.

17. BYRD RB, DIVERTIE MB, SPITTELL JA: Bronchogenic carcinoma and thromboembolic disease. JAMA 202: 1019–1022, 1967.

18. CHRISTENSON LK, SKOVSTED L: Inhibition of drug metabolism by chloramphenicol. Lancet 2: 1397–1399, 1969.

19. CLAGETT GP, SALZMAN EW: Prevention of venous thromboembolism. Prog Cardiovasc Dis 17: 345–366, 1975.

20. COON WW, COLLER FA: Clinicopathologic correlation in thromboembolism. Surg Gynecol Obstet 109: 259–269, 1959.

21. CRANE C, HARTSUCK J, BIRTCH A, COUCH NP, ZOLLINGER R, MATLOFF J, DALEN J, DEXTER L: The management of major pulmonary embolism. Surg Gynecol Obstet 128: 27–36, 1969.

22. CURRY N, BARDANA EJ, PIROFSKY B: Heparin sensitivity. Arch Intern Med 132: 744–745, 1973.

23. DALEN JE, ALPERT JE: Natural history of pulmonary embolism. Prog Cardiovasc Dis 17, 259–270, 1975.

24. DALEN JE, BANAS JS BROOKS HL, EVANS GL, PARASKOS JA, DEXTER L: Resolution rate of acute pulmonary embolism in man. N Engl J Med 280: 1194–1199, 1969.

25. DAVIES JA, MERRICK MV, SHARP AA, HOLT JM: Controlled trial of ancrod and heparin in treatment of deep-vein thrombosis of lower limb. Lancet 1: 113–115, 1972.

26. DAVIS FB, ESTRUCH MT, SAMSON-CORVERA EB, VOIGT GC, TOBIN JD: Management of anticoagulation in outpatients. Experience with an anticoagulation service in a municipal hospital setting. Arch Intern Med 137: 197–202, 1977.

27. DAVIS FB, AND SCZUPAK CA: Outpatient oral anticoagulation. Guidelines for long-term management. Postgrad Med 66: 100–109, 1979.
28. DE SOYZA NDB, MURPHY ML: Persistent post-embolic pulmonary hypertension. Chest 62: 665–668, 1972.
29. DEYKIN D: Warfarin therapy. N Engl J Med 283: 691–694 and 801–803, 1970.
30. DORAN FSA, WHITE M, DRURY M: A clinical trial designed to test the relative value of two simple methods of reducing the risk of venous stasis in the lower limbs during surgical operations, the danger of thrombosis, and a subsequent pulmonary embolus, with a survey of the problem. Br J Surg 57: 20–30, 1970.
31. DOUGLAS AS: Management of thrombotic diseases. Semin. Hematol. 8: 95–139, 1971.
32. EGEBERG O, OWREN, PA: Oral contraception and blood coagulability. Br Med J 1: 220–221, 1963.
33. ELLIOT MS, IMMELMAN EJ, JEFFERY P, BENATAR SR, FUNSTON MR, SMITH JA, SHEPSTONE BJ, FERGUSON AD, JACOBS P, WALKER W, LOUW JH: A comparative randomised trial of heparin versus streptokinase in the treatment of acute proximal venous thrombosis: an interim report of a prospective trial. Br J Surg 66: 838–843, 1979.
34. EMMONS PR, MITCHELL JRA: Postoperative changes in platelet-clumping activity. Lancet 1: 71–75, 1965.
35. ESMON CT, SUTTIE JW, JACKSON CM: The functional significance of vitamin K action. Difference in phospholipid binding between normal and abnormal prothrombin. J Biol Chem 250: 4095–4099, 1975.
36. ESTES JW, POULIN PF: Pharmacokinetics of heparin. Distribution and elimination. Thromb Diath Haemorrh 33: 26–37, 1974.
37. GALLO DG, BAILEY KR, SHEFFNER AL: The interaction between cholestyramine and drugs. Proc Soc Exp Biol Med 120: 60–65, 1965.
38. GALLUS AS, HIRSH J: Antithrombotic Drugs. Drugs 12: 14–68 and 132–157, 1976.
39. GALLUS AS, HIRSH J, O'BRIEN SE, McBRIDE JA, TUTTLE RJ, GENT M: Prevention of venous thrombosis with small subcutaneous doses of heparin. JAMA 235: 1980–1982, 1976.
40. GALLUS AS, HIRSH J, TUTTLE RJ, TREBILCOCK R, O'BRIEN SE, CARROLL JJ, MINDEN JH, HUDECKI SM: Small subcutaneous doses of heparin in prevention of venous thrombosis. N Engl J Med 288: 545–551, 1973.
41. GENTON E: Thrombolytic therapy of pulmonary thromboembolism. Prog Cardiovasc Dis 21: 333–341, 1979.
42. GREEN D, HARRIS K, REYNOLDS N, ROBERTS M, PATTERSON R: Heparin immune thrombocytopenia: evidence for a heparin-platelet complex as the antigenic determinant. J Lab Clin Med 91: 167–175, 1978.
43. GRIFFITH GC, NICHOLS G, ASHER JD, FLANAGAN B: Heparin osteoporosis. JAMA 193: 91–94, 1965.
44. GRINER PF, LAWRENCE GR, RICKLES FR, WESNER, PJ, ODOROFF CL: Chloral hydrate and warfarin interaction: Clinical significance? Ann Intern Med 74: 540–543, 1971.

45. GROOTE SCHUUR HOSPITAL THROMBOEMBOLUS STUDY GROUP: Failure of low dose heparin to prevent significant thromboembolic complications in high-risk surgical patients: interim report of prospective trial. Br Med J 1: 1447–1450, 1979.

46. HALL JG, PAULI RM, WILSON KM: Maternal and fetal sequelae of anticoagulation during pregnancy. Am J Med 68: 122–140, 1980.

47. HALL RJC, SUTTON GC, KERR IH: Long-term prognosis of treated acute massive pulmonary embolism. Br Heart J 39: 1128–1134, 1977.

48. HAN P, AND ARDLIE NG: Heparin, platelets and blood coagulation: implications for low-dose heparin prophylactic regimens in venous thrombosis. Br J Haematol 27: 253–272, 1974.

49. HANDIN RI: Thromboembolic complications of pregnancy and oral contraception. Prog Cardiovasc Dis 16: 395–405, 1974.

50. HANDLEY AJ, EMERSON PA, FLEMING PR: Heparin in the prevention of deep venous thrombosis after myocardial infarction. Br Med J 2: 436–438, 1972.

51. HARRIS WH, SALZMAN EW, ATHANASOULIS C, WALTMAN AC, BAUM S, DESANCTIS RW: Comparison of warfarin, low molecular weight dextran, aspirin and subcutaneous heparin in prevention of venous thromboembolism following total hip replacement. J Bone Joint Surg 56: 1552–1562, 1974.

52. HARVEY WP, AND FINCH CA: Dicumarol prophylaxis of thromboembolic disease in congestive heart failure. N Engl J Med 242: 208–211, 1950.

53. HIRSH J, CADE JF, AND O'SULLIVAN EF: Clinical experience with anticoagulant therapy during pregnancy. Br Med J 1: 270–273, 1970.

54. HIRSH J, VAN AKEN WG, GALLUS AS, DOLLERY CT, CADE JF, YUNG WL: Heparin kinetics in venous thrombosis and pulmonary embolism. Circulation 53: 691–695, 1976.

55. HOWIE PW: Thromboembolism. Clin Obstet Gynaecol 4: 397–417, 1977.

56. HULL R, DELMORE T, GENTON E, HIRSH J, GENT M, SACKETT D, McLOUGHLIN D, ARMSTRONG P: Warfarin sodium versus low dose heparin in the long-term therapy of venous thrombosis. N Engl J Med 301: 855–858, 1979.

57. HUME M, SEVITT S, THOMAS DP: A unified concept of pathogenesis, in Venous Thrombosis and Pulmonary Embolism, Ch. 6, pp. 125–134. Cambridge, Mass.: Harvard University Press, 1970.

58. INNES D, SEVITT S: Coagulation and fibrinolysis in injured patients. J Clin Pathol 17: 1–13, 1964.

59. INTERNATIONAL MULTICENTRE TRIAL: Prevention of fatal postoperative pulmonary embolism by low doses of heparin. Lancet 2: 45–51, 1975.

60. JACOBS J, KLETTER D, SUPERSTINE E, HILL KR, LYNN B, WEBB RA: Intravenous solutions of heparin and penicillins. J Clin Pathol 26: 742–746, 1973.

61. JAQUES LB, MAHADOO JR, KAVANAGH LW: Intrapulmonary heparin. A new procedure for anticoagulant therapy. Lancet 2: 1157–1161, 1976.

62. JICK H, SLONE D, BORDA IT, SHAPIRO S: Efficacy and toxicity of heparin in relation to age and sex. N Engl J Med 279: 284–286, 1968.

63. JOHANSSON L, NYLANDER G, HEDNER U, NILSSON IM: Comparison of streptokinase with heparin: Late results in the treatment of deep venous thrombosis. Acta Med Scand 206: 93–98, 1979.

64. JOIST JH, DOLEZEL G, LLOYD JV, KINLOUGH-RATHBONE RL, MUSTARD JF: Platelet

factor-3 availability and the platelet release reaction. J Lab Clin Med 84: 474–482, 1974.

65. KAKKAR VV: The prevention of acute pulmonary embolism. Br J Hosp Med 18: 32–40, 1977.

66. KAKKAR VV, HOWE CT, FLANC C, CLARKE MB: Natural history of postoperative deep vein thrombosis. Lancet 2: 230–233, 1969.

67. KAKKAR VV, FLANC C, HOWE CT, O'SHEA M, FLUTE PT: Treatment of deep vein thrombosis. A trial of heparin, streptokinase and arvin. Br Med J 1: 806–810, 1969.

68. KAKKAR VV, HOWE CT, LAWS JW, FLANC C: Late results of treatment of deep vein thrombosis. Br Med J 1: 810–811, 1969.

69. KEMP CG, CARRINGTON DW: Pharmacist as member of clinical team. Pharm J 221: 564–565 and 573, 1978.

70. KJELDGAARD NO, PLOUG J: Urokinase. An activator of plasminogen from human urine. II Mechanism of plasminogen activation. Biochim. Biophys 24: 283–289, 1957.

71. KOCH-WESER J, SELLERS EM: Drug interactions with coumarin anticoagulants. N Engl J Med 285: 487–498 and 547–558, 1971.

72. LEE RI, WHITE PD: A clinical study of the coagulation time of blood. Am J Med Sci 145: 495–503, 1913.

73. LEVIN J, CONLEY CL: Thrombocytosis associated with malignant disease. Arch Intern Med 114: 497–500, 1964.

74. LEWIS RJ, TRAGER WF, CHAN KK, BRECKENRIDGE AA, ORME M, ROLAND M, SCHARY W: Warfarin. Stereochemical aspects of its metabolism and the interaction with phenylbutazone. J Clin Invest 53: 1607–1617, 1974.

75. LOWE GD, McKILLOP JH, PRENTICE AG: Fatal retroperitoneal haemorrhage complicating anticoagulant therapy. Postgrad Med J 55: 18–21, 1979.

76. MacDONALD MG, ROBINSON DS, SYLVESTER D, JAFFE JJ: The effects of phenobarbital, chloral betaine and glutethimide administration on warfarin plasma levels and hypoprothrombinemic responses in man. Clin Pharmacol Ther 10: 80–84, 1969.

77. MacLEOD SM, SELLERS EM: Pharmacodynamic and pharmacokinetic drug interactions with coumarin anticoagulants. Drugs, 11: 461–470, 1976.

78. MALCOLM AD: Anticoagulants for heart disease. Br J Hosp Med 23: 606–615, 1980.

79. MANT MJ, THONG KL, BIRTWHISTLE RV, O'BRIEN BD, HAMMOND GW, GRACE MG: Haemorrhagic complications of heparin therapy. Lancet, 1: 1133–1135, 1977.

80. MARDER VJ: Guidelines for thrombolytic therapy of deep-vein thrombosis. Prog Cardiovasc Dis 21: 327–332, 1979.

81. MARDER VJ, SOULEN RL, ATICHARTAKARN V, BUDZYNSKI AZ, PARULEKAR S, KIM JR, EDWARD N, ZAHAVI J, ALGAZY KM: Quantitative venographic assessment of deep vein thrombosis in the evaluation of streptokinase and heparin therapy. J Lab Clin Med, 89: 1018–1029, 1977.

82. MAVOR GE, GALLOWAY JMD: The iliofemoral venous segment as a source of pulmonary emboli. Lancet 1: 871–874, 1967.

83. McAVOY TJ: The biologic half-life of heparin. Clin Pharmacol Ther 25: 372–379, 1979.

84. MᴄNɪᴄᴏʟ GP, Dᴏᴜɢʟᴀs AS: Epsilon-aminocaproic acid and other inhibitors of fibrinolysis. Br Med Bull 20: 233–239, 1964.

85. Mɪʟʟᴇʀ GAH: The management of acute pulmonary embolism. Br J Hosp Med 18: 26–31, 1977.

86. Mɪᴛᴄʜᴇʟʟ JR: Can we really prevent postoperative pulmonary emboli? Br Med J 1: 1523–1524, 1979.

87. Mɪᴛᴄʜᴇʟʟ JF, Bᴀʀɢᴇʀ RC, Cᴀɴᴛᴡᴇʟʟ L: Heparin stability in 5% dextrose and 0.9% sodium chloride solutions. Am J Hosp Pharm 33: 540–542, 1976.

88. Mʟᴄᴢᴏᴄʜ J, Tᴜᴄᴋᴇʀ A, Wᴇɪʀ EK, Rᴇᴇᴠᴇs JT, Gʀᴏᴠᴇʀ RF: Platelet-mediated pulmonary hypertension and hypoxia during pulmonary microembolism. Chest, 74: 648–653, 1978.

89. Mᴏʀʀɪs GK, Mɪᴛᴄʜᴇʟʟ JRA: Prevention and diagnosis of venous thrombosis in patients with hip fractures. A survey of current practice. Lancet 2: 867–869, 1976.

90. Mᴏʀʀɪs GK, Mɪᴛᴄʜᴇʟʟ JRA: Warfarin sodium in prevention of deep venous thrombosis and pulmonary embolism in patients with fractured neck of femur. Lancet 2: 869–872, 1976.

91. Mᴏʀʀɪs GK, Mɪᴛᴄʜᴇʟʟ JRA: The aetiology of acute pulmonary embolism and the identification of high risk groups. Br J Hosp Med 18: 6–12, 1977.

92. Mᴏʀʀɪs GK, Mɪᴛᴄʜᴇʟʟ JRA: Preventing venous thromboembolism in elderly patients with hip fractures: studies of low-dose heparin, dipyridamole, aspirin and flurbiprofen. Br Med J 1: 535–537, 1977.

93. Mᴏʀʀɪs GK, Mɪᴛᴄʜᴇʟʟ JRA: Clinical management of venous thromboembolism. Br Med Bull 34: 169–175, 1978.

94. Mᴜsᴛᴀʀᴅ JF, Kɪɴʟᴏᴜɢʜ-Rᴀᴛʜʙᴏɴᴇ RL, Pᴀᴄᴋʜᴀᴍ MA: Recent status of research in the pathogenesis of thrombosis. Thromb Diath Haemorrh (Suppl 59): 157–188, 1974.

95. Nᴀʟʙᴀɴᴅɪᴀɴ RM, Mᴀᴅᴇʀ IJ, Bᴀʀʀᴇᴛᴛ JL, Pᴇᴀʀᴄᴇ JF, Rᴜᴘᴘ EC: Petechiae, ecchymoses and necrosis of skin induced by coumarin congeners. Rare, occasionally lethal complication of anticoagulant therapy. JAMA 192: 107–112, 1965.

96. Nɪᴄᴏʟᴀɪᴅᴇs AN, Kᴀᴋᴋᴀʀ VV, Fɪᴇʟᴅ ES, Fɪsʜ P: Venous stasis and deep-vein thrombosis. Br J Surg 59: 713–717, 1972.

97. NIH Cᴏɴsᴇɴsᴜs Cᴏɴғᴇʀᴇɴᴄᴇ: Consensus development: Thrombolytic therapy in treatment. Br Med J 2: 1585–1587, 1980.

98. O'Rᴇɪʟʟʏ RA: The streoselective interaction of warfarin and metronidazole in man. N Engl J Med 295: 354–357, 1976.

99. O'Rᴇɪʟʟʏ RA, Aɢɢᴇʟᴇʀ PM: Studies on coumarin anticoagulant drugs: Initiation of warfarin therapy without a loading dose. Circulation, 38: 169–177, 1968.

100. Oʀᴍᴇ M, Bʀᴇᴄᴋᴇɴʀɪᴅɢᴇ A, Cᴏᴏᴋ P: Warfarin and distalgesic interaction. Br Med J 1: 200, 1976.

101. Oʀᴍᴇ ML, Lᴇᴡɪs PJ, ᴅᴇ Sᴡɪᴇᴛ M, Sᴇʀʟɪɴ MJ, Sɪʙᴇᴏɴ R, Bᴀᴛʏ JD, Bʀᴇᴄᴋᴇɴʀɪᴅɢᴇ AM: May mothers given warfarin breast-feed their infants? Br Med J 1: 1564–1565, 1977.

102. Oᴡʀᴇɴ PA: Thrombotest: A new method for controlling anticoagulant therapy. Lancet, 2: 754–758, 1959.

103. Pᴀᴛᴇʀsᴏɴ JC: The pathology of venous thrombi, in Thrombosis, Sherry, S., Brink-

hous, K.M., Genton, E. and Stengle, J.M. (eds.), pp. 321–331. Washington, DC, National Academy of Sciences, 1969.

104. PATERSON JC, McLACHLIN J: Precipitating factors in venous thrombosis. Surg Gynecol Obstet 98: 96–102, 1954.

105. PAULI RM, MADDEN JD, KRANZLER KJ, CULPEPPER W, PORT R: Warfarin therapy initiated during pregnancy and phenotypic chondrodysplasia punctata. J Pediatr 88: 506–508, 1976.

106. PETTIFOR JM, BENSON R: Congenital malformation associated with the administration of oral anticoagulants during pregnancy. J Pediatr 86: 459–462, 1975.

107. PITNEY WR, PETTIT JE, ARMSTRONG L: Control of heparin therapy. Br Med J 4: 139–141, 1970.

108. PIZZO SV, SCHWARTZ ML, HILL RL, McKEE PA: Mechanism of ancrod anticoagulation. A direct proteolytic effect on fibrin. J Clin Invest 51: 2841–2850, 1972.

109. POLLER L, THOMPSON JM: Clotting factors during oral contraception: further report. Br Med J 2: 23–25, 1966.

110. POND SM, GRAHAM GG, WADE DN, SUDLOW G: The effects of allopurinol and clofibrate on the elimination of coumarin anticoagulants in man. Aust NZ J Med 5: 324–328, 1975.

111. POWERS PJ, CUTHBERT D, HIRSH J: Thrombocytopenia found uncommonly during heparin therapy. JAMA 241: 2396–2397, 1979.

112. PUCKETT CL, GERVIN AS, RHODES GR, SILVER D: Role of platelets and serotonin in acute massive pulmonary embolism. Surg Gynecol Obstet 137: 618–622, 1973.

113. ROBIN ED: Overdiagnosis and overtreatment of pulmonary embolism: The emperor may have no clothes. Ann Intern Med 87: 775–781, 1977.

114. ROMANKIEWICZ JA, EHRMAN M: Rifampin and warfarin: A drug interaction. Ann Intern Med 82: 224–225, 1975.

115. ROSENBERG RD: Actions and interactions of antithrombin and heparin. N Engl J Med 292: 146–151, 1975.

116. ROSS JRY, BEELEY L: Interaction between carbamazepine and warfarin. Br Med J 2: 1415–1416, 1980.

117. SALZMAN EW, DEYKIN D, SHAPIRO RM, ROSENBERG R: Management of heparin therapy. Controlled prospective trial. N Engl J Med 292: 1046–1050, 1975.

118. SALZMAN EW, HARRIS WH, DeSANCTIS RW: Anticoagulation for prevention of thromboembolism following fractures of the hip. N Engl J Med 275: 122–130, 1966.

119. SASAHARA AA, SHARMA GVRK, PARISI AF: New developments in the detection and prevention of venous thromboembolism. Am J Cardiol 43: 1214–1224, 1979.

120. SELLERS EM, KOCH-WESER J: Potentiation of warfarin-induced hypoprothrombinemia by chloral hydrate. N Engl J Med 283: 827–831, 1970.

121. SEVITT S, GALLAGHER NG: Prevention of venous thrombosis and pulmonary embolism in injured patients. A trial of anticoagulant prophylaxis with phenindione in middle-aged and elderly patients with fractured necks of femur. Lancet 2: 981–989, 1959.

122. SEVITT S, GALLAGHER NG: Venous thrombosis and pulmonary embolism: a clinico-pathological study in injured and burned patients. Br J Surg 48: 475–489, 1961.

123. SHARP AA, WARREN BA PAXTON AM, ALLINGTON MJ: Anticoagulant therapy with a purified fraction of Malayan pit viper venom. Lancet 1: 493–499, 1968.

124. SIMON TL, HYERS TM, GASTON JP, HARKER LA: Heparin pharmacokinetics: increased requirements in pulmonary embolism. Br J Haematol 39: 111–120, 1978.

125. SPEARING G, FRASER I, TURNER G, DIXON G: Long-term self-administered subcutaneous heparin in pregnancy. Br Med J 1: 1457–1458, 1978.

126. STARR KJ, PETRIE JC: Drug interactions in patients on long-term oral anticoagulant and antihypertensive adrenergic neuron-blocking drugs. Br Med J 4: 133–135, 1972.

127. STEWART GJ: The role of the vessel wall in deep venous thrombosis, in Thromboembolism, Nicolaides, A.N. (ed.), pp. 101–135. Baltimore, University Park Press, 1975.

128. STUART RK, MICHEL A: Monitoring heparin therapy with the activated partial thromboplastin time. Can Med Assoc J 104: 385–388, 1971.

129. TIBBUTT DA, WILLIAMS EW, WALKER MW, CHESTERMAN CN, HOLT JM, SHARP AA: Controlled trial of ancrod and streptokinase in the treatment of deep vein thrombosis of lower limb. Br J Haematol 27: 407–414, 1974.

130. TOW DE, WAGNER HN: Recovery of pulmonary arterial blood flow in patients with pulmonary embolism. N Engl J Med 276: 1053–1059, 1967.

131. TRANZER JP, BAUMGARTNER HR: Filling gaps in vascular endothelium with blood platelets. Nature 216: 1126–1128, 1967.

132. TROWBRIDGE AA, CARAVEO J, GREEN JB, AMARAL B, STONE MJ: Heparin-related immune thrombocytopenia: studies of antibody-heparin specificity. Am J Med 65: 277–283, 1978.

133. UDALL JA: Human sources and absorption of vitamin K in relation to anticoagulation stability. JAMA 194: 107–109, 1965.

134. UROKINASE PULMONARY EMBOLISM TRIAL: Phase 1 results. JAMA 214: 2163–2172, 1970.

135. UROKINASE PULMONARY EMBOLISM TRIAL: Enhancement of fibrinolysis with urokinase. Circulation 47 (Supplement 2): 33–37, 1973.

136. UROKINASE PULMONARY EMBOLISM TRIAL: Morbidity and mortality. Circulation 47 (Supplement 2): 66–72, 1973.

137. UROKINASE-STREPTOKINASE EMBOLISM TRIAL: Phase 2 results. A cooperative study. JAMA 229: 1606–1613, 1974.

138. VERSTRAETE M: The position of long-term stimulation of the endogenous fibrinolytic system: present achievements and clinical perspectives. Thromb Diath Haemorrh 34: 613–622, 1975.

139. VERSTRAETE M: Are agents affecting platelet function clinically useful? Am J Med 61: 897–914, 1976.

140. VESSELL ES, PASSANANTI GT, GREENE FE: Impairment of drug metabolism in man by allopurinol and nortriptyline. N Engl J Med, 283: 1484–1488, 1970.

141. VIEWEG WVR, PISCATELLI RK, HOUSER JJ, PROLX RA: Complications of intravenous administration of heparin in elderly women. JAMA 213: 1303–1306, 1970.

142. VILLASANTA U: Thromboembolic disease in pregnancy. Am J Obstet Gynecol 93: 142–160, 1965.

143. Warlow C, Terry G, Kenmure ACF, Beattie AG, Ogston D, Douglas AS: A double-blind trial of low doses of subcutaneous heparin in the prevention of deep-vein thrombosis after myocardial infarction. Lancet 2: 934–936, 1973.

144. Wessler S: Studies in intravascular coagulation. III. The pathogenesis of serum-induced venous thrombosis. J Clin Invest 34: 647–651, 1955.

145. Wessler S, Freiman DG, Ballon JD, Katz JH, Wolff R, Wolf E: Experimental pulmonary embolism with serum-induced thrombi. Am J Pathol 38: 89–101, 1961.

146. Wessler S, Gitel SN: Rethrombosis—Warfarin or low-dose heparin? N Engl J Med 301: 899–891, 1978.

147. Wessler S, Gitel SN: Heparin: New concepts relevant to clinical use. Blood 53: 525–544, 1979.

148. Wessler S, Yin ET: Experimental hypercoagulable state induced by Factor X: comparison of the non-activated and activated forms. J Lab Clin Med 72: 256–260, 1968.

149. White PW Sadd JR, Nensel RE: Thrombotic complications of heparin therapy: Including six cases of heparin-induced skin necrosis. Ann Surg 190: 595–608, 1979.

150. Wilson JR, Lampman J: Heparin therapy: A randomised prospective study. Am Heart J 97: 155–158, 1979.

151. Wiman B, Collen D: Molecular mechanism of physiological fibrinolysis. Nature 272: 549–550, 1978.

152. Wise PH, Hall AJ: Heparin-induced osteopenia in pregnancy. Br Med J 2: 110–111, 1980.

153. Wright HP: Changes in adhesiveness of blood platelets following parturition and surgical operations. J Pathol Bacteriol 54: 461–468, 1942.

154. Yett HS, Skillman JJ, Salzman EW: The hazards of aspirin plus heparin. N Engl J Med 298, 1092, 1978.

Index

315